CLINICAL PSYCHODERMATOLOGY
A CASEBOOK

CLINICAL PSYCHODERMATOLOGY
A CASEBOOK

By

Mohammad Jafferany, M.D.
Asmahane Souissi, M.D.

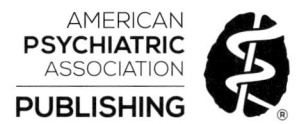

Note: The authors have worked to ensure that all information in this book is accurate at the time of publication and consistent with general psychiatric and medical standards, and that information concerning drug dosages, schedules, and routes of administration is accurate at the time of publication and consistent with standards set by the U.S. Food and Drug Administration and the general medical community. As medical research and practice continue to advance, however, therapeutic standards may change. Moreover, specific situations may require a specific therapeutic response not included in this book. For these reasons and because human and mechanical errors sometimes occur, we recommend that readers follow the advice of physicians directly involved in their care or the care of a member of their family.

Books published by American Psychiatric Association Publishing represent the findings, conclusions, and views of the individual authors and do not necessarily represent the policies and opinions of American Psychiatric Association Publishing or the American Psychiatric Association.

If you wish to buy 50 or more copies of the same title, please go to www.appi.org/specialdiscounts for more information.

Copyright © 2025 American Psychiatric Association Publishing

ALL RIGHTS RESERVED

First Edition

Manufactured in the United States of America on acid-free paper
28 27 26 25 24   5 4 3 2 1

American Psychiatric Association Publishing
800 Maine Avenue SW, Suite 900
Washington, DC 20024-2812
www.appi.org

Library of Congress Cataloging-in-Publication Data
Names: Jafferany, Mohammad, editor. | Souissi, Asmahane, editor.
Title: Clinical psychodermatology : from diagnosis to therapy : a
   case-based approach / edited by Mohammad Jafferany, Asmahane Souissi.
Description: Washington, D.C. : American Psychiatric Association
   Publishing, 2025. | Includes bibliographical references and index.
Identifiers: LCCN 2024020365 (print) | LCCN 2024020366 (ebook) | ISBN
   9781615375400 (paperback ; alk. paper) | ISBN 9781615375417 (ebook)
Subjects: MESH: Skin Diseases--psychology | Skin Diseases--complications |
   Mental Disorders--diagnosis | Mental Disorders--therapy |
   Psychophysiologic Disorders--therapy | Skin Manifestations | Case
   Reports
Classification: LCC RL96 (print) | LCC RL96 (ebook) | NLM WR 140 | DDC
   616.5/0651--dc23/eng/20241004
LC record available at https://lccn.loc.gov/2024020365
LC ebook record available at https://lccn.loc.gov/2024020366

British Library Cataloguing in Publication Data
A CIP record is available from the British Library.

I dedicate this book to my two beautiful daughters Yusra and Maha, whose unwavering support and boundless love have been the cornerstone of my journey. Your encouragement and belief in me have been the guiding light, propelling me through the darkest hours and inspiring me to reach for the stars. Each page is imbued with the warmth of your presence, and every word reflects the values you instilled in me. With heartfelt gratitude, I offer this work as a tribute to the precious moments we've shared and the countless memories yet to be made.

Mohammad Jafferany

I dedicate this book to my family, especially my wonderful daughter Reema, my husband, my parents, and my brother, who were beside me all the time and offered their full support. With my deepest gratitude, I offer this book to my teachers, professors, and colleagues who encouraged me during all my educational and professional life and put trust in me and in my abilities to reach what I want to achieve. Special thanks to my friend, mentor, and coach, Prof. Mohammad Jafferany, who guided me throughout this process and brought me to the world of psychodermatology.

In memory of my inspiring Teacher Prof. Bassem Louzir.

Asmahane Souissi

Contents

Foreword xvii

Foreword xix
Agnes Kalinowski, M.D., Ph.D.
Jacob Ballon, M.D.

Contributors xxiii

Acknowledgments xxxvii

1 Introduction to Psychodermatology 1
Erica Auckerman, B.A.
Chloe Wahl, M.D.
Mohammad Jafferany, M.D.

2 General Principles for Managing Psychocutaneous Disorders 7
Bárbara Roque Ferreira, M.D.

3 Dermatological Side Effects of Psychiatric Drugs and Psychiatric Effects of Dermatological Drugs 19
Ana Carolina Figueiredo, M.D.
Ana Goñi Navarro, M.D.
Bárbara Roque Ferreira, M.D.
Margarida Gonçalo, M.D.

4 Delusional Infestation 31

Samantha Hess, B.S.
Zehra Avan, M.D.
Mohammad Jafferany, M.D.

Case 4–1: Delusional Infestation: Folie à Famille 43
Smitha Prabhu, M.D.
Shrutakirthi D. Shenoi, M.D.
Krishna S. Swathy, N.D.
Priyanka Prabhakaran, M.D.

Case 4–2: A Case of Delusional Parasitosis 45
Asmahane Souissi, M.D.
Meryem Chaabani, M.D.
Rafik Mahmoudi, M.D.

Case 4–3: Delusional Infestation 48
Ilknur Kıvanç Altunay, M.D.
Gül Şekerlisoy Tatar, M.D.

Case 4–4: A Case of Delusional Infestation in a 65-Year-Old Woman..................... 51
Samantha Hess, B.S.
Mohammad Jafferany, M.D.

Case 4–5: Shrimp-Infested Nails: A Rare Side Effect of a Common Drug 56
Reem Al Neyadi, M.D.
Shaden Abdelhadi, M.D.
Dimitre Dimitrov, M.D., Ph.D.

Case 4–6: A Case Report Illustrating How Folie à Deux May Be Managed 59
Allison Kranyak, M.D.
Mitchell Davis, M.D.
John Koo, M.D.

Case 4–7: Delusions of Parasitic Sexually Transmitted Disease in a 71-Year-Old Man 62
Kamila Wala-Zielińska, M.D.
Jacek C. Szepietowski, M.D.

Case 4–8: Morgellons Disease or Delusional Parasitosis? 66
Agnieszka Otlewska, M.D.
Przemysław Pacan, M.D.
Jacek C. Szepietowski, M.D.

Case 4–9: Delusional Infestation of the Scalp and Folie à Deux 69
Mariam Tabka, M.D.
Dorra Mdhaffar, M.D.
Mourad Mokni, M.D.
Asmahane Souissi, M.D.

5 Trichotillomania and Its Variants 75
Asmahane Souissi, M.D.
Mohammad Jafferany, M.D.

Case 5–1: Coexisting Trichotillomania and Onychotillomania in a 10-Year-Old Boy 97
Asmahane Souissi, M.D.
Chaima Kouki, M.D.
Rafik Mahmoudi, M.D.
Mohammad Jafferany, M.D.

Case 5–2: A Journey of Hair Loss: From Alopecia Areata to Trichotemnomania 103
Asmahane Souissi, M.D.
Chaima Kouki, M.D.

Case 5–3: Trichoteiromania of the Beard 109
Asmahane Souissi, M.D.
Dorsaf Elinkichari, M.D.
Mohammad Jafferany, M.D.

Case 5–4: Trichotillomania Associated With Trichotemnomania 114
Tatiana Silyuk, M.D.

Case 5–5: Trichotillomania: More Than Just a Hair-Pulling Disorder 118
Monika Fida, M.D.
Oljeda Kaçani, M.D.
Edri Stafa, M.D.
Ermira Vasili, M.D.

Case 5–6: Trichotemnomania of the Eyebrows . . 122
Emna Chtioui, M.D.
Khadija Sallemi, M.D.
Hamida Turki, M.D.

6 Dermatitis Artefacta 127
Cemre Busra Turk, M.D.
Mohammad Jafferany, M.D.

Case 6–1: Dermatitis Artefacta Mimicking Palmoplantar Keratoderma 136
Gulhima Arora, M.D.
Sandeep Arora, M.D.

Case 6–2: A Case of Dermatitis Artefacta 140
Pavel V. Chernyshov, M.D.

Case 6–3: Dermatitis Artefacta in a 27-Year-Old Woman. 142
İsa An, M.D.
Ayşe Serap Karadag, M.D.

Case 6–4: Dermatitis Artefacta in a 51-Year-Old Woman. 145
Dimitry V. Romanov, M.D.
Anna V. Michenko, M.D.
Andrey N. Lvov, M.D.

Case 6–5: A Case of Dermatitis Artefacta in a 54-Year-Old Man 149
Brunilda Bardhi, M.D.
Monika Fida, M.D.
Arbnore Tafica, M.D.

Case 6–6: Dermatitis Artefacta in a 26-Year-Old Woman. 151
Rozana Cela, M.D.
Etleva Jorgaqi, M.D.

Case 6–7: Dermatitis Artefacta: A Diagnostic and Therapeutic Challenge 154
Ilirjana Zekja, M.D.
Malbora Xhelili, M.D.
Monika Fida, M.D.

Case 6–8: Dermatitis Artefacta as a Complication of Posttraumatic Stress Disorder..................157
Adem Cemerlic, M.D.
Asja Prohić, M.D., Ph.D.

Case 6–9: Giant Facial Ulcer as a Clinical Manifestation of Dermatitis Artefacta..........162
Marta Szepietowska, M.D.
Barbara Białynicka-Birula, M.D.
Jacek C. Szepietowski, M.D.

Case 6–10: Factitious Hand Lymphedema in a 19-Year-Old Female....................165
Maha Lahouel, M.D.
Nour El Imene Ouni, M.D.
Mohamed Denguezli, M.D.

Case 6–11: Occupational Dermatitis Artefacta in a Soldier......................169
Malek Ben Slimane, M.D.
Wafa Kabtni, M.D.
Abdel Aziz Oumaya, M.D.
Mohamed Raouf Dhaoui, M.D.

Case 6–12: Dermatitis Artefacta: A Case Report............................172
Imen Baati, M.D.
Madiha Mseddi, M.D.
Rim Sellami, M.D.
Hamida Turki, M.D.

7 Prurigo Nodularis...................177
Sara Al Janahi, M.D., M.Sc.
Dimitre Dimitrov, M.D., Ph.D.

Case 7–1: Prurigo Nodularis in a 45-Year-Old Woman....................187
Prajwal Pudasaini, M.D.
Sushil Paudel, M.D.
Sadiksha Adhikari, M.D.

Case 7–2: Prurigo Nodularis in a 55-Year-Old Woman................... 193
Atiya Rahman, M.D.
Saadia Tabassum, M.D.
Tazein Amber, M.D.

Case 7–3: Prurigo Nodularis— A Frustrating Malady 199
Usha N. Khemani, M.D.
Neha Fogla, M.D.

Case 7–4: Prurigo Nodularis With Anxiety and Depression................. 203
Varsha Gowda, V.M., M.D. 205
Shrutakirthi D. Shenoi, M.D. 205
Nidhika V. Sorake, M.D. 205

8 Alopecia Areata.................... 209
Zeba H. Hafeez, M.D.

Case 8–1: Alopecia Areata Associated With Trichotillomania 218
Asmahane Souissi, M.D.
Wejden Fakhfekh, M.D.
Mourad Mokni, M.D.

Case 8–2: Alopecia Areata and Psychological Comorbidity 222
Prajwal Pudasaini, M.D.
Sushil Paudel, M.D.
Sadiksha Adhikari, M.D.
Prashanta Pudasaini, M.D.

Case 8–3: Holistic Management of Alopecia Areata—A Case-Based Approach 228
Maria Angeliki Gkini, M.D., M.Sc., Ph.D.

Case 8–4: Alopecia Areata in an Infant Triggered by Admission to Intensive Care Unit 233
Asmahane Souissi, M.D.
Wejden Fakhfekh, M.D.
Zohra Fitouri, M.D.

Case 8–5: Anxiety and Depression Associated
With Alopecia Areata 237
Dipali Rathod, M.D.
Ruchi Hemdani, M.D.

9 Body-Focused Repetitive Behavioral Disorders 243

Usha N. Khemani, M.D.
Neha Fogla, M.D.

Case 9–1: Onychotillomania. 255
Matilde Iorizzo, M.D., Ph.D.
Marcel C. Pasch, M.D., Ph.D.

Case 9–2: A Case of
Treatment-Resistant Onychophagia 263
Mustafa Esen, M.D.
Ayşe Serap Karadag, M.D.

Case 9–3: Pseudo-Knuckle Pads:
A Bridge to Psychodermatology 269
Mezni Line, M.D.
Khallaayoune Mehdi, M.D.
Farah El Hadadi, M.D.
Meziane Mariame, M.D.
Senouci Karima, M.D.

Case 9–4: Chronic Wound Secondary to
Skin Picking Mistaken for Fungal Infection 274
Meera Aladawi, M.D., M.Sc.
Dimitre Dimitrov, M.D., Ph.D.
Tarek Shahrour, M.D.

Case 9–5: Obsessive-Compulsive Disorder
With Repeated Hand Washing and
Onset of Fingernail Onychomycosis 279
Prajwal Pudasaini, M.D.
Sushil Paudel, M.D.
Sadiksha Adhikari, M.D.

Case 9–6: Concomitant Onychophagia
and Dermatotillomania Successfully Treated
With Habit Reversal as Monotherapy 284
    Sara Al Janahi, M.D., M.Sc.
    Dimitre Dimitrov, M.D., Ph.D.
    Shaden Abdelhadi, M.D.

Case 9–7: Long-Term Pathological Skin Picking
Leading to Severe Skin Damage 288
    Mateusz K. Mateuszczyk, M.D.
    Joanna Maj, M.D.
    Jacek C. Szepietowski, M.D.

Case 9–8: Clinical and Medical Treatment
of a Woman With Skin-Picking Disorder 293
    Etleva Jorgaqi, M.D.
    Ermira Vasili, M.D.

10 Cutaneous Sensory Syndrome 295
    Dipali Rathod, M.D.
    Farzana Ansari, M.D.

Case 10–1: The Key Role of Psychodermatology
in the Understanding of Medically
Unexplained Dermatologic Symptoms:
A Case of Glossodynia 302
    Bárbara Roque Ferreira, M.D.

Case 10–2: Vulvodynia:
A Diagnostic Dilemma 304
    Saadia Tabassum, M.D.
    Atiya Rahman, M.D.
    Tazein Amber, M.D.

Case 10–3: Gardner-Diamond Syndrome 308
    İlknur Kıvanç Altunay, M.D.
    İlayda Esna Gülsunay, M.D.

Case 10–4: A Case of Glossodynia
(Burning Mouth Syndrome) 313
    Polina G. Iuzbashian, M.D.
    Andrey N. Lvov, M.D.
    Dimitry V. Romanov, M.D.

Case 10–5: Psychogenic Itch: A Complex Phenomenon 316
Aleksandra Stefaniak, M.D.
Jacek C. Szepietowski, M.D.

Case 10–6: Gardner-Diamond Syndrome in a 5-Year-Old Girl 319
Ines Lahouel, M.D.
Asmahane Souissi, M.D.
Hichem Belhadjali, M.D.
Mohammad Jafferany, M.D.
Jameleddine Zili, M.D.

Case 10–7: A Young Woman With Painful Indurated Erythematous Plaques 323
Meriem Amouri, M.D.
Zeineb Amouri, M.D.
Choumous Kallel, M.D.
Sonia Boudaya, M.D.
Mohammad Jafferany, M.D.
Hamida Turki, M.D.

Case 10–8: Gardner-Diamond Syndrome in an Adolescent Girl..................... 327
Piotr K. Krajewski, M.D.
Jacek C. Szepietowski, M.D.

Case 10–9: Gardner-Diamond Syndrome in an Adult Woman 331
Shahrukh Raza, M.D.
Diptarup Ray, M.D.
Sambit Chatterjee, M.D.
Mohammad Jafferany, M.D.
Anupam Das, M.D.

11 Miscellaneous Case Reports 337

Case 11–1: Hallucinations and Delusions of Vitiligo: A Case Report of Stress-Induced Symptoms................. 337
Tanyo Tanev, M.Sc.

Case 11–2: Pemphigus Vulgaris
and Psychological Percussion 340
   Harrison W. Loftus, B.A.
   Mohammad Jafferany, M.D.

12 Psoriasis, Depression, and Suicide . . . 345
   Harrison W. Loftus, B.A.
   Cemre Busra Turk, M.D.
   Mohammad Jafferany, M.D.

Index 357

Foreword

Anthony Bewley, B.A. (Hons), FRCP

Consultant Dermatologist, Barts Health NHS Trust;
Honorary Professor of Dermatology, Queen Mary College,
University of London; Immediate Past President,
European Society for Dermatology and Psychiatry

It is immensely important to have a psychodermatology text that is illustrated by clinical cases. And until now, there was no such textbook. Psychodermatology is a multidisciplinary subspecialty of dermatology in which dermatologists, psychiatrists, psychologists, primary care physicians, dermatology nurses, pediatricians, and other specialists share knowledge—together with the patient—to develop a diagnosis and treatment plan that is right for the patient. This excellent textbook, *Clinical Psychodermatology: A Casebook* by Dr. Jafferany and Dr. Souissi, provides an evidence-based approach to the management of patients with common psychodermatological conditions, and so facilitates the better practice of psychodermatology by all the members of the multidisciplinary psychodermatology team.

But the book is not just for specialists in psychodermatology. All too often in psychodermatology clinics, trainees from general dermatology, psychiatry, and psychology are surprised how little their training and experience have prepared them to manage patients with psychodermatological disease. So it is particularly brilliant that we now have this practical case-based textbook to guide us all in the management of our patients.

Foreword

Agnes Kalinowski, M.D., Ph.D.

Clinical Instructor, Psychiatry and Behavioral Sciences, Stanford University School of Medicine

Jacob Ballon, M.D.

Associate Professor of Psychiatry and Behavioral Sciences, Division of General Adult Psychiatry and Psychology, Stanford University School of Medicine

This book reflects collaborative efforts in the field of dermatology and psychiatry, preparing clinicians to recognize the psychiatric component in skin conditions. When providing optimal care for our patients, it is crucial to identify and address psychiatric factors influencing the skin—yet those skills are often underappreciated and underdeveloped.

Recognizing the mental health element in skin conditions helps the clinician to provide more *effective* care for patients. Specifically, in *Clinical Psychodermatology: A Casebook*, the compiled case reports have been organized into central themes: 1) general principles, 2) psychosis-spectrum disorders, 3) impulse control disorders, and 4) anxiety- and mood-associated disorders. These themes reflect predominant associations while acknowledging comorbidities with other psychiatric disorders. This framing logic will make the book highly accessible to psychiatrists and help point the clinician to the underlying psychopathology.

Chapters 1–3 address the first central theme of general principles. These chapters introduce the field of psychodermatology, provide basic approaches to patient care, and offer an overview of dermatological side effects of many psychiatric medications.

Examples of the second theme, psychosis-spectrum disorders, are delusional infestation (Chapter 4) and vitiligo (Chapter 11). DSM-5-TR defines psychotic disorders as those with "one or more of the following five domains: delusions, hallucinations, disorganized thinking (speech), grossly disorganized or abnormal motor behavior (including catatonia), and negative symptoms" (American Psychiatric Association 2022, page 101). More simply, psychosis can be defined as unusual choices or behaviors displayed by an individual due to aberrant processing of input: for instance, constantly fumigating owing to a belief that your home is infested. (The behavior would be reasonable if your home were indeed infested but would be considered psychotic in nature if there were no evidence of infestation.) In psychodermatological cases, patients misinterpret sensory input, leading them to believe an abnormality is present that is not. Although antipsychotics are the mainstay of treatment for psychosis, they may not be readily accepted by dermatology patients. In these cases, emerging innovative psychotherapy treatments are particularly useful in people who resist psychiatric medication (Heriot-Maitland et al. 2023; Ridenour et al. 2019).

The majority of the cases described in this book (Chapters 5, 6, 7, and 9) relate to a third central theme, namely, impulse control disorders. DSM-5-TR describes these conditions as characterized by the presence of "problems in the self-control of emotions and behaviors," largely anger and anxiety (American Psychiatric Association 2022, page 521). In the literature, some of these impulse control disorders are called body-focused repetitive behaviors (Sampaio and Grant 2018). The behavior alleviates distress, possibly by causing then alleviating physical pain (as described in nonsuicidal self-injury), which has been shown to decrease negative affective states (Plener et al. 2016). Alternatively, difficulty in controlling motor behaviors due to abnormal connectivity may underlie the repetitive behaviors (Gandhi and Lee 2021). Comorbidity with OCD, autism spectrum disorders, other anxiety disorders, and borderline personality disorder should be considered.

In the fourth central theme, symptoms of depression and anxiety may be a result of or comorbid with the skin condition. Cases appearing in Chapters 8, 10, 11, and 12 fit with this category. For example, visible skin lesions may cause feelings of embarrassment or low self-esteem that then negatively impact a person's social or occupational functioning, leading to a depressive episode or anxiety symptoms. Conversely, stress may lead to the onset or exacerbation of an autoimmune dermatologic condition, such as psoriasis (Zhang et al. 2024). Pain syndromes and itch are thought to be a result of heightened sympathetic nervous system tone that activates immune cells in the skin, making them more sensitive to external stimulation. Undoubtedly, abnormal neurodevelopment due to adverse childhood experiences plays a role: for example, childhood sexual trauma is a well-established risk factor for vulvodynia (Harlow and Stewart 2005; Huber et al. 2022).

The cases in this book highlight the need for an interdisciplinary approach to treating patients with psychodermatological conditions. As a general principle, when a patient has a primary psychiatric disorder and a skin condition, it is vital that the patient receive first-line care such as clinically indicated pharmacotherapy or psychotherapy for the primary condition.

Efforts in clinical research and animal models are revealing the interlacing mechanisms between the brain and the skin. Therefore, it is essential to recognize the comorbidity and take a collaborative approach to diagnosis and treatment. We recommend a focus on alleviating distress and optimizing functioning. Furthermore, while involving a mental health clinician familiar with addressing these conditions is ideal, in areas where such specialists are scarce, an empathic therapist is likely to be worthwhile.

References

American Psychiatric Association: Diagnostic and Statistical Manual of Mental Disorders, 5th Edition, Text Revision. Washington, DC, American Psychiatric Association, 2022

Gandhi T, Lee CC: Neural mechanisms underlying repetitive behaviors in rodent models of autism spectrum disorders. Front Cell Neurosci 14:592710, 2021

Harlow BL, Stewart EG: Adult-onset vulvodynia in relation to childhood violence victimization. Am J Epidemiol 161(9):871–880, 2005

Heriot-Maitland C, Gumley A, Wykes T, et al: A case series study of compassion-focused therapy for distressing experiences in psychosis. Br J Clin Psychol 62(4):762–781, 2023

Huber FA, Kell PA, Kuhn BL, et al: The association between adverse life events, psychological stress, and pain-promoting affect and cognitions in Native Americans: results from the Oklahoma Study of Native American Pain Risk. J Rac Ethn Health Disparities 9(1):215–226, 2022

Plener P, Allroggen M, Kapusta ND, et al: The prevalence of nonsuicidal self-injury (NSSI) in a representative sample of the German population. BMC Psychiatr 16(1):353, 2016

Ridenour JM, Hamm JA, Czaja M: A review of psychotherapeutic models and treatments for psychosis. Psychosis 11(3):248–260, 2019

Sampaio DG, Grant JE: Body-focused repetitive behaviors and the dermatology patient. Clin Dermatol 36(6):723–727, 2018

Zhang H, Wang M, Zhao X, et al: Role of stress in skin diseases: a neuroendocrine-immune interaction view. Brain Behav Immun 116:286–302, 2024

Contributors

Shaden Abdelhadi, M.D.
Professor, Department of Dermatology, Sheikh Khalifa Medical City; Professor, College of Medicine and Health Sciences, Khalifa University, Abu Dhabi, United Arab Emirates

Sadiksha Adhikari, M.D.
Medical Officer, Civil Service Hospital, Government of Nepal, Kathmandu, Nepal

Meera Aladawi, M.D., M.Sc.
Resident Physician, Department of Dermatology, Sheikh Khalifa Medical City, Abu Dhabi, United Arab Emirates

Sara Al Janahi, M.D., M.Sc.
Resident Physician, Department of Dermatology, Khalifa Medical University, Sheikh Khalifa Medical City, Abu Dhabi, United Arab Emirates

Reem Al Neyadi, M.D.
Resident Physician, Dermatology, Sheikh Khalifa Medical City, Abu Dhabi, United Arab Emirates

Ilknur Kıvanç Altunay, M.D.
Professor, Dermatology, University of Health Sciences, Şişli Hamidiye Etfal Training and Research Hospital, Istanbul, Turkiye

Tazein Amber, M.D.
Chief Resident, Dermatology, The Aga Khan University Hospital, Karachi, Pakistan

Meriem Amouri, M.D.
Professor, Dermatology Department, Hedi Chaker University Hospital, Sfax, Tunisia

Zeineb Amouri, M.D.
Professor, Hematology Laboratory Department, Habib Bourguiba University Hospital, Sfax, Tunisia

İsa An, M.D.
Dermatologist, Department of Dermatology, Sanlıurfa Training and Research Hospital, Sanlıurfa, Turkey

Farzana Ansari, M.D.
Assistant Professor, Shree Jagannath Pahadia, Government Medical College, Bharatpur, India

Gulhima Arora, M.D.
Dermatologist, Mehektagul Dermaclinic, New Delhi, India

Sandeep Arora, M.D.
Dermatologist, Mehektagul Dermaclinic, New Delhi, India

Erica Auckerman, B.A.
Resident Physician, Indiana University School of Medicine, Indianapolis, Indiana

Zehra Avan, M.D.
Resident Physician, Necmettin Erbakan University Meram Faculty of Medicine, Konya, Turkey

Imen Baati, M.D.
Associate Professor, Department of Psychiatry A, Hedi Chaker University Hospital, Sfax, Tunisia

Brunilda Bardhi, M.D.
Dermatologist and Aesthetic Surgeon, Venus Derm Clinic, Tirana, Albania

Hichem Belhadjali, M.D.
Professor, Department of Dermatology, Fattouma Bourguiba University Hospital, Monastir, Tunisia

Contributors

Malek Ben Slimane, M.D.
Assistant Professor, Dermatology Department, Military Hospital, Tunis, Tunisia

Barbara Białynicka-Birula, M.D.
Resident Physician, Department of Dermatology, Venereology and Allergology, Wroclaw Medical University, Wroclaw, Poland

Sonia Boudaya, M.D.
Professor, Dermatology Department, Hedi Chaker University Hospital, Sfax, Tunisia

Rozana Cela, M.D.
Consultant Dermatologist, Policlinic of Specialities Nr. 1, Tirana, Albania

Adem Cemerlic, M.D.
Physician, Washington University in St. Louis, St. Louis, Missouri

Meryem Chaabani, M.D.
Specialist Dermatologist, Department of Dermatology, La Rabta University Hospital; Specialist Dermatologist, Faculty of Medicine, University of Tunis El Manar, Tunis, Tunisia

Sambit Chatterjee, M.D.
Department of Dermatology, KPC Medical College and Hospital, Kolkata, India

Pavel V. Chernyshov, M.D.
Professor, Department of Dermatology and Venereology, National Medical University, Kiev, Ukraine

Emna Chtioui, M.D.
Resident Physician, Department of Dermatology, Hedi Chaker University Hospital, Sfax, Tunisia

Anupam Das, M.D.
Assistant Professor, Department of Dermatology, KPC Medical College and Hospital, Kolkata, India

Mitchell Davis, M.D.
Psoriasis Clinical Research Fellow, Department of Dermatology, University of California at San Francisco, San Francisco, California

Mohamed Denguezli, M.D.
Professor, Department of Dermatology, Farhat Hached University Hospital, Sousse, Tunisia

Mohamed Raouf Dhaoui, M.D.
Professor, Dermatology Department, Military Hospital, Tunis, Tunisia

Dimitre Dimitrov, M.D. , Ph.D.
Associate Professor, Department of Dermatology, Sheikh Khalifa Medical City; Associate Professor, College of Medicine and Health Sciences, Khalifa University, Abu Dhabi, United Arab Emirates

Farah El Hadadi, M.D.
Department of Dermatology, Mohammed V University of Rabat, Ibn Sina University Hospital, Rabat, Morocco

Dorsaf Elinkichari, M.D.
Resident Physician, Department of Dermatology, Rabta University Hospital; Resident Physician, Faculty of Medicine, University of Tunis El Manar, Tunis, Tunisia

Mustafa Esen, M.D.
Associate Professor, Fırat University Faculty of Medicine, Department of Dermatology and Venereal Diseases, Elazig, Turkey

Wejden Fakhfekh, M.D.
Resident Physician, Department of Dermatology, La Rabta University Hospital; Resident Physician, Faculty of Medicine of Tunis, University of Tunis El Manar, Tunis, Tunisia

Monika Fida, M.D.
Associate Professor, University Hospital Center "Mother Teresa," University of Medicine of Tirana, Tirana, Albania

Ana Carolina Figueiredo, M.D.
Dermatologist, Department of Dermatology, Coimbra Hospital and University Centre, Coimbra, Portugal

Zohra Fitouri, M.D.
Professor, Faculty of Medicine of Tunis, University of Tunis El Manar; Professor, Emergency Department, Children Hospital Béchir Hamza, Tunis, Tunisia

Contributors

Neha Fogla, M.D.
Resident Physician, Grant Government Medical College and Sir J.J. Group of Hospitals, Mumbai, India

Maria Angeliki Gkini, M.D., M.Sc., Ph.D.
Consultant Dermatologist and Honorary Lecturer, Dermatology Department, Barts Health NHS Trust, London; Dermatology Department, 401 General Army Hospital, Athens, Greece

Margarida Gonçalo, M.D.
Invited Professor of Dermatology, Faculty of Medicine, University of Coimbra, Coimbra, Portugal

Varsha Gowda, V.M., M.D.
Consultant Dermatologist, Department of Dermatology, Kanachur Institute of Medical Sciences, Mangaluru, India

İlayda Esna Gülsunay, M.D.
Resident Physician, University of Health Sciences, Şişli Hamidiye Etfal Training and Research Hospital, Dermatology, Istanbul, Turkey

Zeba H. Hafeez, M.D.
Psychiatrist, Adjunct Assistant Professor, Outpatient Psychiatry Director, Touro University, New York, New York; Kaiser Permanente California, Santa Rosa

Ruchi Hemdani, M.D.
Assistant Professor Dermatology, Himalayan Institute of Medical Sciences, Dehradun, India

Samantha Hess, B.S.
Student, Central Michigan University College of Medicine, Mount Pleasant, Michigan

Matilde Iorizzo, M.D., Ph.D.
Private Dermatology Practice, Lugano/Bellinzona, Switzerland

Polina G. Iuzbashian, M.D.
Assistant Professor, Department of Psychiatry and Psychosomatics, Sechenov University, Moscow, Russia

Mohammad Jafferany, M.D.
Professor, Department of Psychiatry and Behavioral Sciences, Central Michigan University College of Medicine, Saginaw, Michigan

Etleva Jorgaqi, M.D.
Associate Professor, Division of Dermatology, Mother Therezza Hospital, Tirana, Albania

Wafa Kabtni, M.D.
Associate Professor, Psychiatry Department, Military Hospital, Tunis, Tunisia

Oljeda Kaçani, M.D.
University Hospital Center "Mother Teresa," Tirana, Albania

Choumous Kallel, M.D.
Hematology Laboratory Department, Habib Bourguiba University Hospital, Sfax, Tunisia

Ayşe Serap Karadag, M.D.
Professor, Department of Dermatology and Venereal Diseases, İstanbul Arel University Faculty of Medicine, Memorial Health Group Atasehirand Şişli Hospital, İstanbul, Turkey

Senouci Karima, M.D.
Department of Dermatology Mohammed V University of Rabat, Ibn Sina University Hospital, Rabat, Morocco

Usha N. Khemani, M.D.
Associate Professor, Grant Government Medical College and Sir J.J. Group of Hospitals, Mumbai, India

John Koo, M.D.
Professor of Dermatology, Department of Dermatology, University of California at San Francisco; Director, UCSF Psoriasis and Skin Treatment Center, San Francisco, California

Chaima Kouki, M.D.
Resident Physician, Faculty of Medicine of Tunis, University of Tunis El Manar; Resident Physician, Dermatology Department, La Rabta Hospital, Tunis, Tunisia

Contributors

Piotr K. Krajewski, M.D.
Department of Dermatology, Venereology and Allergology, Wroclaw Medical University, Wroclaw, Poland

Allison Kranyak, M.D.
Psoriasis Clinical Research Fellow, Department of Dermatology, University of California San Francisco, San Francisco, California

Ines Lahouel, M.D.
Associate Professor, Department of Dermatology, Fattouma Bourguiba University Hospital, Monastir, Tunisia

Maha Lahouel, M.D.
Associate Professor, Department of Dermatology. Farhat Hached University Hospital, Sousse, Tunisia

Mezni Line, M.D.
Resident Physician, Department of Dermatology, Mohammed V University of Rabat, Ibn Sina University Hospital, Rabat, Morocco

Harrison W. Loftus, B.A.
Medical Student, Central Michigan University, Saginaw, Michigan

Andrey N. Lvov, M.D.
Professor, Department of Dermatovenereology and Cosmetology, Central State Medical Academy, Moscow, Russia; Professor, Medical Research and Educational Center, Lomonosov Moscow State University, Moscow, Russia

Rafik Mahmoudi, M.D.
Resident Physician, Faculty of Medicine, University of Oran 1, Oran, Algeria

Joanna Maj, M.D.
Department of Dermatology, Venereology and Allergology, Wroclaw Medical University, Wroclaw, Poland

Meziane Mariame, M.D.
Department of Dermatology, Mohammed V University of Rabat, Ibn Sina University Hospital, Rabat, Morocco

Mateusz K. Mateuszczyk, M.D.
Resident Physician, Department of Dermatology, Venereology and Allergology, Wroclaw Medical University, Wroclaw, Poland

Dorra Mdhaffar, M.D.
Resident Physician, Department of Dermatology, La Rabta University Hospital, Tunis, Tunisia; Resident Physician, Faculty of Medicine, University of Tunis El Manar, Tunis, Tunisia

Khallaayoune Mehdi, M.D.
Department of Dermatology Mohammed V University of Rabat, Ibn Sina University Hospital, Rabat, Morocco

Anna V. Michenko, M.D.
Professor, Department of Dermatovenereology and Cosmetology, Central State Medical Academy, Moscow, Russia; Professor, Medical Research and Educational Center, Lomonosov Moscow State University, Moscow, Russia

Mourad Mokni, M.D.
Professor, Department of Dermatology, La Rabta University Hospital, Tunis, Tunisia; Professor, Faculty of Medicine, University of Tunis El Manar, Tunis, Tunisia

Madiha Mseddi, M.D.
Professor, Department of Dermatology, Hedi Chaker University Hospital, Sfax, Tunisia

Ana Goñi Navarro, M.D.
Psychiatrist, Hospital Clínico Universitario Lozano Blesa, Zaragoza, España

Agnieszka Otlewska, M.D.
Department of Dermatology, Venereology and Allergology, Medical University, Wroclaw, Poland

Abdel Aziz Oumaya, M.D.
Professor, Psychiatry Department, Military Hospital, Tunis, Tunisia

Nourlimene Ouni, M.D.
Department of Dermatology, Farhat Hached University Hospital, Sousse, Tunisia

Przemysław Pacan, M.D.
Department of Psychiatry, Institute of Medical Sciences, Rzeszow University, Rzeszow, Poland

Marcel C. Pasch, M.D., Ph.D.
Dermatologist, Department of Dermatology, Radboud University MC, Nijmegen, Netherlands

Sushil Paudel, M.D.
Consultant Dermatologist and Head, Department of Dermatology, Civil Service Hospital, Government of Nepal, Kathmandu, Nepal

Priyanka Prabhakaran, M.D.
Consultant Dermatologist, Department of Dermatology and Venereology, Kasturba Medical College; Manipal Academy of Higher Education, Manipal, Karnataka, India

Smitha Prabhu, M.D.
Professor, Department of Dermatology and Venereology, Kasturba Medical College; Manipal Academy of Higher Education, Manipal, Karnataka, India

Asja Prohić, M.D., Ph.D.
Professor of Dermatovenerology, Department of Dermatovenerology, Sarajevo Medical School, University Sarajevo School of Science and Technology, Sarajevo, Bosnia and Herzegovina

Prajwal Pudasaini, M.D.
Consultant Dermatologist, Civil Service Hospital, Government of Nepal, Kathmandu, Nepal

Prashanta Pudasaini, M.D.
Resident Doctor, Kathmandu Medical College and Teaching Hospital, Kathmandu, Nepal

Atiya Rahman, M.D.
Professor of Dermatology, Head, Dermatology Department, PNS Shifa Hospital, Bahria University Medical and Dental College, Karachi, Pakistan

Dipali Rathod, M.D.
Assistant Professor, Department of Dermatology, Seth GS Medical College and KEM Hospital, Mumbai, India

Diptarup Ray, M.D.
Department of Dermatology, KPC Medical College and Hospital, Kolkata, India

Shahrukh Raza, M.D.
Department of Dermatology, KPC Medical College and Hospital, Kolkata, India

Dimitry V. Romanov, M.D.
Professor, Department of Psychiatry and Psychosomatics, Sechenov University; Professor, Department of Boundary Mental Conditions and Psychosomatic Disorders, Mental Health Research Center, Moscow, Russia

Bárbara Roque Ferreira, M.D.
Dermatologist, University of Brest, Laboratoire interactions épithéliums-neurones (LIEN), Brest, France

Khadija Sellami, M.D.
Associate Professor, Department of Dermatology, Hedi Chaker University Hospital, Sfax, Tunisia

Rim Sellami, M.D.
Department of Psychiatry A, Hedi Chaker University Hospital, Sfax, Tunisia

Tarek Shahrour, M.D.
Clinical Professor, Department of Psychiatry, Sheikh Khalifa Medical City; Clinical Professor, College of Medicine and Health Sciences, Khalifa University, Abu Dhabi, United Arab Emirates

Shrutakirthi D. Shenoi, M.D.
Professor and Head, Department of Dermatology, Kanachur Institute of Medical Sciences, Manguluru, Karnataka, India

Tatiana Silyuk, M.D.
Dermatotrichologist, Hair Treatment and Transplantation Center, St. Petersburg, Russian Federation

Nidhika V. Sorake, M.D.
Consultant Dermatologist, Department of Dermatology, Kanachur Institute of Medical Sciences, Mangaluru, India

Contributors

Asmahane Souissi, M.D.
Associate Professor, Department of Dermatology, La Rabta University Hospital; Dermatologist, Department of Internal Medicine, Internal Forces of Security University Hospital, La Marsa; Associate Professor, Faculty of Medicine, University of Tunis El Manar, Tunis, Tunisia

Edri Stafa, M.D.
Assistant Professor, University Hospital Center "Mother Theresa," Tirana, Albania

Aleksandra Stefaniak, M.D.
Resident Physician, Department of Dermatology, Venereology and Allergology, Wroclaw Medical University, Wroclaw, Poland

Krishna S. Swathy, N.D.
Department of Dermatology and Venereology, Kanachur Institute of Medical Sciences, Manguluru, Karnataka, India

Jacek C. Szepietowski, M.D.
Professor, Department of Dermatology, Venereology and Allergology, Wroclaw Medical University, Wroclaw, Poland

Marta Szepietowska, M.D.
Medical Student, Department of Dermatology, Venereology and Allergology, Wroclaw Medical University, Wroclaw, Poland

Saadia Tabassum, M.D.
Assistant Professor, Director, Dermatology Residency Program, The Aga Khan University Hospital, Karachi, Pakistan

Mariam Tabka, M.D.
Assistant Professor, Department of Dermatology, La Rabta University Hospital; Assistant Professor, Faculty of Medicine, University of Tunis El Manar, Tunis, Tunisia

Arbnore Tafica, M.D.
Dermatologist, Anassa Clinic, Tirana, Albania

Tanyo Tanev, M.Sc.
Clinical Psychologist, Yorkville University, Fredericton, New Brunswick, Canada

Gül Şekerlisoy Tatar, M.D.
Resident Physician, University of Health Sciences, Şişli Hamidiye Etfal Training and Research Hospital, Istanbul, Turkiye

Cemre Busra Turk, M.D.
Research Assistant, Massachusetts General Hospital, Boston, Massachusetts

Hamida Turki, M.D.
Professor, Department of Dermatology, Hedi Chaker University Hospital, Sfax, Tunisia

Ermira Vasili, M.D.
Professor, University Hospital Center "Mother Theresa," Tirana, Albania

Chloe Wahl, M.D.
Resident Physician, Southern Illinois University School of Medicine, Springfield, Illinois

Kamila Wala-Zielińska, M.D.
Resident Physician, Department of Dermatology, Venereology and Allergology, Wroclaw Medical University, Wroclaw, Poland

Malbora Xhelili, M.D.
Kavaja Hospital, Kavaja, Albania

Ilirjana Zekja, M.D.
Professor, University Hospital Center "Mother Teresa," Neurology Service, University of Medicine of Tirana, Tirana, Albania

Jameleddine Zili, M.D.
Professor, Department of Dermatology, Fattouma Bourguiba University Hospital, Monastir, Tunisia

Disclosures

The following contributors have indicated a financial interest in or other affiliation with a commercial supporter, manufacturer of a commercial product, and/or provider of a commercial service as listed below:

Barbara Białynicka-Birula, M.D.
Honoraria from Johnson & Johnson Innovative Medicine

Maria Angeliki Gkini, M.D., M.Sc., Ph.D.
Speaking honoraria and travel funds from Pharmaserve-Lilly

Contributors

Harrison W. Loftus, B.A.
Journal of the International Pemphigus and Pemphigoid Foundation

Jacek C. Szepietowski, M.D.
Employment and speaking honoraria from Leo Pharma, Pfizer, and Sanofi-Genzyme; employment, speaking honoraria, and travel funds from Novartis and UCB; speaking honoraria from Abbvie, Janssen, and Almirall

Cemre Busra Turk, M.D.
Grant/research support from the European Academy of Dermatology and Venereology; employment from Wellman Center for Photomedicine, Massachusetts General Hospital

The following contributors stated that they had no competing interests during the year preceding manuscript submission:

Shaden Abdelhadi, M.D.; Sadiksha Adhikari, M.D.; Meera Aladawi, M.D., M.Sc.; Sara Al Janahi, M.D., M.Sc.; Reem Al Neyadi, M.D.; Ilknur Kıvanç Altunay, M.D.; Tazein Amber, M.D.; Meriem Amouri, M.D.; Zeineb Amouri, M.D.; İsa An, M.D.; Farzana Ansari, M.D.; Gulhima Arora, M.D.; Sandeep Arora, M.D.; Erica Auckerman, B.A.; Zehra Avan, M.D.; Imen Baati, M.D.; Brunilda Bardhi, M.D.; Hichem Belhadjali, M.D.; Malek Ben Slimane, M.D.; Sonia Boudaya, M.D.; Rozana Cela, M.D.; Adem Cemerlic, M.D.; Meryem Chaabani, M.D.; Sambit Chatterjee, M.D.; Pavel V. Chernyshov, M.D.; Emna Chtioui, M.D.; Anupam Das, M.D.; Mitchell Davis, M.D.; Mohamed Denguezli, M.D.; Mohamed Raouf Dhaoui, M.D.; Dimitre Dimitrov, M.D., Ph.D.; Farah El Hadadi, M.D.; Dorsaf Elinkichari, M.D.; Mustafa Esen, M.D.; Wejden Fakhfekh, M.D.; Monika Fida, M.D.; Ana Carolina Figueiredo, M.D.; Zohra Fitouri, M.D.; Neha Fogla, M.D.; Margarida Gonçalo, M.D.; Varsha Gowda, V.M., M.D.; İlayda Esna Gülsunay, M.D.; Zeba H. Hafeez, M.D.; Ruchi Hemdani, M.D.; Samantha Hess, B.S.; Matilde Iorizzo, M.D., Ph.D.; Polina G. Iuzbashian, M.D.; Mohammad Jafferany, M.D.; Etleva Jorgaqi, M.D.; Wafa Kabtni, M.D.; Oljeda Kaçani, M.D.; Choumous Kallel, M.D.; Ayşe Serap Karadag, M.D.; Senouci Karima, M.D.; Usha N. Khemani, M.D.; John Koo, M.D.; Chaima Kouki, M.D.; Piotr K. Krajewski, M.D.; Allison Kranyak, M.D.; Ines Lahouel, M.D.; Maha Lahouel, M.D.; Mezni Line, M.D.; Andrey N. Lvov, M.D.; Rafik Mahmoudi, M.D.; Joanna Maj, M.D.; Meziane Mariame, M.D.; Mateusz K. Mateuszczyk, M.D.; Dorra Mdhaffar, M.D.; Khallaayoune Mehdi, M.D.; Anna V. Michenko, M.D.; Mourad Mokni, M.D.; Madiha Mseddi, M.D.; Ana Goñi Navarro, M.D.; Abdel Aziz Oumaya, M.D.; Nourlimene Ouni, M.D.; Przemysław Pacan, M.D.; Marcel C. Pasch, M.D., Ph.D.; Sushil Paudel, M.D.; Priyanka Prabhakaran, M.D.; Smitha Prabhu, M.D.; Asja Prohić, M.D., Ph.D.; Prajwal Pudasaini,

M.D.; Prashanta Pudasaini, M.D.; Atiya Rahman, M.D.; Dipali Rathod, M.D.; Diptarup Ray, M.D.; Shahrukh Raza, M.D.; Dimitry V. Romanov, M.D.; Bárbara Roque Ferreira, M.D.; Rim Sellami, M.D.; Tarek Shahrour, M.D.; Shrutakirthi D. Shenoi, M.D.; Tatiana Silyuk, M.D.; Nidhika V. Sorake, M.D.; Asmahane Souissi, M.D.; Edri Stafa, M.D.; Aleksandra Stefaniak, M.D.; Krishna S. Swathy, N.D.; Marta Szepietowska, M.D.; Saadia Tabassum, M.D.; Mariam Tabka, M.D.; Arbnore Tafica, M.D.; Tanyo Tanev, M.Sc.; Gül Şekerlisoy Tatar, M.D.; Ermira Vasili, M.D.; Chloe Wahl, M.D.; Malbora Xhelili, M.D.; Ilirjana Zekja, M.D.; Jameleddine Zili, M.D.

The following contributors did not supply information regarding disclosures:

Agnieszka Otlewska, M.D.; Khadija Sellami, M.D.; Hamida Turki, M.D.; Kamila Wala-Zielińska, M.D.

Acknowledgments

A heartfelt thank you to Samantha Hess and Harrison Loftus, who provided administrative assistance for this book. Your dedication and expertise were invaluable, ensuring this project's success. We are deeply grateful for your unwavering support behind the scenes. Together, we brought this vision to life, and we are forever thankful for your contributions.

Readers are advised that terminology used in dermatology may differ somewhat from diagnoses in DSM-5-TR.

Introduction to Psychodermatology

Erica Auckerman, B.A.
Chloe Wahl, M.D.
Mohammad Jafferany, M.D.

Psychodermatology, also referred to as psychocutaneous medicine, lies at the intersection of two medical specialties: psychiatry and dermatology. Psychiatry is the study of mental illness, an internal process, whereas dermatology is the study of skin disease, an external process. The practice of psychodermatology highlights the mind-skin connection. The field is relatively new, although the basic principles of psychodermatology can be traced back thousands of years. Hippocrates mentioned the impact of stress on his skin several times, and Aristotle described the mind and body as complementary entities rather than separate (Dalgard et al. 2015). Since ancient times, philosophers have commented on the phenomenon of people pulling their hair out in response to stress, a common condition now known as trichotillomania (Jafferany and Franca 2016).

The interplay between the psyche, the skin, and the nervous system can be traced back to their embryological origins. The ectoderm, the outermost of the three germ layers, gives rise to both the nervous system and the epidermis, the uppermost skin layer. Cutaneous nerve endings are responsible for the numerous skin sensations we experience, including itching and burning. These nerves weave through the dermal layer of our skin and transmit signals from the external environment back to the brain. Specific cells in our skin also release neurotransmitters and neuropeptides that relay important signals to the nervous system. Each system relies on the other to function optimally. When there is a disturbance to a system, it can manifest externally or internally.

Certain internal states, such as high stress, can present externally on the skin. High stress levels are associated with excess secretion of glucocorticoids, such as cortisol, and catecholamines, such as epinephrine. These hormones impact the immune system by selectively increasing the production of mast cells and eosinophils, which are heavily involved in the body's allergic inflammatory response. This is just one example of how an internal imbalance can aggravate a skin condition, as in atopic dermatitis.

The practice of psychodermatology acknowledges that the mind and skin are tightly intertwined. The field includes the study of psychocutaneous conditions and the psychosocial implications of skin disease. A primarily psychiatric condition can present with dermatologic symptoms, and many dermatologic conditions have profound psychological impacts. It is important for providers to recognize and address problems at both ends of the spectrum for comprehensive, holistic patient care.

The term *psychocutaneous condition* refers to a broad range of disorders. These disorders can be classified into several subgroups, including psychophysiological disorders, psychiatric disorders with dermatologic symptoms, and dermatologic disorders with psychiatric symptoms (Koo and Lee 2003). Psychophysiological disorders are skin diseases that flare with psychological stress. Patients usually acknowledge a chronological association between stress and exacerbation of their symptoms (Jafferany and Franca 2016). Conditions such as alopecia areata, atopic dermatitis, psoriasis, rosacea, and urticaria often fall into this category. Psychiatric disorders with dermatologic symptoms have no primary cutaneous process—all skin manifestations are self-inflicted. These disorders include delusions of infestation, neurotic excoriations, and trichotillomania. Dermatological disorders with psychiatric symptoms include skin conditions with adverse psychological effects. Conditions such as alopecia areata, atopic dermatitis, ichthyosis, vitiligo, psoriasis, and epidermolysis bullosa can have severely damaging psychosocial consequences. Often, the psychological impact associated with these disorders is more debilitating than the physical process itself.

The key to treating patients with psychocutaneous conditions is developing good rapport. Many patients do not want to admit to the underlying psychological turmoil that may be connected to their physical symptoms. It is often emotionally difficult for patients to discuss the psychosocial impact of their skin disease. A good doctor-patient relationship paves the way for open communication and improved treatment adherence down the road.

The treatment of psychocutaneous conditions often warrants both pharmacological and psychological intervention. Pharmacological interventions include a vast array of medications, including antidepressants, anxiolytics, antipsychotics, and antihistamines. Certain medications, such as naltrexone, have been shown to have off-label success in treating physical symptoms such as pruritus. Pimozide and *N*-acetylcysteine have shown promise in the treatment of delusions of infestation. Commonly used psychological interventions include psychodynamic therapy, CBT, stress management, guided imagery, and biofeedback. A multidisciplinary approach is often the most successful. Collaboration between dermatologists, psychologists, psychiatrists, and social services leads to higher patient satisfaction and improved outcomes. Unfortunately, the bias against mental illness serves as a barrier. Patients who present to dermatology clinics are generally not looking for a psychological referral. As mentioned earlier, good patient rapport is key to having success with these difficult conversations. Normalizing the mind-skin connection can help patients rationalize what they are experiencing from a physiological standpoint.

When treating patients with psychocutaneous conditions, it is important to conduct a functional assessment. This assessment ought to give insight into how the patient's presenting condition is impacting their daily life. Mental health struggles as well as sleep problems are extremely important to discuss, given their association with major depression and even suicidality. Certain conditions, such as psoriasis, hidradenitis suppurativa, and atopic dermatitis, can severely impair social or occupational functioning. These impairments can go on to cause serious interpersonal or occupational problems and eventual social isolation and withdrawal. In a society that correlates flawless skin with beauty, it is easy to understand why visible blemishes perpetuate a negative self-image. Stigmatization of certain skin conditions certainly exacerbates their psychosocial impact.

When treating patients with psychocutaneous conditions, the goal is to improve day-to-day functioning by reducing psychological and physical distress. Ultimately, this should improve self-esteem and reduce psychiatric symptoms. Many skin conditions are associated with increased rates of anxiety and depression. Anxiety is the most common psychiatric disorder in patients with chronic skin disease.

Dermatology clinics often screen for psychological symptoms by administering questionnaires. Written screening tools can elucidate psychological distress in patients who would otherwise have seemed fine. Commonly used instruments include the Hospital Anxiety and Depression Scale, Dermatology Life Quality Index, Skindex Questionnaire, and Generalized Anxiety Disorder-7. It is important to have these measures in place in dermatology clinics because of the high rates of comorbid psychological conditions.

As the field of psychodermatology gains momentum, psychodermatology clinics continue to arise across the world. These clinics, composed of dermatologists, psychiatrists, psychologists, and social services, have been shown to improve patients' quality of life, streamline care, and reduce overall health care costs (Mostaghimi 2021). Although there are multiple well-established psychodermatology centers in Europe, they have not yet gained the same traction in the United States. Common diagnoses warranting referral to a psychodermatology clinic include skin-picking disorder, pruritus, delusions of infestation, trichotillomania, vulvodynia, and the full gamut of common skin conditions. In one psychodermatology clinic in particular, skin-picking disorder made up more than 50% of total referrals (Mostaghimi 2021). Patients who present with skin-picking behavior are at high risk of developing concomitant trichotillomania, onychotillomania, and a variety of psychiatric symptoms (Picardi et al. 2000). Early intervention is key in preventing progression and potentially irreversible self-inflicted damage. The benefit of a psychodermatology clinic is that patients can receive dermatologic and psychiatric care in just one visit.

Multiple associations exist, including the Association for Psychoneurocutaneous Medicine of North America (APMNA), the European Society for Dermatology and Psychiatry (ESDaP), and the European Academy of Dermatology and Venereology (EADV) psychodermatology task force, dedicated to advancing research in the field and bringing awareness to its importance. ESDaP offers courses for dermatology residents that highlight the management of psychocutaneous conditions.

To say that this is an important area of concern is an understatement. We know that 30%–40% of patients who present to outpatient dermatology clinics suffer from underlying psychological issues (Picardi et al. 2000). Ensuring that patients are referred to appropriate psychological support services is of utmost importance. Collaboration between dermatologists, psychiatrists, and psychologists should be highly encouraged. When certain psychological conditions go unaddressed, it can be difficult to successfully treat the dermatologic condition. The mind and skin function in tandem, and to achieve satisfactory outcomes, clinicians must acknowledge this.

References

Dalgard FJ, Gieler U, Tomas-Aragones L, et al: The psychological burden of skin diseases: a cross-sectional multicenter study among dermatological out-patients in 13 European countries. J Invest Dermatol 135(4):984–991, 2015 25521458

Jafferany M, Franca K: Psychodermatology: basics concepts. Acta Derm Venereol 96(217):35–37, 2016 27282585

Koo JY, Lee CS: General approach to evaluating psychodermatological disorders, in Psychocutaneous Medicine. Edited by Koo JY, Lee CS. New York, Marcel Dekker, 2003, pp 1–29

Mostaghimi L: Psychocutaneous medicine clinic: Wisconsin experience. J Acad Consult Liaison Psychiatry 62(5):522–527, 2021 33975073

Picardi A, Abeni D, Melchi CF, et al: Psychiatric morbidity in dermatological outpatients: an issue to be recognized. Br J Dermatol 143(5):983–991, 2000 11069507

2

General Principles for Managing Psychocutaneous Disorders

Bárbara Roque Ferreira, M.D.

Introduction

Psychocutaneous (or psychodermatological) disorders include a wide spectrum of skin conditions linked with psychological stress and psychiatric illness. These disorders can present with visible skin lesions commonly associated with pruritus (such as atopic dermatitis), but some psychodermatological disorders (such as psychogenic pruritus and vulvodynia) are characterized by the presence of pruritus or dysesthesia without visible skin lesions. The adequate management of psychocutaneous disorders requires appropriate knowledge of both dermatology and mental health assessment. In fact, some of the most important challenges in the clinical practice of dermatology are the recognition and correct approach of psychosocial features and psychiatric illness linked with skin diseases (Marshall et al. 2016).

Skin disorders commonly have a significant impact on quality of life. Chronic dermatoses and their visibility are deeply linked with the concept of stigma. For instance, in psoriasis, the presence of lesions on the hands seems to be significantly associated with stigma, possibly because it resembles a contagious disease (Hawro et al. 2017) (see also Chapter 12, "Psoriasis, Depression, and Suicide"). In turn, skin disorders that do not have visible skin lesions, such as burning mouth syndrome and psychogenic pruritus, can be underappreciated and not sufficiently addressed (Ferreira et al. 2018).

This chapter highlights the relevance of psychodermatology and reviews key concepts of practical interest in psychodermatology, including classification, basic principles of dermatology and psychopathology, and therapeutic intervention, to guide and improve patient management.

Classification and Terminology of Psychocutaneous Disorders

To correctly treat a patient with a psychocutaneous disorder, it is important to recognize the wide spectrum of disorders as well as their differences and similarities (Table 2–1). Although no universal classification yet exists, these disorders are commonly classified into four main categories: psychophysiological, primary psychiatric, secondary psychiatric, and cutaneous sensory disorders (Koo and Lee 2003).

The first group, *psychophysiological disorders*, concerns primary dermatoses that are triggered or worsened by psychological stress. *Primary psychiatric disorders* include conditions whose skin symptoms directly result from a psychiatric diagnosis. Dermatoses or disfiguring skin disorders with *secondary psychiatric* illness concern the psychiatric consequences, commonly symptoms of anxiety and depression, that result from having a chronic and disfiguring skin disease. *Cutaneous sensory disorders* include conditions that also have a physiopathological link with psychological stress, but that are characterized by chronic pruritus or dysesthesia without primary skin lesions.

In this classification, overlaps can occur. For instance, the dysfunction of itch processing observed in cutaneous sensory disorders may result from a psychiatric illness, whereas in other patients, that cause-effect relationship is less clear. Therefore, psychogenic pruritus along with some cases of vulvodynia and burning mouth syndrome could also be classified as primary psychiatric disorders. In turn, most chronic skin diseases (namely, psychophysiological disorders) can lead to significant secondary psychiatric comorbidities; thus they also may be classified as secondary psychiatric disorders (Roque Ferreira et al. 2020b).

TABLE 2–1. Classification of psychodermatological disorders

Psychophysiological	Primary psychiatric	Secondary psychiatric	Cutaneous sensory
Acne vulgaris	Body dysmorphic disorder	Alopecia areata	Burning mouth syndrome
Alopecia areata	Delusion of infestation	Chronic urticaria	Penodynia
Atopic dermatitis	Factitious disorders	Hidradenitis suppurativa	Psychogenic itch
Chronic urticaria	Malingering	Ichthyosis	Sensitive skin
Psoriasis	Olfactory reference syndrome	Psoriasis	Scrotodynia
Vitiligo	Skin-picking syndromes	Vitiligo	Vulvodynia

A classic subgroup under primary psychiatric disorders concerns skin-picking syndromes, which can be considered an example of *nonsecret* self-inflicted skin lesions (the behavior that is responsible for the somatic damage is not denied or kept secret by the patient). Some terms that were previously used as synonyms for skin-picking syndromes, such as "dermatitis para-artefacta" and "neurotic excoriation," should be avoided, as the former may incorrectly suggest that inflammation is present as a primary mechanism in skin picking, and the latter may lead to stigmatization of patients as neurotic. Similarly, the term *factitious disorder* should be preferred to "dermatitis artefacta" (Gieler et al. 2013).

Finally, skin-picking syndromes should be clearly differentiated from *secret* self-inflicted skin lesions—namely, those observed in factitious disorders and other examples of nonsecret self-inflicted skin lesions that can be observed in other psychodermatological disorders, such as delusion of infestation, psychogenic pruritus, and other etiologies of chronic pruritus.

Basic Principles of Mental Health Assessment in Psychodermatology

Although more complex details regarding mental health assessment should be explored and managed by psychiatrists, some basic principles of psychopathology and mental health assessment should be familiar to all who deal with patients with psychodermatological disorders (Reichenberg et al.

2018). The prevalence of psychiatric comorbidity in dermatology is ~30%, and increasing scientific evidence has supported the role of psychiatry in the etiopathogenesis of several skin disorders, along with the deep impact psychiatric illness may have on quality of life (Connor 2017; Goyal et al. 2018).

The most common psychiatric comorbidities in dermatology are anxiety, depression, and sleep disorders (Ferreira et al. 2019). It is important to highlight that most patients do not exhibit a severe psychiatric diagnosis, although they may still present with less severe symptoms that are underdiagnosed and undertreated, with significant impact on quality of life. Therefore, dermatologists may play a very important role in addressing these comorbidities and may place referrals to a psychiatrist, depending on the severity of the symptoms. Taking all these factors into account, knowing the basic principles of mental health assessment of a patient with a psychocutaneous disorder is of utmost importance in dermatology.

Broadly, it is important to analyze the appearance and the behavior of the patient and ask about their experience with the current skin symptoms. Another important topic concerns biological functions, such as sleep. It is relevant to explore whether sleep patterns have changed, how, and since when. Sleep disorders are typically linked with several psychiatric comorbidities and are quite common in psychodermatology. Furthermore, psychosocial aspects are also deeply linked with psychiatric illness and thus with psychocutaneous disorders: it is important to ask the patient about the most relevant past and current relationships. Additionally, coping strategies should be explored along with the risk assessment: it is important to ask whether the patient has suicidal thoughts, actions, or plans in place. Other relevant topics are mood, the capacity the patient has to recognize and accept that symptoms can be a consequence of a psychiatric illness (insight), cognitive functions, perception, thought, and speech. Essentially, most of these aspects can be evaluated during the clinical interview, but some questionnaires and scales may be useful to evaluate psychiatric comorbidities such as anxiety and depression (Roque Ferreira et al. 2020d; Reichenberg et al. 2018) (Table 2–2).

Other relevant psychiatric diagnoses in psychodermatology include delusional beliefs (absence of insight), which define patients with a delusion of infestation, which can also be observed in body dysmorphic disorder (Phillips and Kelly 2021; Torales et al. 2020). Obsessive-compulsive symptoms are associated with body dysmorphic disorder and skin-picking syndromes (Grant and Chamberlain 2022). Increasing research has documented the role of personality disorders and personality traits in several psychocutaneous disorders (Holmes et al. 2022; Jafferany et al. 2020a). It is important to note that more than one psychiatric comorbidity may be present.

TABLE 2–2. Mental health assessment in psychodermatology: useful questionnaires and scales

Condition	Tool
Alexithymia	20-item Toronto Alexithymia Scale
Anxiety	Hospital Anxiety and Depression Scale
Cognitive function	Mini Mental Status Examination
Depression	Hospital Anxiety and Depression Scale
Obsessive symptoms	Dimensional Obsessive-Compulsive Scale
Somatic symptoms	Patient Health Questionnaire-15
Substance use	CAGE (cut down, annoyed, guilty, eye-opener)

Source. Adapted from Roque Ferreira et al. 2020d.

Basic Principles of Dermatologic Examination in Psychodermatology

Basic principles of dermatologic examination are required to correctly treat a patient with a psychocutaneous disorder. These concepts are particularly relevant considering that not all patients with psychocutaneous disorders will present to a dermatologist. Basic aspects of clinical history and examination in dermatology with relevance in psychodermatology include the presence or absence of skin lesions, type of lesions (primary and secondary), distribution of lesions, the presence or absence of pruritus or unpleasant cutaneous sensation (dysesthesia), the duration and frequency of skin symptoms, factors that trigger or worsen the symptoms (including the role of psychological stress), factors that improve the symptoms, current treatments for the psychocutaneous disorder (or other comorbidities), social context, family history, and clinical examination. Further details that are more specific for a dermatology consultation may eventually be required, depending on the disorder, including dermoscopy, trichoscopy, and dermatopathological examination (Roque Ferreira et al. 2020c).

Of particular importance to specialists in psychodermatology who are not dermatologists is the recognition that some psychocutaneous disorders present with visible skin lesions, but others do not.

Visible skin lesions can be primary or secondary. Primary skin lesions are those that arise de novo, meaning they are present at the onset of a primary skin disease (also called primary dermatosis). Some examples of primary skin diseases that are also psychocutaneous disorders are atopic dermatitis, chronic spontaneous urticaria, vitiligo, psoriasis, and alopecia areata (Figure 2–1). Secondary skin lesions are visible skin lesions that oc-

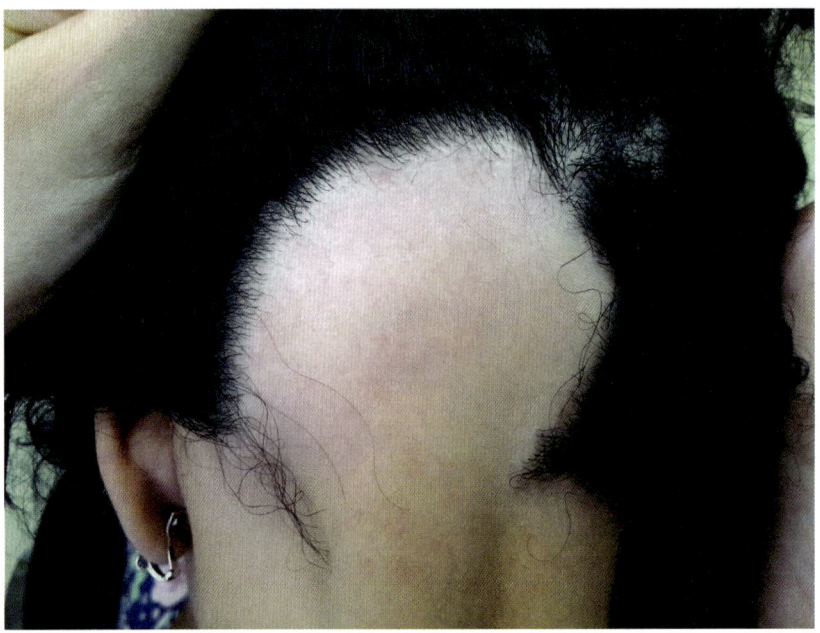

FIGURE 2–1. Alopecia areata: a round patch of hair loss.
Source. Dr. Asmahane Souissi.

cur over time through disease progression or skin manipulation (Holmes et al. 2022; Roque Ferreira et al. 2020c). Secondary skin lesions that result from skin manipulation are characteristic of several psychocutaneous disorders, namely, self-inflicted skin lesions, such as excoriations in skin-picking syndromes (Figure 2–2) (Bolognia et al. 2014; Roque Ferreira et al. 2020a).

Therapeutic Intervention

The adequate management of psychodermatological disorders requires awareness of a wide spectrum of skin disorders as well as the physiopathological link with psychological stress and interrelated mental illness; it may require the intervention of several fields of knowledge (Figure 2–3).

An appropriate therapeutic intervention may involve the collaboration of dermatologists, psychiatrists, psychologists, and other medical specialties (such as aesthetic medicine and surgery) (Jafferany et al. 2020b; Marshall et al. 2016). Although psychodermatology is of utmost importance in general dermatology practice, specialized psychodermatological care usu-

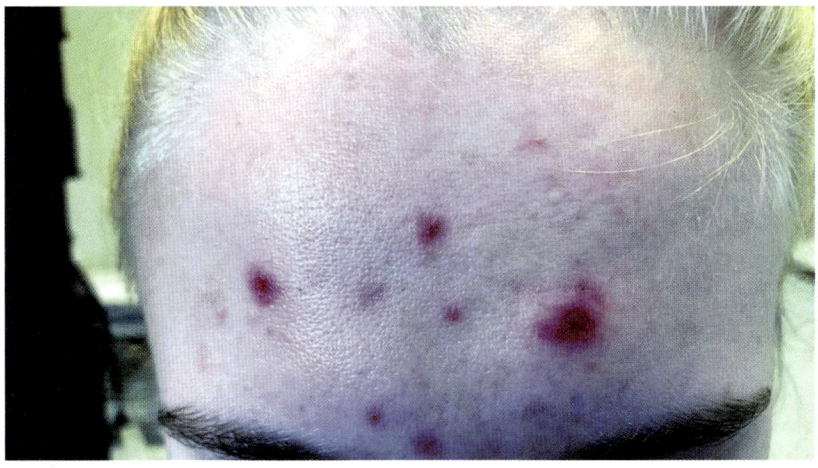

FIGURE 2–2. Skin-picking syndrome: acne excoriée.
Source. Dr. Bárbara Roque Ferreira.

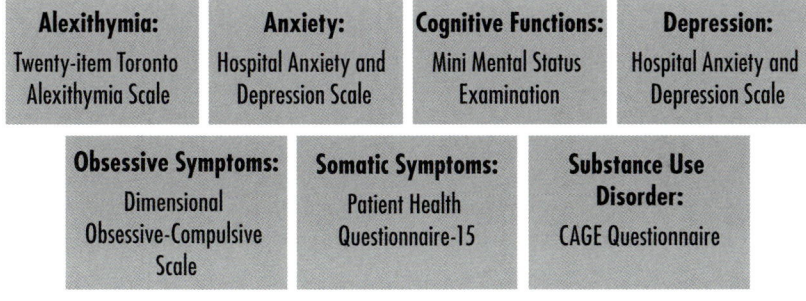

FIGURE 2–3. The adequate management of psychodermatological disorders may involve several fields of knowledge.

ally conforms to one of three models: dermatologist alone (and for selected cases, with referral to or discussion with a psychiatrist or clinical psychologist who works in a separate consultation); dermatologist and psychiatrist in the same consultation; and dermatologist and psychologist in the same consultation (Ferreira et al. 2019).

In psychodermatology, the therapeutic approach should consider specific dermatological characteristics related to the skin disorder, the type and severity of the associated psychopathology, the patient's uniqueness, and the understanding of patient expectations. Thus, this therapeutic intervention may include the following (Patel et al. 2020; Roque Ferreira et al. 2020b):

- General dermatological treatment
- Therapeutic education
- Psychoeducation about the dermatosis and the skin symptoms
- Psychotherapy (such as cognitive-behavioral therapy, mindfulness, biofeedback, hypnosis)
- Psychotropic treatment
- Psychobiotics

In some dermatoses, the combination of dermatology treatments with psychotherapy may improve the outcome. For instance, in a case-control study involving patients with psoriasis, treatment with CBT and biofeedback combined with narrow-band ultraviolet B administration was associated with significant improvement of disease severity and quality of life over narrow-band ultraviolet B alone (Piaserico et al. 2016). Moreover, psychotherapy helps improve coping strategies in visible dermatoses, with a positive impact on quality of life. For example, in a prospective study, mindfulness-based interventions significantly improved coping strategies related to the disease and the quality of life in patients with moderate to severe alopecia areata (Gallo et al. 2017).

Psychotropic medications can be useful in psychodermatological disorders. Depending on the severity of symptoms and the associated psychopathology, multiple psychotropics can be combined; they should also be considered in combination with dermatology treatments (Roque Ferreira et al. 2020b):

- Antidepressants (e.g., selective serotonin reuptake inhibitors [SSRIs], serotonin and norepinephrine reuptake inhibitors [SNRIs])
  - To treat depression, chronic anxiety, obsessive-compulsive symptoms, somatic symptom disorders, and sleep disorders
  - SSRIs are commonly used in the treatment of cutaneous sensory disorders, body dysmorphic disorder, and skin-picking syndromes
- Benzodiazepines and hydroxyzine
  - For acute anxiety and sleep disorders
- Antipsychotics (e.g., risperidone, aripiprazole)
  - To treat delusional infestation, some cases of body dysmorphic disorder, burning mouth syndrome, and self-inflicted skin lesions associated with impulsive behavior and dissociative symptoms
- Antiepileptics (e.g., gabapentin, pregabalin, topiramate)

- If anxiety is present, can be used as mood stabilizers, or in combination with antidepressants in some obsessive-compulsive and impulsive spectrum disorders
- Used in the treatment of cutaneous sensory disorders, such as glossodynia and vulvodynia, prurigo nodularis, lichen simplex chronicus, and in some cases of skin-picking syndromes

Finally, the interconnection of central nervous system disorders with gut microbiota dysfunction bolsters the relevance of psychobiotic treatment for psychiatric illness. Some studies have documented involvement of an alteration of commensal intestinal microflora in the etiopathogenesis of depression and anxiety disorders. Psychobiotics are bacteria (e.g., *Lactobacillus*, *Bifidobacterium*) or prebiotics that modulate a bacteria-mediated effect and have effects on the central nervous system through the modulation of neurotransmitters involved in psychiatric illness. Therefore, they have potential relevance in psychodermatology, particularly in disorders that have a close link with anxiety and depression, such as psychophysiological dermatoses (Palepu and Dandekar 2022; Roque Ferreira et al. 2020b).

Conclusion

The skin has a multifaceted role in our lives, including the development of our identity, being a physiologically privileged place for the expression of our emotions. Psychodermatology highlights the clinical relevance of what is less visible in dermatology (a medical specialty classically associated with what is more objective or visible), improving the knowledge of skin disorders without visible lesions (Ferreira et al. 2018). Moreover, significant research in psychodermatology has highlighted the relevance of subjective aspects related to chronic and visible skin disorders and their involvement in clinical evolution and quality of life. For instance, the health-related quality of life of a psoriasis patient (as assessed by the Dermatology Life Quality Index) is not closely associated with their psoriasis severity (as assessed by the Psoriasis Symptom Inventory), nor with the dermatologist's assessment of psoriasis severity (as assessed by the Psoriasis Area and Severity Index [PASI]). An objective method to assess disease severity, such as PASI, does not represent all the aspects of the disease that may interfere with quality of life—the more subjective aspects (Lacour et al. 2020). These findings, along with the significant prevalence of psychiatric illness in dermatology, strengthen the relevance of considering both patient- and physician-reported outcomes in the management of psoriasis, other chronic primary dermatoses, and cutaneous sensory disorders (Ferreira et al. 2018; Lacour et al. 2020). Psychosocial and psychiatric aspects are, indeed, a crosscutting issue in most skin disorders, underscoring the importance of general principles of psychodermatology in general dermatology practice.

References

Bologna JL, Schaffer JV, Duncan KO, Ko CJ: Basic principles of dermatology, in Dermatology Essentials, 3rd Edition. Edited by Bologna JL, Schaffer JV, Duncan KO, Ko CJ. Oxford, UK, Saunders/Elsevier, 2014, pp 39–49

Connor CJ: Management of the psychological comorbidities of dermatological conditions: practitioners' guidelines. Clin Cosmet Investig Dermatol 10:117–132, 2017 28458571

Ferreira BR, Pio-Abreu JL, Reis JP, Figueiredo A: Medically unexplained dermatologic symptoms and psychodermatology. J Eur Acad Dermatol Venereol 32(12):e447–e448, 2018 29633356

Ferreira BR, Pio-Abreu JL, Reis JP, Figueiredo A: First psychodermatology clinic in a Portuguese department of dermatology. J Eur Acad Dermatol Venereol 33(3):e119–e120, 2019 30357953

Gallo R, Chiorri C, Gasparini G, et al: Can mindfulness-based interventions improve the quality of life of patients with moderate/severe alopecia areata? A prospective pilot study. J Am Acad Dermatol 76(4):757–759, 2017 28325394

Gieler U, Consoli SG, Tomás-Aragones L, et al: Self-inflicted lesions in dermatology: terminology and classification—a position paper from the European Society for Dermatology and Psychiatry (ESDaP). Acta Derm Venereol 93(1):4–12, 2013 23303467

Grant JE, Chamberlain SR: The role of compulsivity in body-focused repetitive behaviors. J Psychiatr Res 151:365–367, 2022 35551067

Goyal N, Shenoi S, Prabhu SS, et al: Psychodermatology liaison clinic in India: a working model. Trop Doct 48(1):7–11, 2018 29041838

Hawro M, Maurer M, Weller K, et al: Lesions on the back of hands and female gender predispose to stigmatization in patients with psoriasis. J Am Acad Dermatol 76(4):648–654.e2, 2017 28069297

Holmes A, Marella P, Rodriguez C, et al: Alexithymia and cutaneous disease morbidity: a systematic review. Dermatology 238(6):1120–1129, 2022 35636409

Jafferany M, Afrin A, Mkhoyan R, et al: Therapeutic implications of personality disorders in dermatology. Dermatol Ther 33(6):e13910, 2020a 32594602

Jafferany M, Ferreira BR, Abdelmaksoud A, Mkhoyan R: Management of psychocutaneous disorders: a practical approach for dermatologists. Dermatol Ther 33(6):e13969, 2020b 32621633

Koo JYM, Lee CS, Eds: General approach to evaluating psychodermatological disorders, in Psychocutaneous Medicine. New York, Marcel Dekker, 2003, pp 1–12

Lacour JP, Bewley A, Hammond E, et al: Association between patient- and physician-reported outcomes in patients with moderate-to-severe plaque Psoriasis Treated with Biologics in Real Life (PSO-BIO-REAL). Dermatol Ther (Heidelb) 10(5):1099–1109, 2020 32761560

Marshall C, Taylor R, Bewley A: Psychodermatology in clinical practice: main principles. Acta Derm Venereol 96(217):30–34, 2016 27283859

Palepu MSK, Dandekar MP: Remodeling of microbiota gut-brain axis using psychobiotics in depression. Eur J Pharmacol 931:175171, 2022 35926568

Patel A, Jafferany M, Roque Ferreira B: Principles of psychotherapy applied to the psychodermatologic disorders, in The Essentials of Psychodermatology. Edited by Jafferany M, Roque Ferreira, B, Patel A. Cham, Switzerland, Springer International, 2020, pp 105–110

Phillips KA, Kelly MM: Body dysmorphic disorder: clinical overview and relationship to obsessive-compulsive disorder. Focus Am Psychiatr Publ 19(4):413–419, 2021 35747292

Piaserico S, Marinello E, Dessi A, et al: Efficacy of biofeedback and cognitive-behavioural therapy in psoriatic patients: a single-blind, randomized and controlled study with added narrow-band ultraviolet B therapy. Acta Derm Venereol 96(217):91–95, 2016 27283367

Reichenberg JS, Kroumpouzos G, Magid M: Approach to a psychodermatology patient. G Ital Dermatol Venereol 153(4):494–496, 2018 29667793

Roque Ferreira B, Jafferany M, Patel A, Eds: Basic principles of dermatology applied to psychodermatology, in The Essentials of Psychodermatology. Cham, Switzerland, Springer International, 2020a, pp 19–28

Roque Ferreira B, Jafferany M, Patel A, Eds: Common psychotropic treatments used in dermatology, how and when to use, in The Essentials of Psychodermatology. Cham, Switzerland, Springer International, 2020b, pp 91–103

Roque Ferreira B, Jafferany M, Patel A, Eds: How to classify and to use adequate terminology in psychodermatology, in The Essentials of Psychodermatology. Cham, Switzerland, Springer International, 2020c, pp 37–43

Roque Ferreira B, Jafferany M, Patel A, Eds: Screening questionnaires, scales and approach to patients with psychodermatologic disorders, in The Essentials of Psychodermatology. Cham, Switzerland, Springer International, 2020d, pp 47–54

Torales J, García O, Barrios I, et al: Delusional infestation: clinical presentations, diagnosis, and management. J Cosmet Dermatol 19(12):3183–3188, 2020 33098221

# 3

Dermatological Side Effects of Psychiatric Drugs and Psychiatric Effects of Dermatological Drugs

Ana Carolina Figueiredo, M.D.
Ana Goñi Navarro, M.D.
Bárbara Roque Ferreira, M.D.
Margarida Gonçalo, M.D.

Introduction

Psychiatric drugs (PsyDs) have been associated with a variety of cutaneous adverse drug reactions (CADRs) ranging from mild to life-threatening. PsyDs have also been identified as the exacerbating or inducing factor of

---

Ana Carolina Figueiredo and Ana Goñi Navarro contributed equally to this chapter.

specific dermatosis in predisposed patients. The range of dermatologic manifestations of PsyDs should be recognized by clinicians who prescribe them.

Many reactions are not severe enough to discontinue the drug, but the patient's self-esteem and compliance with therapy are aspects to consider. For more severe reactions, early diagnosis takes a significant role, as prompt drug withdrawal is associated with better survival. In these patients, a thorough analysis is mandatory, to identify the causal drug and avoid further exposure to related chemicals.

Drugs used for the treatment of dermatologic diseases, particularly systemic drugs, may be associated with disturbing psychiatric adverse effects that need to be recognized by psychiatrists, dermatologists, and primary care providers. It is very important to recognize these adverse events and distinguish them from primary psychiatric disorders.

Cutaneous Adverse Reactions From Psychiatric Drugs

The prevalence of PsyD-related CADRs has been estimated at 0.1% (Greil et al. 2019) to 5% (Litvak and Kaelbling 1972), with reported higher rates linked to mood stabilizers and lower rates for neuroleptics. Females and older patients seem to be more affected (Greil et al. 2019). The reactions may be immune-mediated (immediate or nonimmediate hypersensitivity reactions) or result from other mechanisms, such as abnormal pharmacological effect or drug/metabolite accumulation (Friedmann et al. 2003). Immediate reactions, presenting as urticaria or angioedema, are characterized by a rapid onset of transient migratory pruritic erythematous wheals or deeper cutaneous or mucosal edema, and may rarely progress to anaphylaxis. Maculopapular exanthema, the most common pattern of all CADRs, typically develops within 2 weeks of treatment, with few associated systemic symptoms. It usually starts on the upper chest and progresses symmetrically and distally, disappearing within 1–3 weeks.

Severe immune-mediated CADRs such as drug reaction with eosinophilia and systemic symptoms (DRESS), Stevens-Johnson syndrome (SJS), and toxic epidermal necrolysis (TEN) are relatively rare. DRESS usually develops after a long latency period (≤8 weeks), and resolution is slow (>3 weeks), presenting with exanthema associated with facial edema, enlarged lymph nodes, fever, eosinophilia, and multiorgan involvement, usually in the form of hepatitis. SJS and TEN are acute life-threatening CADRs with exanthematic necrolysis varying from 1% to the entire body surface area. After a prodrome of fever and flu-like symptoms, mucositis and exanthema are noted, consisting of dusky red macules resembling atypical targets, often with central bullae that coalesce in large sheets of detached epidermis.

Other CADRs include fixed drug eruptions, with lesional recurrence at the same sites shortly after drug exposure, as well as photosensitivity reactions (presenting as exaggerated sunburn or eczema on photo-exposed areas), cutaneous and mucosal pigmentary changes, monomorphic acneiform eruptions of the face and trunk, psoriasis aggravation or de novo, alopecia (mostly diffuse nonscarring alopecia due to telogen effluvium), and lichenoid reactions, characterized by late-onset violaceous flat-topped papules and plaques affecting the trunk and extremities symmetrically and generally sparing the mucosae.

Skin Reactions Associated With Specific Psychotropics

Mood Stabilizers

The highest reported rates of PsyD-related severe CADRs (Lange-Asschenfeldt et al. 2009) are in the context of aromatic anticonvulsants and other types of mood stabilizers, especially when used in combination. DRESS occurs more frequently in patients taking aromatic anticonvulsants such as carbamazepine (Figure 3–1), phenytoin, or phenobarbital but also can occur with non-aromatic anticonvulsants such as lamotrigine. A carbamazepine-induced rash, either mild or severe, occurs in 3%–17% of patients. European patients carrying the HLA-A*31:01 haplotype or Han Chinese with HLA-B*15:02 have a higher risk of carbamazepine-induced DRESS or SJS/TEN, respectively (Bertulyte et al. 2014). Lamotrigine-induced CADRs occur in 5%–10% of patients and may be severe, particularly when there is a rapid dose titration, simultaneous use of valproic acid, or a history of anticonvulsant-associated rash or in very young patients (Hirsch et al. 2006). SJS/TEN has also been reported in patients taking valproic acid, gabapentin, and oxcarbazepine (Warnock and Morris 2003). Frequent cross-reactivity between aromatic anticonvulsants and lamotrigine should be considered when starting a new drug (Warnock and Morris 2003). Valproic acid is usually considered a good alternative for patients with carbamazepine-induced DRESS (Bommersbach et al. 2016).

Lithium is associated with dermatologic complications in 3%–45% of patients (Jafferany 2008), most commonly presenting as a maculopapular exanthema, acneiform eruptions, psoriasis, folliculitis, or alopecia. Lithium induces or exacerbates dermatosis associated with neutrophilic inflammation (acne and psoriasis), likely through the inhibition of adenylate cyclase

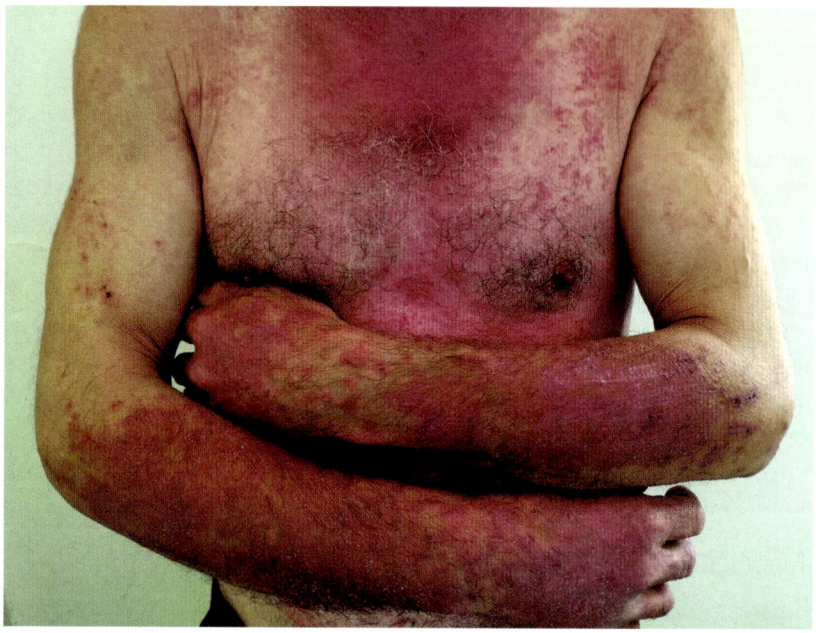

FIGURE 3–1. Carbamazepine-induced drug reaction with eosinophilia and systemic symptoms (DRESS) syndrome
Source. Dr. Mariam Tabka.

that causes prolonged neutrophil survival and an increased number of circulating neutrophils (Jafferany 2008). Lithium-induced psoriasis, presenting mostly as plaque-type psoriasis and seldom as pustular psoriasis or psoriatic arthropathy, appears in 1.8%–6% of treated individuals (Jafferany 2008), usually within weeks to months of therapy onset. Hair loss, observed mainly in females after several months of treatment, has been reported with mood stabilizers such as lithium, with rates as high as 10%–19% (Druschky et al. 2018).

Other CADRs caused by mood stabilizers include fixed drug eruptions (reported with carbamazepine, lithium, and gabapentin), drug-induced pigmentation (reported with carbamazepine, topiramate, lamotrigine, and gabapentin), photosensitivity (reported with carbamazepine, valproic acid, topiramate, gabapentin, and oxcarbazepine), erythema multiforme (reported with carbamazepine, valproic acid, lamotrigine, gabapentin, and oxcarbazepine), lupus erythematosus (reported with carbamazepine, lithium, valproic acid, lamotrigine, and oxcarbazepine), and hyperhidrosis (reported with carbamazepine, topiramate, lamotrigine, gabapentin, and oxcarbazepine) (Warnock and Morris 2003).

Antidepressants

Exanthematous reactions are more common with bupropion and less frequent with selective serotonin reuptake inhibitors (SSRIs) (Warnock and Morris 2002a). Urticaria can occur with any antidepressant, and angioedema has been particularly associated with paroxetine and bupropion (Krasowska et al. 2007). Serum sickness–like reactions (fever, urticaria, angioedema, arthralgia, and lymphadenopathy) have been reported in patients taking fluoxetine and bupropion (Warnock and Morris 2002a). SSRIs are commonly associated with phototoxicity in the first days of treatment, and as these drugs block serotonin reuptake in platelets, they can increase bleeding, enhancing spontaneous ecchymoses and petechiae (Krasowska et al. 2007).

Fixed drug eruptions have been reported particularly with nefazodone. Alopecia has been associated with all antidepressants, with the antimitotic activity of SSRIs likely playing a role (Etminan et al. 2018); paradoxically, hypertrichosis has also been described (Warnock and Morris 2002a).

SJS/TEN and DRESS are rare side effects of antidepressants. SJS/TEN has been reported with bupropion, amoxapine, and fluoxetine; DRESS has been reported with desipramine, amitriptyline, and imipramine (Warnock and Morris 2002a).

Vasculitis presenting as palpable purpura, rash, and fever has been reported with maprotiline and trazodone (Krasowska et al. 2007).

Other reactions include erythema multiforme (fluoxetine, paroxetine, and bupropion), exfoliative dermatitis (desipramine, nortriptyline, amitriptyline, and doxepin), psoriasiform reactions (fluoxetine, citalopram, and bupropion), and hyperhidrosis (nortriptyline, clomipramine, and maprotiline) (Warnock and Morris 2002a).

Antipsychotics

Antipsychotics can cause cutaneous reactions in ~5% of patients (Warnock and Morris 2002b), most frequently exanthematous eruptions, but newer antipsychotics appear to induce fewer CADRs. Urticarial eruptions have been described with clozapine, olanzapine, risperidone, and phenothiazines; angioedema may occur in patients taking loxapine, ziprasidone, risperidone, and clozapine (Warnock and Morris 2002b). Pigmentary changes are a common side effect of antipsychotics, specifically phenothiazines, whose metabolites may bind to melanin, impairing its degradation (Warnock and Morris 2002b). A blue-grayish pigmentation in sun-exposed areas occurs most commonly in women and after prolonged and high-dose therapy; it generally fades slowly after drug discontinuation. Photosensitive reactions, mostly phototoxic, have been described in 3% of patients taking chlorpromazine, promethazine, and mepazinortrimepazine (Warnock and Morris 2002b).

DRESS, a rare adverse effect of antipsychotics, has been reported with olanzapine and clozapine (de Filippis et al. 2022), the latter also associated with hypersensitivity vasculitis and SJS/TEN (Warnock and Morris 2002b).

Other reported CADRs include fixed drug eruption (chlorpromazine, haloperidol, olanzapine, prochlorperazine, quetiapine, and risperidone), alopecia (olanzapine, risperidone, ziprasidone, loxapine, and haloperidol), exfoliate dermatitis (risperidone, quetiapine, and ziprasidone), erythema multiforme (clozapine and risperidone), acneiform eruptions (quetiapine and haloperidol), psoriasiform eruptions (quetiapine and risperidone), and hyperhidrosis (olanzapine, quetiapine, and pimozide) (Warnock and Morris 2002b).

Anxiolytics

Benzodiazepines are very occasionally associated with cutaneous eruptions, most commonly exanthematous eruptions, with a few reported cases of erythema multiforme, and lichenoid eruptions caused by clonazepam or tetrazepam (Mitkov et al. 2014).

Psychiatric Adverse Effects From Dermatological Drugs

Systemic treatments used in dermatology can induce psychiatric side effects (Liu et al. 2016). Regardless of etiology (primary mental health disorder or psychiatric disorder induced by medication), the clinical approach of a patient with mental illness requires a holistic approach, in which it is essential to perform a complete clinical history and explore personal and family psychiatric history, along with physical and mental examination, including risk factors for mental health. Moreover, it is necessary to establish a temporal relationship between drug exposure and the side effect and support the diagnostic hypothesis in evidence (Raju et al. 2022).

Regarding management, in many cases, it will be enough to stop the suspected drug and switch to another drug with similar indications. If necessary, antipsychotics and mood stabilizers can be used, keeping in mind that it is better to start at a minimal effective dose. Nonpharmacological measures such as regular reorientation of the patient, regular visits by the family, and psychoeducation might be useful in decreasing side effects (Raju et al. 2022).

Dermatological Drugs and Psychiatric Side Effects

The aim of this section is to review the psychiatric effects of FDA-approved medications. The most important neuropsychiatric reactions according to the literature are found with drugs for psoriasis, especially nonbiological treatments, namely cyclosporine and methotrexate (Liu et al. 2016). The following text summarizes the main psychiatric side effects of dermatologic systemic medications as discussed in the literature; those for which a cause-effect relationship has been suggested are summarized in Table 3–1.

Antihistamines

First-generation anti-H_1 antihistamines have sedative-hypnotic actions that can be used accessorily for insomnia treatment, although sleep induced by these drugs is not repairing and can limit daily activities on the following days. This adverse effect is much less frequent with second-generation anti-H_1 antihistamines (Stahl 2008).

Apremilast

The literature warns of depressive mood disorder in patients treated with apremilast compared with patients receiving placebo, but there is no evidence-based link between apremilast treatment and mood changes (Haber et al. 2016; Liu et al. 2016).

Cyclosporine

Adverse effects of cyclosporine depend on dose and treatment duration and are reversible with treatment cessation. Headache, paresthesia, and tremor are the most common. In a few cases, psychosis, mania, and seizures have been reported (Liu et al. 2016; Raju et al. 2022).

Hydroxychloroquine

A recent systematic review warns of the risk of developing short-term psychiatric effects (such as anxiety or mental distress) after hydroxychloroquine treatment, effects that are not dependent on the drug dose (Talarico et al. 2022).

TABLE 3–1. Medications prescribed in dermatology and possible psychiatric side effects

Drug	Side effects
Antihistamines (anti-H$_1$)	Sedative-hypnotic
Cyclosporine	Psychosis Mania Seizures
Hydroxychloroquine	Anxiety Mental distress
Interferon α2β	Depression Suicidal ideation Mania, hypomania
Intravenous immunoglobulin	Anxiety, irritability Nervousness Tremor
Methotrexate	Psychosis Mania
Oral dapsone	Psychosis Mania
Systemic corticosteroids	Depression Mania Psychosis Delirium Sleep disorders Cognitive effects
Tetracyclines	Anxiety Depersonalization symptoms Suicidal ideation
Tumor necrosis factor α inhibitors (infliximab, etanercept, adalimumab)	Psychosis Mania

Interferon α2β

The most common adverse effects of interferon α2β (IFNα2β) are fatigue and flu-like symptoms. Neuropsychiatric manifestations include depression and mania. There is literature warning of patients developing depression while treated with IFNα2β; thus, treatment with SSRIs can be considered to decrease the severity of the major depressive disorder, and SSRIs can be useful as a prophylactic strategy. There are case reports of mania and hypomania related to IFNα2β dose changes (Liu et al. 2016).

Interleukin Inhibitors

The literature warns of the risk of depression and mood changes related to ixekizumab, but there is no strong evidence confirming this warning (Liu et al. 2016). Brodalumab was suggested to be associated with depression and increased risk for suicidal ideation and behavior. According to recent studies, however, there is no causal association between brodalumab and increased risk of suicide (Reich et al. 2022), but it is recommended to consider each case, also considering that psoriasis is associated with depression and suicide. Therefore, monitoring psychiatric symptoms during treatment and increasing frequency of follow-up reviews are recommended with this treatment.

Intravenous Immunoglobulin

Treatment with immunoglobulin G antibodies is associated with anxiety, tremor, and irritability (Liu et al. 2016; Raju et al. 2022).

Isotretinoin and Acitretin

Isotretinoin has been associated with an increased risk of depression and suicide, although a meta-analysis published in 2017 (Huang and Cheng 2017) concluded that isotretinoin treatment for acne does not appear to be associated with an increased risk for depression. In the setting of history of a mental health disorder, however, it is recommended to monitor psychiatric symptoms and increase frequency of follow-up reviews (Huang and Cheng 2017). Moreover, there is literature that warns of stiff-person syndrome with oral isotretinoin therapy. Stiff-person syndrome produces muscle rigidity and musculature spasms. Acitretin has fewer neuropsychiatric adverse effects, although there are case reports of peripheral neuropathy (Liu et al. 2016).

Methotrexate

Cases of psychosis and mania have been reported with methotrexate use (Liu et al. 2016; Raju et al. 2022), which resolved with drug cessation and adequate therapeutic management. Neurologic toxicity is related to overdose (Liu et al. 2016).

Oral Dapsone

Although it is controversial, there is literature that warns of psychosis and depression that resolved days after withdrawal from oral dapsone (Liu et al. 2016).

Systemic Corticosteroids

Adverse effects of systemic corticosteroids are dose dependent and include depression, mania, psychosis, and delirium. Moreover, systemic corticosteroids can be associated with sleep disorders and behavioral and cognitive effects (Gable and Depry 2015; Liu et al. 2016; Raju et al. 2022).

Tetracyclines

Depersonalization symptoms have been reported in the literature as a potentially severe side effect of minocycline (Shamout et al. 2019). There are some reports of psychiatric adverse events, including suicidal ideation, related to doxycycline (Atigari et al. 2013).

Tumor Necrosis Factor α Inhibitors

There are case reports of psychosis and mania linked with etanercept and infliximab; these side effects resolved with drug suspension and antipsychotic treatment (Austin and Tan 2012; Liu et al. 2016).

References

Atigari OV, Hogan C, Healy D: Doxycycline and suicidality. BMJ Case Rep 2013:bcr2013200723, 2013 24347450

Austin M, Tan YC: Mania associated with infliximab. Aust N Z J Psychiatry 46(7):684–685, 2012 22735640

Bertulyte I, Schwan S, Hallberg P: Identification of risk factors for carbamazepine-induced serious mucocutaneous adverse reactions: a case-control study using data from spontaneous adverse drug reaction reports. J Pharmacol Pharmacother 5(2):100–138, 2014 24799813

Bommersbach TJ, Lapid MI, Leung JG, et al: Management of psychotropic drug-induced DRESS syndrome: a systematic review. Mayo Clin Proc 91(6):787–801, 2016 27126302

de Filippis R, Kane JM, Kuzo N, et al: Screening the European pharmacovigilance database for reports of clozapine-related DRESS syndrome: 47 novel cases. Eur Neuropsychopharmacol 60:25–37, 2022 35635994

Druschky K, Bleich S, Grohmann R, et al: Severe hair loss associated with psychotropic drugs in psychiatric inpatients—data from an observational pharmacovigilance program in German-speaking countries. Eur Psychiatry 54:117–123, 2018 30193142

Etminan M, Sodhi M, Procyshyn RM, et al: Risk of hair loss with different antidepressants: a comparative retrospective cohort study. Int Clin Psychopharmacol 33(1):44–48, 2018 28763345

Friedmann PS, Lee MS, Friedmann AC, Barnetson RS: Mechanisms in cutaneous drug hypersensitivity reactions. Clin Exp Allergy 33(7):861–872, 2003 12859440

Gable M, Depry D: Sustained corticosteroid-induced mania and psychosis despite cessation: a case study and brief literature review. Int J Psychiatry Med 50(4):398–404, 2015 26644319

Greil W, Zhang X, Stassen H, et al: Cutaneous adverse drug reactions to psychotropic drugs and their risk factors—a case-control study. Eur Neuropsychopharmacol 29(1):111–121, 2019 30424913

Haber SL, Hamilton S, Bank M, et al: Apremilast: a novel drug for treatment of psoriasis and psoriatic arthritis. Ann Pharmacother 50(4):282–290, 2016 26783350

Hirsch LJ, Weintraub DB, Buchsbaum R, et al: Predictors of lamotrigine-associated rash. Epilepsia 47(2):318–322, 2006 16499755

Huang YC, Cheng YC: Isotretinoin treatment for acne and risk of depression: a systematic review and meta-analysis. J Am Acad Dermatol 76(6):1068–1076.e9, 2017 28291553

Jafferany M: Lithium and skin: dermatologic manifestations of lithium therapy. Int J Dermatol 47(11):1101–1111, 2008 18986438

Krasowska D, Szymanek M, Schwartz RA, Mysinski W: Cutaneous effects of the most commonly used antidepressant medication, the selective serotonin reuptake inhibitors. J Am Acad Dermatol 56(5):848–853, 2007 17147971

Lange-Asschenfeldt C, Grohmann R, Lange-Asschenfeldt B, et al: Cutaneous adverse reactions to psychotropic drugs: data from a multicenter surveillance program. J Clin Psychiatry 70(9):1258–1265, 2009 19538904

Litvak R, Kaelbling R: Dermatological side effects with psychotropics. Dis Nerv Syst 33(5):309–311, 1972 4146745

Liu M, Huang YYM, Hsu S, Kass JS: Neurological and neuropsychiatric adverse effects of dermatologic medications. CNS Drugs 30(12):1149–1168, 2016 27832476

Mitkov MV, Trowbridge RM, Lockshin BN, Caplan JP: Dermatologic side effects of psychotropic medications. Psychosomatics 55(1):1–20, 2014 24099686

Raju NN, Kumar KSVRNP, Nihal G: Management of medication-induced psychiatric disorders. Indian J Psychiatry 64(Suppl 2):S281–S291, 2022 35602361

Reich K, Thaçi D, Stingl G, et al: Safety of brodalumab in plaque psoriasis: integrated pooled data from five clinical trials. Acta Derm Venereol 102:adv00683, 2022 35191512

Shamout Y, Sigal A, Litvinov IV: Minocycline-induced transient depersonalization: a case report. SAGE Open Med Case Rep 7:2050313X18823827, 2019 30719316

Stahl SM: Selective histamine H1 antagonism: novel hypnotic and pharmacologic actions challenge classical notions of antihistamines. CNS Spectr 13(12):1027–1038, 2008 19179941

Talarico F, Chakravarty S, Liu YS, et al: Systematic review of psychiatric adverse effects induced by chloroquine and hydroxychloroquine: case reports and population studies. Ann Pharmacother 57(4):463–479, 2022 35927939

Warnock JK, Morris DW: Adverse cutaneous reactions to antidepressants. Am J Clin Dermatol 3(5):329–339, 2002a 12069639

Warnock JK, Morris DW: Adverse cutaneous reactions to antipsychotics. Am J Clin Dermatol 3(9):629–636, 2002b 12444805

Warnock JK, Morris DW: Adverse cutaneous reactions to mood stabilizers. Am J Clin Dermatol 4(1):21–30, 2003 12477370

4

Delusional Infestation

Samantha Hess, B.S.
Zehra Avan, M.D.
Mohammad Jafferany, M.D.

Delusional infestation (previously known as delusional parasitosis) is an uncommon, monosymptomatic, psychocutaneous disorder in which an individual has the fixed, false belief that they have an infestation of parasites in their body (Reich et al. 2019). Delusional infestation is a historically well-described condition that is known by multiple previous names including psychogenic parasitosis, Ekbom syndrome, and Morgellons disease (Reich et al. 2019). Although delusional infestation is largely a psychiatric disorder, it is important that all health care providers have the knowledge base to correctly identify it so that the patient can receive psychiatric assistance in a timely manner.

Patients with delusional infestation are very disturbed by their perceived symptoms. Thoughts of infestation are usually limited to the skin but can also extend to other areas of the body such as the gastrointestinal tract (Mumcuoglu et al. 2018). A patient with delusional infestation may show their provider samples of bodily tissues, such as nails or skin, or other belongings that they believe are infected with a parasite to prove their infestation (Mumcuoglu et al. 2018); this is called *matchbox sign* or *specimen sign*. Modern patients present videos or digital images depicting areas they believe are affected by infestation (Torales et al. 2020). Despite clear medical evidence proving a lack of parasitic infestation, patients with delusional infestation will continue to develop their complex delusional thoughts associated with the perceived infestation (Laidler 2018; Rosales Santillan et al. 2018). Therefore, these patients may attempt to consult multiple health care practices to find a provider who will assist them with perceived infestation (Mumcuoglu et al. 2018; Reich et al. 2019). Patients will also spend significant amounts of their time and money to attempt to rid themselves of the infestation.

Patients with delusional infestation are also capable of welcoming a second individual who is close to the patient into their delusion. This very rare process is called *folie à deux*, when an individual who is close to the patient with the delusion adopts the same delusion (Mumcuoglu et al. 2018; Reich et al. 2019; Sawant and Vispute 2015). Inclusion of even more individuals may be termed *folie à trois*, *folie à plusieurs*, or *folie à famille*.

Delusional infestation can be further classified into either primary or secondary diagnoses (Reich et al. 2019). Primary delusional infestation is characterized by the patient having the monosymptomatic delusion of an infestation with parasites with a lack of any other medical or psychiatric disorders. The delusion of infestation will be accompanied by unusual cutaneous sensations that further the individual's belief of an infestation. In secondary delusional infestation, the delusion of an infestation with parasites is accompanied by an additional medical condition, psychiatric disorder, pharmacological adverse effect, or use of illicit substances (Katsoulis et al. 2020).

Etiology and Epidemiology

The prevalence and incidence of delusional infestation are not well established, and it has a wide reported range. Data from varying studies show potential ranges from 1.9 to 27.3 cases per 100,000 individuals per year (Kohorst et al. 2018; Laidler 2018). The mean age at diagnosis of delusional infestation is 57 to 61.4 years, suggesting that the prevalence of the disease increases in that age range (Kohorst et al. 2018); however, a bimodal distribution has been described. Multiple studies have also reported a higher incidence in women than men (Ansari and Bragg 2023). Secondary delusional infestation occurs more frequently than primary delusional infestation and is often associated with the disorders described in Table 4–1.

TABLE 4–1. Causes of secondary delusional infestation

Psychiatric condition	Medical condition	Medication	Illicit substance
Bipolar disorder	Alcohol use disorder	Antibiotics	Benzodiazepines
Delirium	Cancer	Antifungals	Cannabis
Generalized anxiety disorder	Cardiovascular disease	Parkinson's disease treatments (levodopa, pramipexole, ropinirole, entacapone, decarboxylase inhibitors, amantadine)	Cocaine
Major depressive disorder	Cholestasis		Heroin (withdrawal)
Obsessive-compulsive disorder	Cysticercosis		Methadone
Schizophrenia	Diabetes		Methamphetamine
	Lupus erythematous		Opiates
	Neuropathies		
	Parkinson's disease	NSAIDs	
	Renal failure	Steroids	
	Stroke		
	Thyroid disorders		
	Vascular encephalopathy		
	Vitamin deficiencies		

Note. NSAID=nonsteroidal anti-inflammatory drug.
Source. Katsoulis et al. 2020.

Pathophysiology

The pathophysiology of delusional infestation is not precisely known (Katsoulis et al. 2020). It is hypothesized that increased extracellular dopamine levels occur as a result of a dysfunctional dopamine transporter (Huber et al. 2007). The symptomatic response of many delusional infestation patients to dopamine antagonists serves to support this theory (Laidler 2018). Additionally, a recent study used magnetic resonance imaging (MRI) to measure the cortical thickness of patients with delusional infestation compared with healthy individuals. Researchers found atrophy in the frontal cortex, dorsal striatum, parietal and temporal cortices, and thalamus, suggesting that various neural circuits responsible for perception, visuospatial control, and self-awareness were affected (Huber et al. 2007). Further investigation is required.

Evaluation

Two clinical features are required for proper diagnosis of delusional infestation: the persistence of a delusion of infestation lasting for more than a month and the accompaniment of cutaneous symptoms (Reich et al. 2019) (see next section for more details). In concert with the patient, the clinician should collect a complete and comprehensive history, including recent travels, contact with family members or friends with similar symptoms, or any history of parasites in pets. The clinician should first aim to exclude organic parasitosis through the patient's medical history.

If the patient brings in samples for inspection (matchbox sign), they should be properly examined by the clinician and appropriate laboratory technicians if indicated. The clinician should then perform a complete and comprehensive physical examination, including a complete body inspection. Any associated laboratory tests, such as eosinophil count, should be performed as needed. If there is any doubt as to what physical findings are pertinent during examination, it is appropriate to consult a dermatologist.

Upon ruling out an organic cause of delusional infestation, the clinician should interview the patient further about the delusion. It is crucial to ascertain how unshakable the delusion is for the patient. If it is determined that there is no present delusion, other causes of pruritus should be investigated. However, if the patient presents with cutaneous symptoms and a delusion of infestation, then it can be determined that the patient has delusional infestation and it will be necessary to determine whether it is primary or secondary in nature. Primary delusional infestation will ultimately be a diagnosis of exclusion following the ruling out of all possible psychiatric, pharmacological, and medical causes of delusional infestation (Reich et al. 2019). If the delusional infestation is determined to be secondary, the treatment focus should be on treating the causative condition (Rosales Santillan et al. 2018).

When evaluating a patient with delusional infestation, it is important to remember that it is extremely difficult for the patient to accept the diagnosis and appropriate treatment plan owing to their delusion (Rosales Santillan et al. 2018). Showing the patient their test results can increase patient compliance, although this is not always successful. The clinician should always express empathy and work as a team with the patient to ensure the best outcomes.

Clinical Features

Patients with delusional infestation can present with a variety of psychological and dermatological symptoms. To be classified as delusional infestation, the following symptoms must be present:

1. The patient should have a fixed, false belief that they have an infestation lasting for more than a month (Mumcuoglu et al. 2018; Reich et al. 2019). The infestation can be from any form of organism, microscopic or macroscopic. Most patients with delusional infestation will identify macroscopic organisms as the cause of their infestation. The patient is not required to have delusions outside of the belief of an infestation.
2. The patient should have cutaneous symptoms that further their belief in the presence of an infestation (Mumcuoglu et al. 2018). The symptoms usually include itching, tingling, prickling, and burning.

The cutaneous manifestations of delusional infestation often result in the patient scratching their skin (Reich et al. 2019). This can lead to varying degrees of skin damage and sequelae. Skin damage can present as erosions (Figures 4–1 and 4–2), ulcers, and hair loss, as a few examples. For this reason, patients may present with scratches and scars at varying degrees of healing (Figure 4–3), with the degree of damage being more severe on the areas of the body the patient can reach with their dominant hand (Freudenmann and Lepping 2009).

Matchbox sign is seen in ~70% of cases (Kalovidouri et al. 2022; Laidler 2018). The items patients collect are often lint, pieces of plants, skin flakes, or small bugs from their surroundings. Patients with delusional infestation can have ocular involvement (believing the infestation is within their eyes), leading to ocular damage (Katsoulis et al. 2020). Patients can present with a variety of psychiatric involvements, such as isolation out of fear of contaminating their loved ones, anxiety, depression, suicidal ideation, and suicide attempt. Approximately 8%–12% of cases of delusional infestation can lead to folie à deux, in which a loved one is also convinced of the delusion (Katsoulis et al. 2020).

Differential Diagnosis

When a clinician suspects delusional infestation, all other potential causes of the patient's symptoms must be thoroughly investigated and ruled out before making a diagnosis. The clinician should use anamnesis, thorough physical examination, imaging, and appropriate laboratory tests (Kalovidouri et al. 2022). Physical examination should be used to reveal whether the

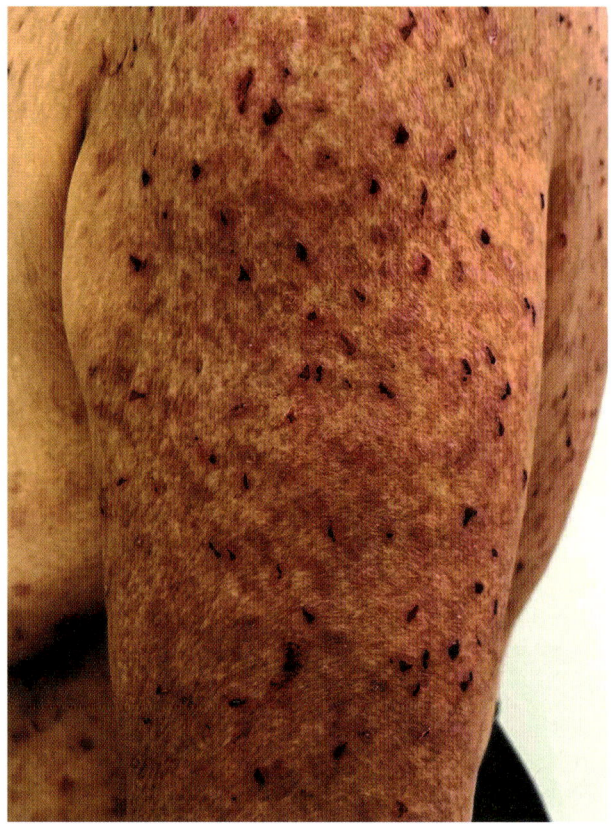

FIGURE 4–1. Multiple erosions on the arm in a patient with delusional infestation.
Source. Dr. Asmahane Souissi.

skin findings reported by the patient are caused by the presence of a parasite or the patient's own manipulation of their skin (the lesions are present only in areas within reach of the patient's hand). Laboratory tests, including eosinophil count, white blood cell count, and C-reactive protein concentration, should be within normal range to exclude the presence of true parasitosis.

After excluding true parasitosis, possible causes of pruritus should be investigated. Many systemic diseases, including renal insufficiency and cholestasis, have pruritus as a clearly described symptom. The investigation should also include a thorough review of medications, as many medications can cause itching and tingling in the extremities (Campbell et al. 2019).

When working through the differential diagnosis, the precise type of delusional infestation should be defined to guide treatment options (Reich

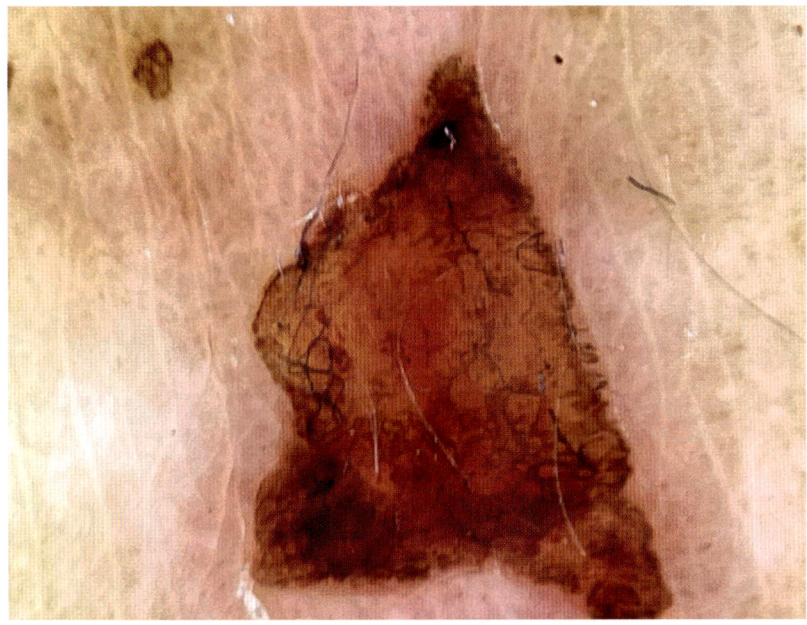
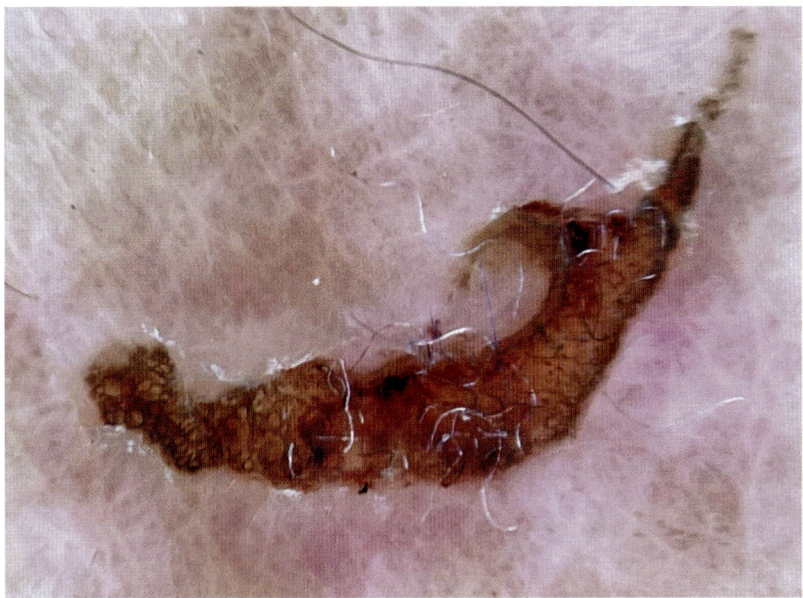

FIGURE 4–2. Dermoscopic images of erosions in a patient with delusional infestation.
Source. Dr. Asmahane Souissi.

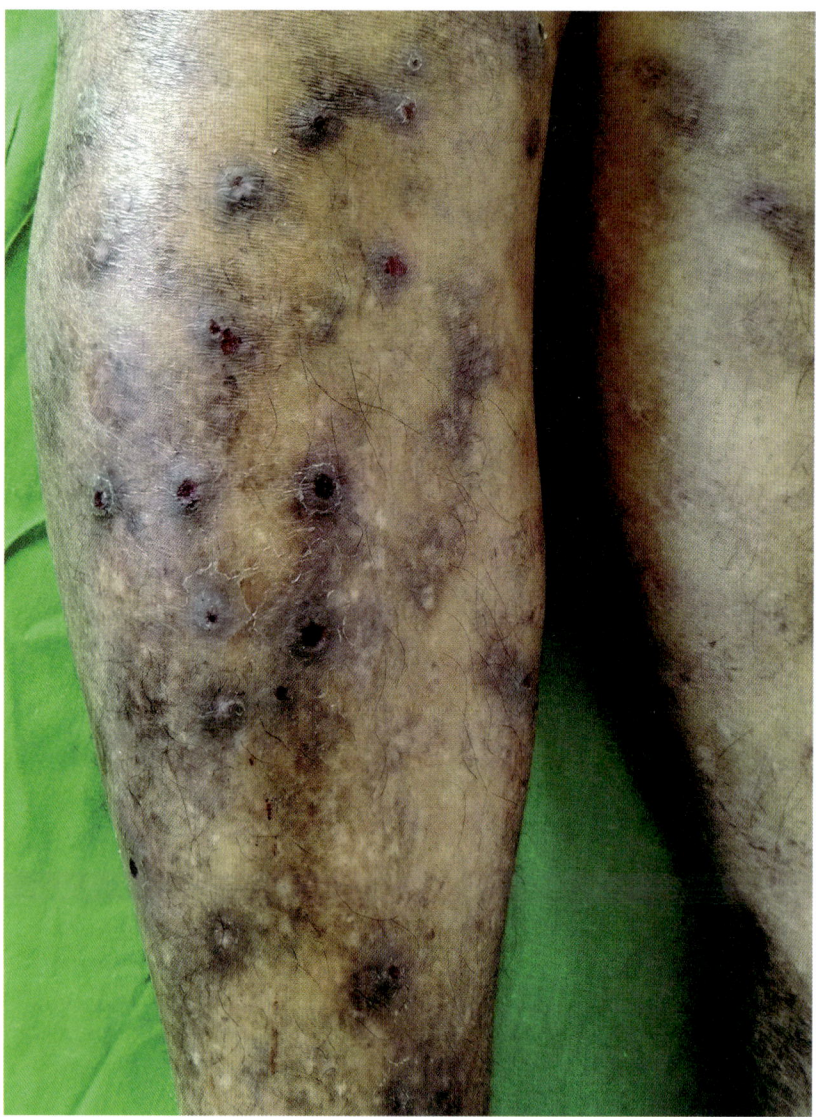

FIGURE 4–3. Hyper- and hypopigmented lesions in different stages of healing in a patient with delusional infestation.
Source. Dr. Asmahane Souissi.

et al. 2019; Rosales Santillan et al. 2018). Primary delusional infestation is largely a diagnosis of exclusion (Huber et al. 2007); therefore, it is essential that the presence of a delusion of parasitic infestation is the only positive finding in the patient, with no accompanying psychiatric disorders. Alternatively, delusional infestation can be secondary to many psychiatric disorders, neurological diseases, nutritional deficiencies, infections, and substance or medication consumption (Mumcuoglu et al. 2018). Therefore, for diagnosis, all conditions that are known to cause secondary delusional infestation should be ruled out in the traditional manner. Once every diagnosis has been effectively ruled out, a patient-stated parasitic infestation alongside the matchbox sign supports a diagnosis of delusional infestation (Ansari and Bragg 2023). An algorithm for the diagnosis of delusional infestation is shown in Figure 4–4.

Treatment

Secondary Delusional Infestation

If a patient is diagnosed with secondary delusional infestation, the medical or psychiatric condition causing the delusion must be treated appropriately. All previous medications must be discontinued, and the cessation of all substance use should be highly recommended (Ansari and Bragg 2023). In individuals using illicit substances, cessation usually eliminates the patient's complaints of a parasitic infestation. Additionally, in cases such as delirium and medication intoxication, the delusion will cease upon resolution of the delirium and toxicity. Therefore, if a patient is diagnosed with delusional infestation secondary to any of the previously listed causes, it is recommended to wait and follow up on the patient's complaints of parasitic infestation, as they may be eliminated spontaneously (Huber et al. 2007).

Primary Delusional Infestation

Any patient being treated for primary delusional infestation should be treated by both a psychiatrist and a dermatologist (Reich et al. 2019). If possible, all care providers should be within the same health care system and should be able to easily and quickly communicate between themselves and the patient. Additionally, it is essential to establish rapport with the patient. A patient diagnosed with primary delusional infestation will not be disposed to taking antipsychotic medications, because they believe their condition is not of a psychiatric origin. However, a clinician should always attempt to encourage the patient to take antipsychotic medication before any other treatment avenues. Moreover, adherence to treatment may be an issue. This is an area in which patient rapport is essential (Reich et al. 2019). Struggling to convince the patient that their symptoms are in fact delusions is often inconclusive and even detrimental to patient care; it may lead to discontinuation of follow-up and referral to another clinician for a second opinion. Instead, the

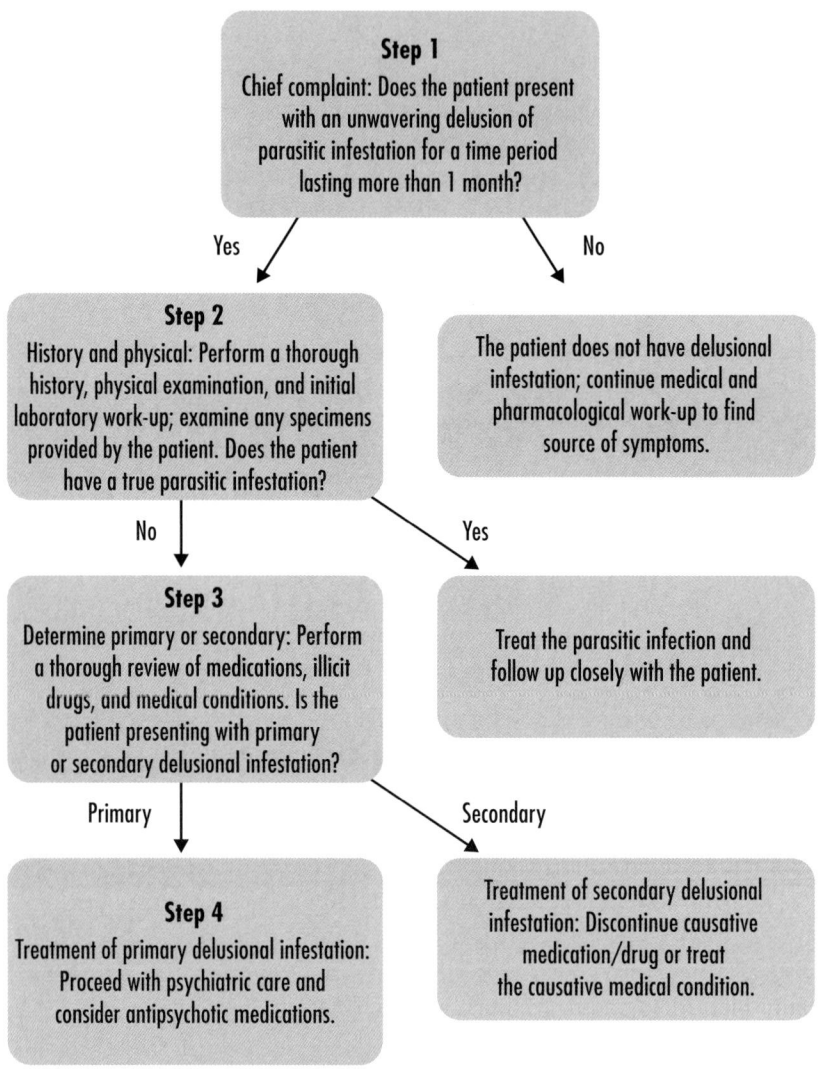

FIGURE 4–4. Algorithm of delusional infestation diagnosis.
Source. Adapted from Katsoulis et al. 2020.

clinician should be objective and attempt to understand the emotions of the patient. A kind, nonjudgmental approach will have higher success rates in treatment. For patients who fear the stigma associated with mental illness, and to increase compliance with treatment, the clinician should educate the patient that such symptoms occur as a result of changing chemicals in the brain.

Overall, the clinician should be aware that the patient's symptoms are disturbing, and treatment plans should be symptom oriented and not diagnosis oriented. As mentioned earlier, the first-line treatment for primary delusional infestation is antipsychotic medication (Campbell et al. 2019; Rosales Santillan et al. 2018). There is no one specific medication indicated for treatment; many have led to positive results, and the choice of treatment should be made by looking at the side-effect profile of available medications. Although first-generation antipsychotics (especially pimozide) have been used as first-line therapy (Katsoulis et al. 2020), they are now restricted because of side effects including postural hypotension, QT prolongation, extrapyramidal symptoms, weight gain, and other metabolic effects. To minimize these effects, atypical, second-generation antipsychotic medications should be preferred to typical, first-generation antipsychotics (Kalovidouri et al. 2022). The chosen treatment should be prescribed at a low dosage over an extended period, which both minimizes side effects and reduces the possibility of recurrence when treatment is discontinued. If the disease recurs after the treatment course is complete, the medication should be started again.

Prognosis

Delusional infestation usually does not restrict a patient's ability to function in daily life, but it does cause unnecessary obstacles. The delusion can significantly reduce the quality of some patients' lives and leave them feeling disappointed and hopeless. Patients with primary delusional infestation have a high response rate to second-generation antipsychotic medications. Patients may have their medication dosage reduced after just weeks of treatment, and a good response can be obtained by restarting treatment if symptoms reappear. Studies have shown that the success rate of antipsychotic treatment of delusional infestation is 60%–100%. In patients with secondary delusional infestation, although the focus should be on treating the condition causing the disease, additional antipsychotic therapy may be used to manage symptoms (Kalovidouri et al. 2022).

Complications

Delusional infestation has several associated complications. Failure to treat skin wounds in a timely manner can lead to scarring and reduced skin function. Self-induced keratoconjunctivitis can occur.

Enhancing Health Care Team Outcomes

Delusional infestation is seen most frequently by health care departments outside of psychiatry. Therefore, it is essential that dermatologists and general practitioners have a clear understanding of the disease and the process of accurate diagnosis. Additionally, it is essential that health care departments are interconnected and have efficient and professional communication to ensure the best possible patient outcomes.

Effective treatment can be achieved with a good doctor-patient relationship. Treatment will progress much more effectively when a doctor gains the patient's trust by assuring them that their symptoms are being taken seriously. A prescription written by a dermatologist rather than a psychiatrist will be more accepted by patients, so the treatment should be directed by the dermatologist. Patients may be unwilling to see a psychiatrist for treatment. To persuade patients to start treatment with antipsychotics, explain that antipsychotics are used not only in psychiatric diseases but also in many dermatological applications because they contain antihistamines. Delusions are mostly eliminated when the patient receives psychopharmacological treatment. However, there is always a risk of recurrence in delusional infestation (Kalovidouri et al. 2022).

References

Ansari MN, Bragg BN: Delusions of parasitosis, in StatPearls [Internet]. Treasure Island, FL, StatPearls Publishing, updated May 22 2023. Available at: www.ncbi.nlm.nih.gov/books/NBK541021. Accessed April 30, 2024.

Campbell EH, Elston DM, Hawthorne JD, Beckert DR: Diagnosis and management of delusional parasitosis. J Am Acad Dermatol 80(5):1428–1434, 2019 30543832

Freudenmann RW, Lepping P: Delusional infestation. Clin Microbiol Rev 22(4):690–732, 2009 19822895

Huber M, Kirchler E, Karner M, Pycha R: Delusional parasitosis and the dopamine transporter: a new insight of etiology? Med Hypotheses 68(6):1351–1358, 2007 17134847

Kalovidouri C, Kowalewski L, Mos DV, Waqar MU: A case of delusional parasitosis with folie à deux treated with low-dose quetiapine. Cureus 14(5):e25344, 2022 35774659

Katsoulis K, Rutledge KJ, Jafferany M: Delusional infestation: a prototype of psychodermatological disease. Int J Dermatol 59(5):551–560, 2020 31773724

Kohorst JJ, Bailey CH, Andersen LK, et al: Prevalence of delusional infestation—a population-based study. JAMA Dermatol 154(5):615–617, 2018 29617524

Laidler N: Delusions of parasitosis: a brief review of the literature and pathway for diagnosis and treatment. Dermatol Online J 24(1):13030/qt1fh739nx, 2018 29469757

Mumcuoglu KY, Leibovici V, Reuveni I, Bonne O: Delusional parasitosis: diagnosis and treatment. Isr Med Assoc J 20(7):456–460, 2018 30109800

Reich A, Kwiatkowska D, Pacan P: Delusions of parasitosis: an update. Dermatol Ther (Heidelb) 9(4):631–638, 2019 31520344

Rosales Santillan M, Taylor DL, Reichenberg JS: Delusional infestation in psychodermatology. G Ital Dermatol Venereol 153(4):497–505, 2018 29667798

Sawant NS, Vispute CD: Delusional parasitosis with folie à deux: a case series. Ind Psychiatry J 24(1):97–98, 2015 26257494

Torales J, García O, Barrios I, et al: Delusional infestation: clinical presentations, diagnosis, and management. J Cosmet Dermatol 19(12):3183–3188, 2020 33098221

Case 4-1
Delusional Infestation: Folie à Famille

Smitha Prabhu, M.D.
Shrutakirthi D. Shenoi, M.D.
Krishna S. Swathy, N.D.
Priyanka Prabhakaran, M.D.

Case Description

A 46-year-old woman presented to the dermatology clinic with recurrent intractable pruritus with sensation of crawling of insects of 1.5 years' duration. During that time, she was repeatedly treated for dermatophytosis and scabies, with no apparent improvement. Pest control of her house and premises was undertaken multiple times. The patient had hypertension on treatment, was living with her husband, and had no history of mental illness. She was not adherent to oral amitriptyline and olanzapine prescribed by a psychiatrist (for current symptoms). She reported aggravation of symptoms for the past 2 months. Her son and daughter who were living independently also reported generalized itching with crawling sensation, which started after visiting their parents a year ago. They too had undergone multiple treatments, including scabies treatment, and showed moderate improvement with sporadic worsening. The husband did not have any symptoms, although he believed that his wife and children were affected.

On examination, there were a few excoriation marks over the legs and the lower abdomen, but there was no sign suggestive of any infestation in either the patient or her son (the daughter had not accompanied the patient). At their insistence, skin scrapings from various sites were subjected to light microscopy, which showed normal stratum corneum cells.

Differential Diagnosis

Scabies and ectoparasitic infestation were ruled out by clinical examination and microscopy.

Diagnosis

The patient was diagnosed with delusional infestation with folie à famille; she was admitted as an inpatient and referred to the psychodermatology clinic. After admission to a semispecial ward, the patient had repeated crying spells. She scared the adjacent patients by "revealing" the highly contagious nature of her skin condition. The other patients had to be separately counseled regarding the noncontagiousness of the condition.

Management

Clinical psychologists opined that psychological intervention was not possible for the patient as there was no insight, and the patient was highly concerned about the symptoms. Psychiatrists started her on oral risperidone 3 mg along with oral trihexyphenidyl 2 mg daily for 4 weeks. Dermatological treatment consisted of cetirizine 10 mg orally in the evening and liberal application of antipruritic emollient lotions. At 4 weeks' follow-up, she had subjectively improved by ~60%.

Discussion

Folie à deux, or shared psychotic disorder, is a rare presentation with delusional infestation in which the patient's belief is shared by another person, and in folie à famille, the whole family persists in the belief. Patients with delusional infestation tend to show obsessive cleansing of their body to get rid of the pathogen. They may also spray pesticides in their house, which was noted here. Shared psychotic disorder is seen in 5%–15% of delusional infestation patients (Trabert 1995). The primary case triggers symptoms in the other patients, most often close associates and relatives.

Genetic factors—depression or dementia in the primary case and abnormal personality traits in the secondary case—and disturbed interpersonal relationships may be predisposing factors. This case was a classic example of shared psychotic behavior (folie à famille).

The first-line therapy for the folie à deux is separation of secondary cases from the dominant case. If the symptoms do not abate, antipsychotic drugs are needed (Friedmann et al. 2006). However, in this case, neither of the patient's two children who shared the delusional belief agreed to any treatment. As they were staying apart, the patient alone was treated, with hope that once the mother improved, the children would as well.

TEACHING POINTS

- Delusional infestation can present as "folie à famille," involving multiple family members.
- Clinical and laboratory investigations to rule out ectoparasitic infestations such as scabies, pediculosis, deficiency disorders such as vitamin B_{12} deficiency, and endocrine and neurological abnormalities should be performed before labeling as delusional infestation.
- An approach combining psychodermatology with psychopharmacology is essential for good treatment response.
- Prolonged follow-up and treatment are the norm.

References

Friedmann AC, Ekeowa-Anderson A, Taylor R, Bewley A: Delusional parasitosis presenting as folie à trois: successful treatment with risperidone. Br J Dermatol 155(4):841–842, 2006 16965440

Trabert W: 100 years of delusional parasitosis: meta-analysis of 1,223 case reports. Psychopathology 28(5):238–246, 1995 8559947

Case 4-2
A Case of Delusional Parasitosis

Asmahane Souissi, M.D.
Meryem Chaabani, M.D.
Rafik Mahmoudi, M.D.

Case Description

A 50-year-old woman with a history of glaucoma presented with complaints of chronic pruritus reportedly caused by the presence of parasites on her

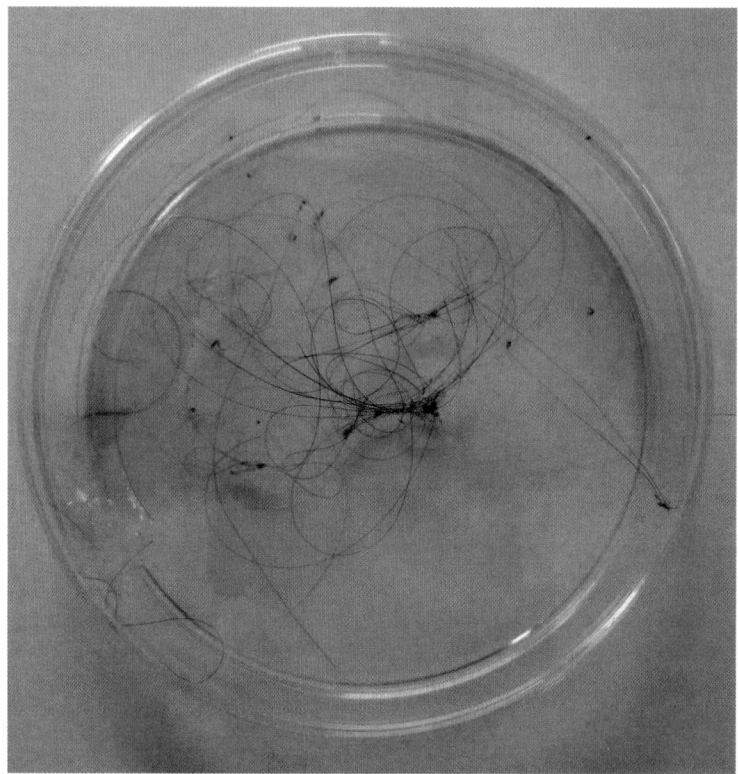

FIGURE 4–5. Matchbox sign: the patient supplied a Petri dish containing hair.
Source. Dr. Asmahane Souissi.

body, especially her scalp, following a renovation of her apartment 6 months prior. She reported that she had changed her house furniture and bought new clothes to get relief from the parasites. She stopped working out of fear of contagiousness, and she has been spending a lot of time cleaning her apartment.

The patient brought a Petri dish containing some hair that she considered infected by the parasite (Figure 4–5). Parasitological examination of the content of the Petri dish was negative. She consulted several dermatologists, who conducted many laboratory investigations, which were all normal. Careful examination of the body and the scalp revealed no visible skin lesions.

The patient showed a high level of anxiety related to the perceived feeling of parasites crawling on her skin. At times, she was very paranoid about her itching and thought that no dermatologist would be able to diagnose her suffering.

Differential Diagnosis

- Idiopathic scalp itching
- Seborrheic dermatitis
- Parasitic infestation
- Delusional infestation

Diagnosis

Given the normal clinical examination and laboratory investigations, the diagnosis of delusional infestation was made.

Management

The patient was referred to a psychiatrist, but she appeared very apprehensive about the stigma of going to see a psychiatrist. The patient then was lost to follow-up.

Discussion

Delusional infestation has a major impact on the social and professional life of a patient. This patient changed her apartment and furniture, bought new clothes, and contacted multiple companies specializing in pest control.

Patients usually tend to consult a dermatologist rather than see a psychiatrist because they are convinced that their skin is infested by parasites, and therefore, only dermatologists can treat their affliction. The patients don't feel the need to see a mental health provider (Jafferany 2021). In this case, the patient was misdiagnosed by several dermatologists because of lack of awareness.

A patient with delusional infestation is difficult to reason with. They will frequently change consultants when they have the feeling of not being heard, which is what occurred with this patient. It is also very difficult to maintain follow-up with delusional infestation patients, as many do not return. They often decline to see a psychiatrist.

Many cases of delusional infestation respond to antipsychotics and antidepressants. The role of psychotherapy is very limited, except in intellectual and highly educated patients (Jafferany 2021).

TEACHING POINTS

- Delusional infestation may have a huge impact on social and professional life. Patients may isolate themselves from friends and family out of fear that they may be contagious.

- Patients with delusional infestation frequently change their doctors. When a psychiatric referral is discussed, they usually decline.

References

Jafferany M: Handbook of Psychodermatology: Introduction to Psychocutaneous Disorders. Cham, Switzerland, Springer Nature, 2021

Case 4–3
Delusional Infestation

Ilknur Kıvanç Altunay, M.D.
Gül Şekerlisoy Tatar, M.D.

Case Description

The patient was a 58-year-old woman with a 2-year history of itching supposedly caused by insects, causing uncomfortable feeling and scratching of the skin. The patient reported that "flies and their larvae" were coming out of her skin and believed that her complaints were due to a parasitic infection. The woman's complaints started 2 years prior when she saw insects coming out of the air conditioner ducts when her son cleaned the air conditioner. She believed that these insects caused parasitic infection on her body. They crawled on her body surface, reproduced their larvae, and caused itching. As a result, she had to scrape her skin to get rid of the insects. Her complaints increased when her father died.

She had a history of diabetes mellitus type 2, hypertension, coronary artery disease, dyslipidemia, and meningioma in the frontal region for 10 years. There was no significant family history. She did not smoke or use any substance. She had previous sudden speech difficulties, which started about 20 years ago when her son was involved in a serious car accident; she later recovered from that problem. For the last 6 months, she was treated with topical permethrin lotions, antihistamines, and antidepressants (trazodone,

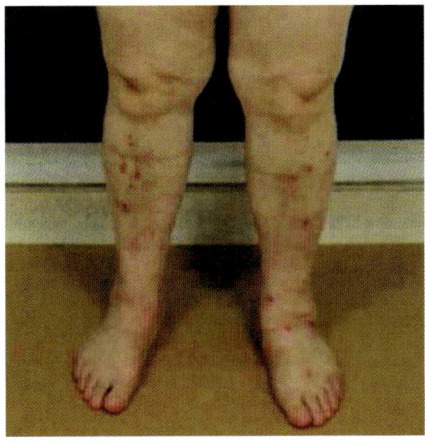

FIGURE 4–6. Erythematous, eczematous patches in various stages of healing, involving the legs and feet.

Source. Prof. Ilknur Altunay.

escitalopram), with minimal resolution of symptoms. She developed erosions, excoriations, and postlesional hyperpigmentation on her upper and lower extremities, abdomen, and upper part of her back, secondary to scratching and attempting to extract the presumed pathogen (Figures 4–6 and 4–7).

On dermatological examination, the patient presented with erythematous, eczematous patches in various stages of healing, involving the scalp, face, abdomen, back, legs, arms, and feet, as well as excoriated papules and generalized xerosis.

On laboratory examination, glycated hemoglobin was 6.7%, and all other tests including biochemistry, complete blood count, vitamin B_{12}, and iron deficiency were within normal limits. Skin biopsy demonstrated chronic spongiotic dermatitis and nonspecific changes. Bacterial, mycobacterial, and fungal cultures were negative. Serologic studies failed to provide evidence of infection. Neurological consultation was uneventful.

Differential Diagnosis

- Ectoparasitic infestation, secondary delusional infestation related to diabetes mellitus, vitamin B_{12} deficiency.

Diagnosis

In the light of all evaluations, the patient was diagnosed with primary delusional parasitosis.

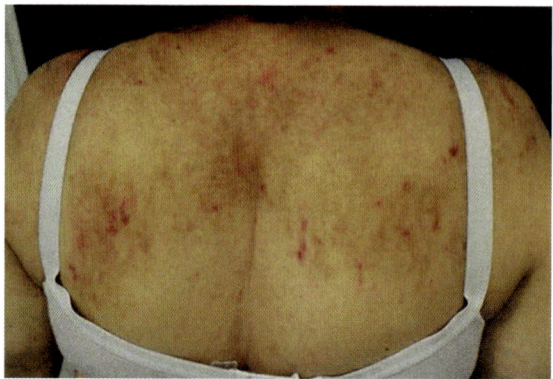

FIGURE 4–7. Erythematous, eczematous patches and excoriated papules at various healing stages on the back (only areas reached by the patient's hands).
Source. Prof. Ilknur Altunay.

Management

The patient was referred to a psychiatrist. On psychiatric examination, the patient was found to have significant anxiety. She was treated with 2 mg pimozide daily with electrocardiogram follow-up. The patient is in remission in the third month of treatment.

Discussion

Because of the tactile sensations associated with delusional infestation, patients injure themselves to remove organisms and relieve their symptoms. The lesions they cause are usually in different healing stages and in areas that their hands can reach (Freudenmann and Lepping 2009), as shown in Figure 4–7. In this case, incidental meningioma gave the patient the feeling that the symptoms were related to meningioma. In some cases, patients link the onset of symptoms to a particular event, such as the exposure to air conditioning pipes reported by this patient.

TEACHING POINTS

- The presence of lesions of different healing stages in only areas reached by the patient's hands is highly suggestive of the diagnosis of delusional infestation.

- Primary delusional infestation needs to be distinguished from secondary delusional infestation, because the main treatment for primary delusional infestation includes antipsychotic and antidepressant drugs, whereas secondary delusional infestation can be treated only by treating the medical conditions that cause it.

References

Freudenmann RW, Lepping P: Delusional infestation. Clin Microbiol Rev 22(4):690–732, 2009 19822895

Case 4–4
A Case of Delusional Infestation in a 65-Year-Old Woman

Samantha Hess, B.S.
Mohammad Jafferany, M.D.

Case Description

The patient is a 65-year-old woman who presented to her provider with multiple papules and erosions of varying sizes along the forearms bilaterally for ~6 months, as displayed in Figure 4–8. The patient stated that unspecified parasites were crawling out of her skin, and she had been attempting to pick at the parasites to remove them from her skin manually. The erosions along the forearms presented with associated symptoms of pruritus, itching, and skin picking. Displaying matchbox sign, she brought in perceived samples of parasites.

The patient had used multiple lotions and creams, with no perceived improvement to her presenting symptoms. No oral treatments or prescription lotions were used. Her lack of symptomatic improvement led to her using pesticides within her home.

The patient also presented with associated psychiatric symptoms. She was openly frustrated and endorsed symptoms of both depression and anxiety, including difficulty sleeping. Additionally, she displayed signs of paranoid thoughts regarding the perceived parasites in her skin. She stated that nobody believed her symptoms were real, and she was not easily trusting of those around her. Overall, the patient's psychological presentation was psychotic in nature and consistent with the presence of delusions.

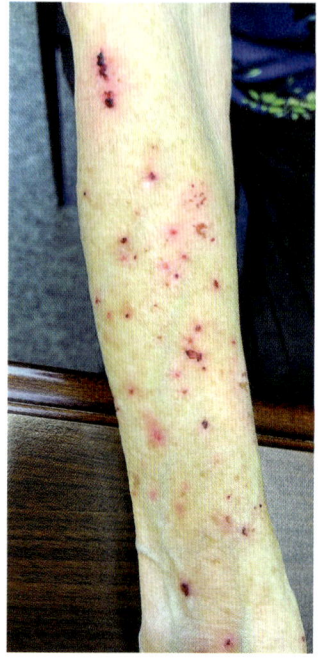

FIGURE 4–8. Patient's forearm before treatment.
Source. Prof. Mohammad Jafferany.

Differential Diagnosis

- Delusional infestation
- True parasitic infestation
- Dermatillomania
- Medication side effect
- Drug intoxication

Other differential diagnoses to consider include a multitude of acute and chronic diseases that may lead to pruritus and skin picking.

It is important to remember that delusional infestation is a diagnosis of exclusion, and all potential causes of the patient's symptoms must be thoroughly investigated.

Diagnosis

In the patient's evaluation, a basic laboratory work-up was conducted to rule out potential causes of pruritus. The patient's complete blood count (CBC), comprehensive metabolic panel, and vitamin B_{12} levels were unremarkable.

The physical examination and evaluation of the perceived parasitic samples were consistent with a lack of parasites in the patient's body. Therefore, the presence of a true parasitic infestation could be ruled out.

The patient's symptoms were consistent for skin picking, pruritus, and delusional infestation (Freudenmann and Lepping 2009). The patient displayed no signs consistent with impulsivity or obsessive behavior. Therefore, it was further concluded that the psychiatric manifestations were solely psychotic and delusional in nature.

Additionally, the patient was not taking any medications or diagnosed with any chronic illnesses that may be a cause of secondary delusional infestation. Therefore, through the process of elimination, the patient was diagnosed with primary delusional infestation (Bewley et al. 2010).

Management

At the time of treatment, first-generation antipsychotics were first-line treatments for individuals with primary delusional infestation. The patient was initially given pimozide 1 mg at bedtime, which was subsequently increased to pimozide 1 mg twice a day for a 6-week course. Throughout the treatment course, the patient's pruritus, difficulty sleeping, and paranoia decreased. As the delusion of parasitosis waned, the patient's skin picking decreased, leading to improvement in the papules and erosions, as seen in Figure 4–9. Along with the stated symptoms, the patient's endorsement of depression and anxiety symptoms decreased as well.

Discussion

To diagnose a patient with delusional infestation, the patient must present with two characteristic symptoms:

1. Delusions of infestation: the patient must present with a false, fixed belief that they have a parasitic infestation lasting for a period longer than a month. The parasite identified by the patient can be microscopic or macroscopic.
2. Cutaneous symptoms: the patient must present with a form of cutaneous manifestation that deepens their belief in the presence of a parasitic infection. The cutaneous manifestations may present as pruritus, tingling, burning, and associated skin picking and itching.

As previously stated, however, delusional infestation is a diagnosis of exclusion, and extensive testing must be performed by the patient's primary care team, dermatological team, and psychiatric team to come to the diagnosis. It is of utmost importance that both a dermatologist and a psychiatrist are on the care team of an individual suspected to have delusional infestation. Without integration of a dermatologist properly investigating

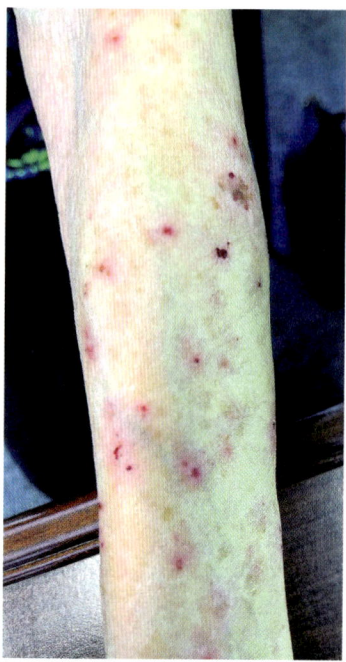

FIGURE 4–9. Patient's forearm after treatment.
Source. Prof. Mohammad Jafferany.

the body for cutaneous parasites and a psychiatrist properly evaluating and treating the patient's delusional state, the patient will have less chance of a proper recovery. Routine laboratory tests and a thorough history of symptoms can quickly rule out the presence of actual parasites and lead the providers to the diagnosis of delusional infestation.

Through proper evaluation and work-up, it will be apparent whether a patient is suffering from primary or secondary delusional infestation. If a patient is diagnosed with secondary delusional infestation, the treatment plan should consist of treating the causative factor, including cessation of all medications and illicit substances. If a patient is diagnosed with primary delusional infestation, they will be treated with an antipsychotic therapy regimen with close monitoring for side effects and cessation of symptoms. It is important to note that the patients do not believe their symptoms are psychiatric in nature, and it may be difficult to get them to start an antipsychotic regimen. Therefore, one of the most important aspects of treatment for a patient with delusional infestation is trust and open communication between the provider and the patient. Patients' delusions should not be validated, and the approach should be nonjudgmental.

In addition to a trusting relationship between the patient and the provider, it is important to involve the patient's family and support system in the treatment process. Delusional infestation, by definition, directly interferes with the patient's ability to understand the state of their health. By involving those who are trustworthy and respected within the patient's life, there is a higher chance of a smooth recovery.

TEACHING POINTS

- Any patient presenting for health care assistance should not have their delusions directly confronted. When confronted, the patient is more likely to lose trust in their provider and will seek assistance elsewhere, delaying treatment.

- Psychiatry and dermatology should both be brought into the care team of a patient with delusional infestation.

- Inclusion of the family in treatment of the patient is critical to increasing positive outcomes in the treatment of delusional infestation.

References

Bewley AP, Lepping P, Freudenmann RW, Taylor R: Delusional parasitosis: time to call it delusional infestation. Br J Dermatol 163(1):1–2, 2010 20645978

Freudenmann RW, Lepping P: Delusional infestation. Clin Microbiol Rev 22(4):690–732, 2009 19822895

Case 4–5

Shrimp-Infested Nails: A Rare Side Effect of a Common Drug

Reem Al Neyadi, M.D.
Shaden Abdelhadi, M.D.
Dimitre Dimitrov, M.D., Ph.D.

Case Description

An 86-year-old man with multiple comorbidities, including dyslipidemia, coronary artery disease, diabetes mellitus type 2, and atrial fibrillation, was brought by his family to the dermatology clinic with the complaint of irritation and stinging sensation around his fingertips, gradually progressing over a period of 9 months, due to the patient seeing shrimps creeping out of his fingertips.

He presented with prominent periungual erosions resulting from picking his skin and attempting to "catch the shrimp." Multiple stages of development of these lesions were present, from fresh bleeding erosions to crusting, postinflammatory hyperpigmentation (Figure 4–10).

A psychiatric assessment revealed a constant low mood status that was associated with crying spells. He also expressed feelings of worthlessness without suicidal ideation. His son reported deterioration of short-term memory and difficulties dealing with money. The patient was alert, oriented, and cooperative and had preserved language.

Differential Diagnosis

- Contact dermatitis (irritant or allergic)
- Nutritional deficiency
- Delusion of parasitosis
- Formication

Diagnosis

The diagnosis of drug-induced delusion of parasitosis was made after reviewing the patient's medication list. Three of the patient's medications may cause hallucinations (metoprolol, clopidogrel, and esomeprazole).

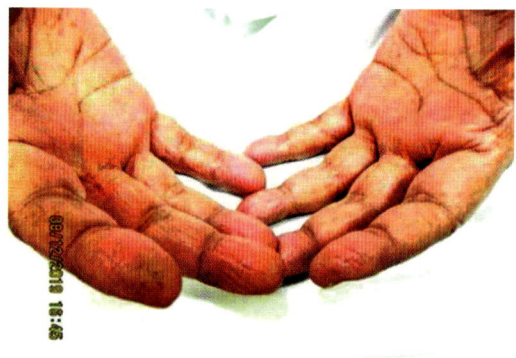

FIGURE 4–10.   Erosions and crusting on fingertips.
Source.   Dr. Dimitre Dimitrov.

Management

A multidisciplinary approach was applied. Discontinuing esomeprazole for 2 weeks did not provide any improvement. Next, clopidogrel was suspended, and the family noticed significant improvement within 2 weeks. The patient stopped picking his nails and did not mention the shrimp as often. He continued to improve in the ensuing 4 months until achieving a complete resolution.

Later, a resumption of clopidogrel (with a different brand name) in another health care facility resulted in recurrence of the shrimp hallucination. All symptoms resolved again upon cessation of the drug, further confirming the causality.

Discussion

Delusional infestation is characterized by a fixed, false, unshakable belief by a person that they are infested with living or inanimate pathogens, despite a lack of medical evidence for such an infestation (Bewley et al. 2010).

Delusional infestation occurs in primary and secondary forms. In primary form, no cause is known; secondary form, as in this case, is always associated with secondary causes such as drug intake. Clinically, patients report sensations of crawling, biting, or stinging. This patient developed symptoms after many months of being on clopidogrel, whereas in two other cases reported in the literature, the onset of symptoms was within days of starting the medication, and the patients developed auditory as well as visual hallucinations (Founztopoulous et al. 2007; Osuagwu et al. 2016).

TEACHING POINTS

- Drug-induced secondary causes of delusional infestation must be considered in idiopathic delusion of parasitosis.

- Clopidogrel-induced hallucination has been reported in the literature, albeit rarely.

- Vigilance about drug-induced hallucination could prevent long-term unnecessary pharmacological interventions.

With this case, we aim to highlight delusional infestation and the importance of recognition of secondary causes of this condition. It is noteworthy that this side effect is rarely noted or reported. Furthermore, we highlight the importance of multidisciplinary collaboration to achieve the best patient care and management.

References

Bewley AP, Lepping P, Freudenmann RW, Taylor R: Delusional parasitosis: time to call it delusional infestation. Br J Dermatol 163(1):1–2, 2010 20645978

Founztopoulous E, Mavroudis C, Nadar SK, Gunning MG: Case report: an unusual complication of clopidogrel. Int J Cardiol 115(1):e27–e28, 2007 17049649

Osuagwu FC, Parashar S, Amalraj B, et al: Clopidogrel-induced auditory and visual hallucinations. Prim Care Companion CNS Disord 18(3):10.4088/PCC.15l01894, 2016 27722029

Case 4–6
A Case Report Illustrating How Folie à Deux May Be Managed

Allison Kranyak, M.D.
Mitchell Davis, M.D.
John Koo, M.D.

Case Description

A 65-year-old man presented to our clinic with the chief complaint of being "infested by parasites." In August 2022, both the patient and his wife were diagnosed with scabies, which was treated with permethrin and ivermectin. Approximately 3–4 months later, although he specifically clarified that they were no longer concerned about scabies, he and his wife developed concerns for a "new species" of parasite infection. The couple reportedly had spent more than $30,000 for investigation and treatment for this parasitosis without lasting benefit. Failed treatment included four additional courses of permethrin and ivermectin, albendazole, and praziquantel. He was currently taking albendazole that was not prescribed to him. Prior skin biopsies were unrevealing for parasites. Upon physical examination, excoriations were appreciated, but no primary skin lesion or evidence of infestation could be found. Dermatologic history included nonmelanoma skin cancer; other medical history was unremarkable. He denied recreational drug use. Laboratory examination (complete blood count; comprehensive metabolic panel; thyroid-stimulating hormone, vitamin D, and vitamin B_{12} levels; and urinary toxin screen) were unremarkable. For reasons unknown, the patient reported to us without his wife.

Differential Diagnosis

- Primary delusional infestation with folie à deux
- Psychiatric disorder causing secondary delusional infestation
- Neurological disorder, such as new-onset multiple sclerosis
- Delusional infestation-like symptoms secondary to internal medical problem
- Substance-induced delusional infestation

Diagnosis

The patient lacked history or complaints consistent with an underlying psychiatric disorder. His overall presentation was not consistent with a neurologic etiology (no weakness, vision changes, or neuropathic symptoms), so a neurologic cause of his symptoms was thought to be exceedingly unlikely. His normal laboratory evaluation ruled out an underlying medical cause or substance use. Thus, he was given the diagnosis of primary delusional infestation with folie à deux (which translates from French to "madness for two").

Management

Because this was likely a case of folie à deux, the primary objective was to determine which person was the primary driver of the ideation of parasitosis and who was merely the passive participant. After interviewing him for multiple sessions, it was our judgment that he was not the primary driver. He had reported repeatedly that his wife was "much more into the parasites" than he was. In fact, when discussing the possibility of trying pimozide on a trial-and-error basis, he was informed of the mechanism of action of the medication, and he spontaneously stated, "I better not tell my wife some of these details, because she would object if she knew that this isn't an antiparasitic." However, the patient expressed continued interest in medical therapy with pimozide despite knowing that fact. Therefore, the patient was initiated on a course of pimozide. At the time of writing, the patient had been taking pimozide for less than 1 week and thus an update on treatment response is not available.

Discussion

Even though this case's outcome is not determined, it was selected for its multiple teaching points. Delusional infestation presenting as folie à deux is relatively rare. However, when a situation of folie à deux does present itself, the clinician needs to decide based on the available information which of the two individuals is the driver of the parasitic ideation and which is the passive participant. In an extremely rare case, when more than two people are involved (folie à famille), it is still likely that one person is the main driver of the process and others are passively following.

This determination is clinically important for two reasons. First, in an ideal setting, a provider can direct the treatment deliberately to the driver of the delusion. If the driver improves, with lessening or resolution of the delusional ideation, the passive participants may improve even without treatment. The second reason is that in a situation like the one here, where the primary driver is not the one seeking medical expertise, the very recognition that this patient is the passive participant lets the provider talk openly, or at least with less caution. The primary driver tends to be more intensely delusional and is unlikely to tolerate a point of view that differs

Delusional Infestation 61

TABLE 4–2. Koo-Brownstone staging system

Koo-Brownstone stage	Name
1	Formication only (patient has insight)
2	Overvalued ideation of parasitosis (patient has mild decline in insight)
3	Predelusional (patient has moderate decline in insight)
4	Delusional (patient has very severe decline in insight)
5	Terminally delusional (patient has absolutely no insight)

Source. Brownstone and Koo 2022 with permission from Taylor and Francis.

from their own. Even a hint that implies that there is no parasite can set them off into an antagonistic, hostile mood, and the conversation may become oppositional. Passive followers are able to better engage in a normal dialog without becoming intensely displeased.

TEACHING POINTS

- It is important to recognize folie à deux. A shared delusional system is a rare occurrence but a real clinical phenomenon.
- Once folie à deux is recognized, it is important to determine which of the two individuals is the driver and which is the passive participant.
- When caring for the driver, it is important to not antagonize the patient and to recognize that they may not be capable of engaging in a normal dialog about the topic of infestation given the intensity of the delusion.
- When caring for a passive participant, there is a greater likelihood that the patient is not fully delusional and may be capable of a normal dialog, allowing for easier communication.
- If the patient is judged to not be fully delusional and retains some flexibility, then we recommend trying to characterize the intensity of their delusion by applying the Koo-Brownstone staging system (stages 1–3 are not fully delusional; stages 4

and 5 are fully delusional and therefore require great caution) (Table 4–2) (Brownstone and Koo 2022).

- Even though in this case the primary driver did not seek care from our clinic, ideally one would make an effort to engage her for treatment for the maximum potential benefit for two (or more, in cases of folie à famille).

References

Brownstone N, Koo J: The Koo-Brownstone staging system as a tool to assist in the management of patients with a possible diagnosis of dermatological delusions: an experts suggestion. J Dermatolog Treat 33(8):3199–3201, 2022 35950783

Case 4–7
Delusions of Parasitic Sexually Transmitted Disease in a 71-Year-Old Man

Kamila Wala-Zielińska, M.D.
Jacek C. Szepietowski, M.D.

Case Description

A 71-year-old man was admitted for suspicion of a sexually transmitted disease (STD). He reported pruritus for about 5 years, linking the onset of symptoms to sexual contact with his wife. He denied risky sexual contacts and believed that he contracted the disease from his wife, who he said had an affair. He denied other symptoms of STDs such as urethral discharge or ulcers in the genital area. The patient stated pruritus occurring mainly in the evening and at night. He claimed that "itching intensifies during the full moon"; he said that during the day and while working, he had no symptoms. Pruritus occurred all over the body and was most severe in the genital area. The patient believed that the germs that caused his STD were walking around his body and biting him, which was the cause of pruritus. Moreover, he claimed that he constantly found "small black balls" all over his body, which he believed were parasites. The patient had visited several doctors and was prescribed oral antihistamines, steroid ointments, and anti-scabies drugs without any improvement. He denied any history of psychiatric or chronic medical disorders and was not taking any medications.

Differential Diagnosis

Differential diagnosis included scabies and pubic lice, substance-induced or senile pruritus, venereophobia, and other causes of secondary delusions, including substance-induced delusions, and mental and physical disorders (e.g., schizophrenia, psychotic depression, Parkinson disease, dementia, stroke, HIV infection, anemia, diabetes).

Diagnosis

The patient underwent a thorough physical examination including dermoscopic examination. There were no skin lesions, no erosions or scabies burrows, and no evidence of lice. Microscopic examination of skin scrapings was negative. Laboratory tests including routine blood count, comprehensive metabolic panel, and tests for HIV and hepatitis B and C were normal. The mental status examination revealed the presence of a firm, fixed belief of having parasitic STD. Visual hallucinations were related to the theme of delusions. Mood and affect were consistent with delusional content. Speech, eye contact, cognition, and psychomotor activity stayed unchanged.

Management

The patient received risperidone (an atypical antipsychotic) at 2 mg/day, which improved his delusions.

Discussion

Per DSM-5-TR (American Psychiatric Association 2022) (Box 4–1), delusional disorder is defined as the presence of one or more delusions that persist for at least a month and are not caused by any substance, chronic disease, or psychiatric disorder such as schizophrenia. One of the specifiers of delusional disorder is somatic subtype. Delusional disorder can be divided into primary type, when there is no underlying disorder or medical illness, and secondary type, when associated with psychiatric or organic diseases and effects of drugs or substance of abuse (González-Rodríguez and Seeman 2020).

Box 4–1. Diagnostic Criteria for Delusional Disorder

A. The presence of one (or more) delusions with a duration of 1 month or longer.
B. Criterion A for schizophrenia has never been met.
   Note: Hallucinations, if present, are not prominent and are related to the delusional theme (e.g., the sensation of being infested with insects associated with delusions of infestation).

C. Apart from the impact of the delusion(s) or its ramifications, functioning is not markedly impaired, and behavior is not obviously bizarre or odd.
D. If manic or major depressive episodes have occurred, these have been brief relative to the duration of the delusional periods.
E. The disturbance is not attributable to the physiological effects of a substance or another medical condition and is not better explained by another mental disorder, such as body dysmorphic disorder or obsessive-compulsive disorder.

Specify whether:

Erotomanic type: This subtype applies when the central theme of the delusion is that another person is in love with the individual.

Grandiose type: This subtype applies when the central theme of the delusion is the conviction of having some great (but unrecognized) talent or insight or having made some important discovery.

Jealous type: This subtype applies when the central theme of the individual's delusion is that his or her spouse or lover is unfaithful.

Persecutory type: This subtype applies when the central theme of the delusion involves the individual's belief that he or she is being conspired against, cheated, spied on, followed, poisoned or drugged, maliciously maligned, harassed, or obstructed in the pursuit of long-term goals.

Somatic type: This subtype applies when the central theme of the delusion involves bodily functions or sensations.

Mixed type: This subtype applies when no one delusional theme predominates.

Unspecified type: This subtype applies when the dominant delusional belief cannot be clearly determined or is not described in the specific types (e.g., referential delusions without a prominent persecutory or grandiose component).

Specify if:

With bizarre content: Delusions are deemed bizarre if they are clearly implausible, not understandable, and not derived from ordinary life experiences (e.g., an individual's belief that a stranger has removed his or her internal organs and replaced them with someone else's organs without leaving any wounds or scars).

Source. Reprinted from American Psychiatric Association: *Diagnostic and Statistical Manual of Mental Disorders*, 5th Edition, Text Revision. Washington, DC, American Psychiatric Association, 2022. Copyright © 2022 American Psychiatric Association. Used with permission.

The main symptom of primary delusional disorder is isolated delusions, which in the case of the somatic form, may be accompanied by bizarre tactile sensations or itching of the skin (Opjordsmoen 2014). In delusional infestation, patients are rigidly convinced that bugs are crawling on the body despite the lack of evidence. Other areas in patients' life are unchanged.

STD delusions are less common (Freudenmann and Lepping 2009). Isolated STD delusions are often related to HIV infection. In the description of three cases of men with delusional HIV infection, each had depressive disorder (Nash 1996). Similarly, another case of a man with delusions of HIV infection also presented with a depressive disorder, and his delusions and guilt led him to genital self-mutilation (Mishra et al. 2014).

Most often, cases of delusional STD are not accompanied by itchy skin or the belief that worms are crawling on the skin, as in this case. The patient here was convinced that he was infected through sexual contact and believed that parasites resided in the genital area, spreading throughout the body, causing pruritus and a strange sensation on the skin.

The treatment of delusional disorder includes both psychotherapy and pharmacotherapy; in the case of secondary delusional disorder, treatment of the underlying disease is attempted (Jalali Roudsari et al. 2015; Moriarty et al. 2019). The first-line treatment is antipsychotics, especially second-generation (atypical) drugs, such as risperidone and olanzapine (Opjordsmoen 2014). However, first-generation (typical) antipsychotics such as pimozide can also be considered. Antidepressants (e.g., SSRIs) are used for comorbid depressive disorders, whereas antipruritics, such as antihistamines, can be used for pruritus. CBT can be particularly beneficial in patients whose delusions lead to anxiety, insomnia, and faulty logic (Jalali Roudsari et al. 2015). In addition, if necessary, topical treatment of skin lesions should be implemented, including antibiotic therapy for infections. As in this case, risperidone at 1–2 mg/day has been found to have a beneficial effect.

In conclusion, taking care of a patient with delusional disorder, including delusional infection, requires an interdisciplinary approach involving a dermatologist, psychiatrist, and psychologist. Making the correct diagnosis and implementing the appropriate treatment of delusional disorder will allow patients to avoid unnecessary testing and ineffective therapy. Antipsychotics, including risperidone, are first-line therapy for delusional disorder.

TEACHING POINTS

- Delusional infestation as a cause of STDs is a rare presentation and is classified as delusional disorder, somatic type.
- The condition must be distinguished from venereophobia, where the patient expresses a phobia of having an STD.

- Antipsychotics, including risperidone, are first-line therapy for delusional disorder, and may be combined with psychotherapy.

References

American Psychiatric Association: Diagnostic and Statistical Manual of Mental Disorders, 5th Edition, Text Revision. Washington, DC, American Psychiatric Association, 2022

Freudenmann RW, Lepping P: Delusional infestation. Clin Microbiol Rev 22(4):690–732, 2009 19822895

González-Rodríguez A, Seeman MV: Addressing delusions in women and men with delusional disorder: key points for clinical management. Int J Environ Res Public Health 17(12):4583, 2020 32630566

Jalali Roudsari M, Chun J, Manschreck TC: Current treatments for delusional disorder. Curr Treat Options Psychiatry 2:151–167, 2015

Mishra KK, Reddy S, Khairkar P: Genital self-mutilation in a suicide attempt: a rare sequela of a hypochondriacal delusion of infection with HIV. Int J STD AIDS 25(4):312–314, 2014 24021211

Moriarty N, Alam M, Kalus A, O'Connor K: Current understanding and approach to delusional infestation. Am J Med 132(12):1401–1409, 2019 31295443

Nash L: The delusion of infection with HIV. Aust N Z J Psychiatry 30(4):467–471, 1996 8887696

Opjordsmoen S: Delusional disorder as a partial psychosis. Schizophr Bull 40(2):244–247, 2014 24421383

Case 4–8
Morgellons Disease or Delusional Parasitosis?

Agnieszka Otlewska, M.D.
Przemysław Pacan, M.D.
Jacek C. Szepietowski, M.D.

Case Description

A 58-year-old married woman presented to the clinic for evaluation of suspicion of Morgellons disease. The patient stated that for more than a year, she had been observing different types of fibers growing out from her skin with punctate "black dots" on its surface. According to the patient's report, the lesions first appeared on the soles of her feet and then subsequently progressed to different parts of her body, including palms, buttocks, arms, and trunk. The lesions were accompanied by a stinging sensation. The patient reported that the release of threads and fibers from the skin as well as the stinging sensation were intensified under pressure, such as during walking. She suspected that the cause of her symptoms was "some infection of the skin of unknown origin."

Since the first symptoms appeared, she has been treated as an outpatient for about a year. She was prescribed anti-scabies treatment without any benefit. The patient also reported that she asked for skin samples, which allegedly contained threads, to be taken to the laboratory, but her requests were refused.

During the admission and throughout her hospitalization, no skin lesions were observed, but the patient was frequently seen examining her skin through a magnifying glass and showing the caregivers small black dots on her fingers, which on dermoscopy appeared to be artifacts. Routine laboratory work was within normal limits.

Differential Diagnosis

- Delusional parasitosis
- Morgellons disease
- Scabies infestation

Diagnosis

The patient was referred to the consultant psychiatrist, who reported normal mental status examination except for the thought content that was significant for delusions of fibers and threads coming out of the skin. Based on negative laboratory results and clinical and morphological examination, the diagnosis of delusional infestation was made.

Management

The patient was recommended risperidone 1 mg twice a day, but as she lacked insight into her condition, she did not consent to the prescribed medication, it being a psychotropic medication. As a result, she was discharged home and was lost to follow-up.

Discussion

Delusional infestation is a rare psychodermatological disorder. It has two types: primary, which occurs when there are no other underlying psychiatric or organic conditions, and secondary, where an underlying pathology may cause symptoms such as psychiatric causes (e.g., depression, dementia, or schizophrenia) or organic causes (e.g., anemia, vitamin B_{12} deficiency, diabetes, infections, or hypothyroidism). The secondary form can also be associated with substance abuse (Alhendi and Burahmah 2023; Freudenmann and Lepping 2009).

The disorder is characterized by tactile hallucinations such as tingling, prickling, and itching sensations, resulting from the erroneous and strong belief of patients about creeping of parasites on or under their skin (Hylwa and Ronkainen 2018). Not infrequently, this persistent belief can lead to self-inflicted injuries, causing ulcerations, as patients often attempt to eliminate the perceived parasite (Alhendi and Burahmah 2023). A common behavior among patients with delusional infestation is the collection of samples of suspected parasites or other materials from the infested skin as evidence of parasitic infestation, called matchbox sign or specimen sign (Reszke et al. 2021).

Another psychodermatologic condition (and perhaps a form of delusional infestation) is Morgellons disease. This has not been classified in any standard nomenclature. It shares similarities with delusional infestation, as it is characterized by a strong belief in the emergence of various fibers, filaments, or threads from the skin. Patients often spend a significant amount of time observing their skin and become obsessively focused on their symptoms (Mohandas et al. 2018).

Both delusional infestation and Morgellons disease are psychodermatologic disorders in which delusions play a crucial role in pathogenesis. In general, patients lack insight into their condition and frequently refuse psychiatric treatment (Reszke et al. 2021). The presented case illustrates the similarities between the two disorders. The study of this case shows the importance of considering whether these are truly two separate disease entities or closely related conditions.

TEACHING POINTS

- Patients with delusional infestation experience tactile hallucinations and delusions of the presence of parasites on or under their skin, which can lead to self-inflicted injuries.

- Morgellons disease is a related condition, not classified in the standard nomenclature, characterized by a belief in the emergence of fibers or threads from the skin.

Delusional Infestation 69

- Patients with delusional infestation or Morgellons disease often lack insight into their condition and may resist psychiatric treatment.
- This case raises questions about the relationship between delusional infestation and Morgellons disease and whether they represent separate entities or stages of the same condition.

References

Alhendi F, Burahmah A: Delusional parasitosis or Morgellons disease: a case of an overlap syndrome. Case Rep Dent 2023:3268220, 2023 37152271

Freudenmann RW, Lepping P: Delusional infestation. Clin Microbiol Rev 22(4):690–732, 2009 19822895

Hylwa SA, Ronkainen SD: Delusional infestation versus Morgellons disease. Clin Dermatol 36(6):714–718, 2018 30446193

Mohandas P, Bewley A, Taylor R: Morgellons disease: experiences of an integrated multidisciplinary dermatology team to achieve positive outcomes. J Dermatolog Treat 29(2):208–213, 2018 28665169

Reszke R, Pacan P, Reich A, Szepietowski JC: Delusional infestation in clinical practice over a period of two decades. Postepy Dermatol Alergol 38(2):144–150, 2021 34408581

Case 4–9
Delusional Infestation of the Scalp and Folie à Deux

Mariam Tabka, M.D.
Dorra Mdhaffar, M.D.
Mourad Mokni, M.D.
Asmahane Souissi, M.D.

Case Description

A 50-year-old married woman presented to the clinic with a 2-year history of intermittent scalp pruritus. She complained of worms crawling underneath her skin, but mainly on her scalp. No history of psychiatric disorders or psychoactive substance use was reported, and she was not taking any

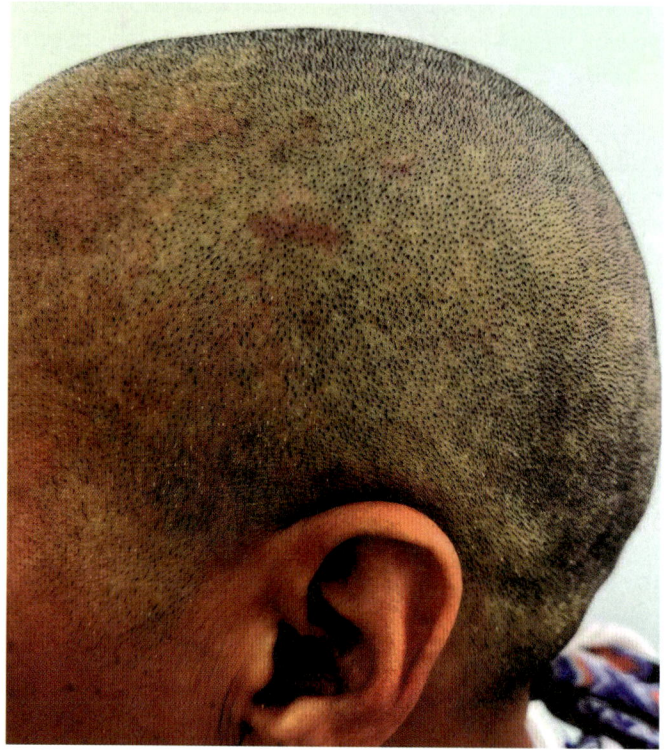

FIGURE 4–11. A completely shaven scalp.
Source. Dr. Asmahane Souissi.

medications. The patient consulted several dermatologists and was repeatedly treated with ivermectin and dimethicone, with no improvement. Dermatological examination revealed generalized hair loss with no evidence of scaling, atrophy, or scarring (Figure 4–11). The patient had shaved her hair attempting to extract the suspected worms. She stated that she removed "insects" from her skin daily, which she brought to us in a jar; they appeared to be dead skin debris (Figure 4–12). She had isolated herself from her husband and children for fear of contaminating them. Her husband also reported similar symptoms of being infected with worms under his skin.

Differential Diagnosis

- True parasite infestation
- Delusional infestation
- Trichotemnomania
- Fungal infection of scalp

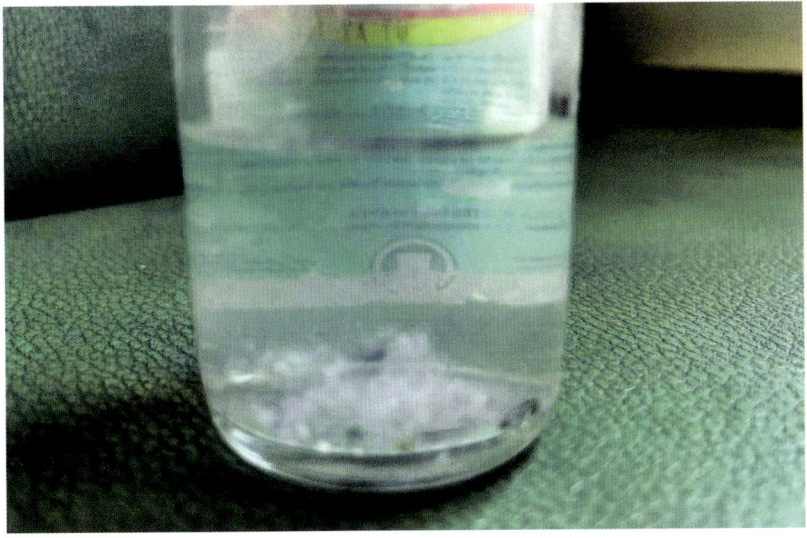

FIGURE 4–12. The specimen sign.
Source. Dr. Asmahane Souissi.

Diagnosis

Trichoscopy revealed short, uniformly broken hair without any evidence of lice or nits (Figure 4–13). Routine lab work and mycological examination were normal. Further investigations were conducted, including laboratory tests for thyroid-stimulating hormone, urine analysis for illicit substances testing, and computed tomography of the brain. These tests ruled out any secondary delusional infestation.

Psychiatric evaluation revealed hypochondriacal delusional ideas focused on the hair and scalp and affective lability. She had tactile hallucination and delusion of parasitosis. The diagnosis of delusional infestation was established.

Management

The patient was reassured during the consultation, and dermatopsychiatric follow-up was scheduled on an outpatient basis.

Discussion

Delusional infestation can be categorized into primary and secondary forms, depending on the presence or absence of another underlying cause (physical, toxic, or psychiatric). The primary delusional infestation, an isolated, monosymptomatic delusional disorder, meets criteria for a delusional disorder, somatic type, according to DSM-5-TR (American Psychiatric As-

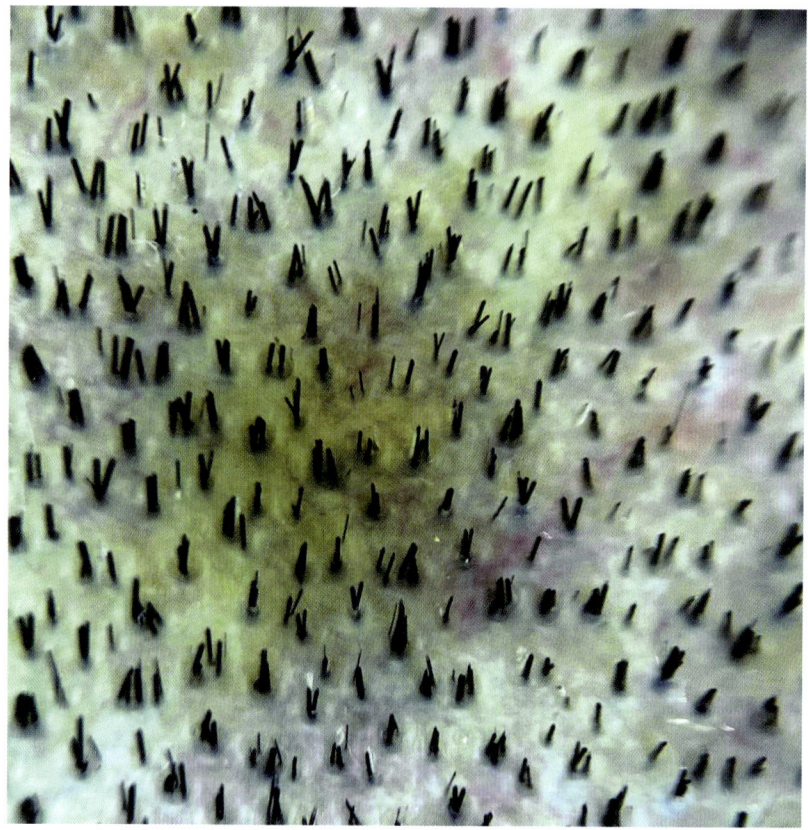

FIGURE 4–13. Trichoscopy showed short, uniformly broken hair without any evidence of lice or nits.
Source. Dr. Asmahane Souissi.

sociation 2022) (see Box 4–1). This implies that patients with delusional disorders do not meet diagnostic criteria for schizophrenia or other psychiatric disorders, although hallucinations secondary to the delusional theme (e.g., tactile hallucinations) may be present. de Portugal et al. (2013) reported that 64% of patients had at least one premorbid personality disorder, with paranoid premorbid personality disorder being the most common (38.4%), followed by schizoid premorbid personality disorder. Secondary delusional infestation may occur in the context of psychiatric disorders (such as schizophrenia, depression, dementia, anxiety, and phobia) or substance abuse (cocaine, amphetamines, cannabis) and be linked to other medical disorders (Reich et al. 2019).

This patient fulfills the diagnostic criteria for primary delusional infestation. The onset of delusional infestation can be sudden or progressive, typically characterized by intense pruritus and abnormal sensations on or underneath the skin such as crawling, itching, stinging, biting, tingling, and formication (Torales et al. 2020). These abnormal tactile sensations are interpreted as illusions or hallucinations, as a true cause for tactile symptoms is difficult to prove or disprove. Patients claim that pathogens including parasites, bacteria, viruses, worms, insects, and both organic and nonorganic fibers are living, eating, breeding, and building nests in their body (Lepping et al. 2015). As a result of their persistent belief in parasitic infestation, they exhibit self-inflicted skin lesions of varying severity in an attempt to remove the presumed pathogen. They often provide the physician with samples of these pathogens as proof of infestation, known as the specimen sign (Freudenmann and Lepping 2009). Increasingly, modern patients present videos or digital images depicting areas they believe are affected by infestation (Torales et al. 2020). The psychosis may selectively involve specific areas of the body, such as natural orifices, gastrointestinal tract, or the scalp, as seen in this patient. Sometimes, the delusional ideas spread to a shared belief involving two or more individuals of the family: folie à deux (two people), folie à trois (three people), and folie à plusieurs or folie à famille (many people or the entire family) (Yang et al. 2019). This patient's husband reported similar symptoms. Patients usually require antipsychotic treatment, which should be part of a multidisciplinary approach.

TEACHING POINTS

- Differentiating primary from secondary delusional infestation is a crucial step that guides subsequent management.
- Detailed history regarding any family member involvement should be part of screening.
- A therapeutic bond with the patient is important in the subsequent recommendation for psychotropic medication.

References

American Psychiatric Association: Diagnostic and Statistical Manual of Mental Disorders, 5th Edition, Text Revision. Washington, DC, American Psychiatric Association, 2022 de Portugal E, Díaz-Caneja CM, González-Molinier M, et al: Prevalence of pre-morbid personality disorder and its clinical correlates in patients with delusional disorder. Psychiatry Res 210(3):986–993, 2013 23993136

Freudenmann RW, Lepping P: Delusional infestation. Clin Microbiol Rev 22(4):690–732, 2009 19822895

Lepping P, Huber M, Freudenmann RW: How to approach delusional infestation. BMJ 350:h1328, 2015 25832416

Reich A, Kwiatkowska D, Pacan P: Delusions of parasitosis: an update. Dermatol Ther (Heidelb) 9(4):631–638, 2019 31520344

Torales J, García O, Barrios I, et al: Delusional infestation: clinical presentations, diagnosis, and management. J Cosmet Dermatol 19(12):3183–3188, 2020 33098221

Yang EJ, Beck KM, Koo J: Folie à famille: a systematic review of shared delusional infestation. J Am Acad Dermatol 81(5):1211–1215, 2019 31002848

5

Trichotillomania and Its Variants

Asmahane Souissi, M.D.
Mohammad Jafferany, M.D.

Trichotillomania (TTM) is an obsessive-compulsive spectrum disorder characterized by recurrent urges to pull hair, causing hair loss and significant functional impairment; it may lead to a negative impact on quality of life in patients. TTM is associated with several psychiatric comorbidities, such as anxiety, depression, and OCD. Many cultures stigmatize hair loss, so patients generally have low self-esteem and avoid social situations. TTM can be challenging to manage and usually requires a multidisciplinary approach.

Epidemiology

The lifetime prevalence of TTM is 1%–3% (Panza et al. 2013). Because patients with TTM are often ashamed and embarrassed about their disorder, they usually do not seek help from health providers; therefore, the real prevalence of TTM is often underestimated. Subclinical TTM is estimated to be present in 11% of the general population (Woods et al. 1996). Compulsive hair pulling generally begins in childhood or early adolescence. Sex distribution seems to be equal in childhood. A large female preponderance has been found in some studies (female/male=4/1) (Christenson et al. 1994), but other series showed no differences in rates among men and women (Grant et al. 2020).

Etiology and Pathogenesis

Data are limited concerning the pathogenesis of TTM, and its etiology is not well understood. TTM may result from a combination of multiple factors, including genetics, neurobiology, and social environments. Animal model research has shown that *Hoxb8*, *Sapap3*, and *Slitrk5* genes are associated with TTM. Mice with these genes have been shown to display markedly elevated grooming behaviors similar to those observed in humans with TTM (Greer and Capecchi 2002; Shmelkov et al. 2010; Welch et al. 2007).

Neuroimaging studies have shown abnormalities in neuropsychological functioning in patients with TTM compared with control subjects. MRI has revealed reduced right amygdala and left putamen volumes and gray matter abnormalities in patients with TTM, and increased density in brain regions playing a role in motor habits and affect regulation (Chamberlain et al. 2008). Increased cortical thickness has also been noted in the right inferior frontal gyrus of patients with TTM. One study showed that 91% of patients with TTM experienced trauma, especially during childhood, such as verbal, physical, or sexual abuse (Boughn and Holdom 2003). In terms of psychoanalytic theory, TTM is regarded as a symbolic manifestation of unconscious conflicts that occurred in childhood. Therefore, pulling hair may serve as a coping mechanism to release tension and feelings of frustration. Nevertheless, temporary relief from these negative emotions maintains a reinforcement cycle of repetitive behavior.

Psychopathological Features

There are two distinguishable types of hair pulling: automatic and focused. In the automatic type, the patient is not fully aware of their pulling behaviors. For example, younger children usually pull hair outside of their awareness, as if they were playing with it. In the focused type, hair pulling is intentionally performed to regulate negative emotions. Older children and a majority of adults tend to pull hair in response to negative emotions such as anger, sadness, anxiety, or frustration. They usually pull out hairs that seem different from the rest (white, kinky, coarse, etc.) to release tension generated by stressful events (Fernandes et al. 2021; Henkel et al. 2019). Most patients with TTM engage in both focused and automatic hair-pulling. It is also documented that children with TTM become aware of re-

Trichotillomania and Its Variants

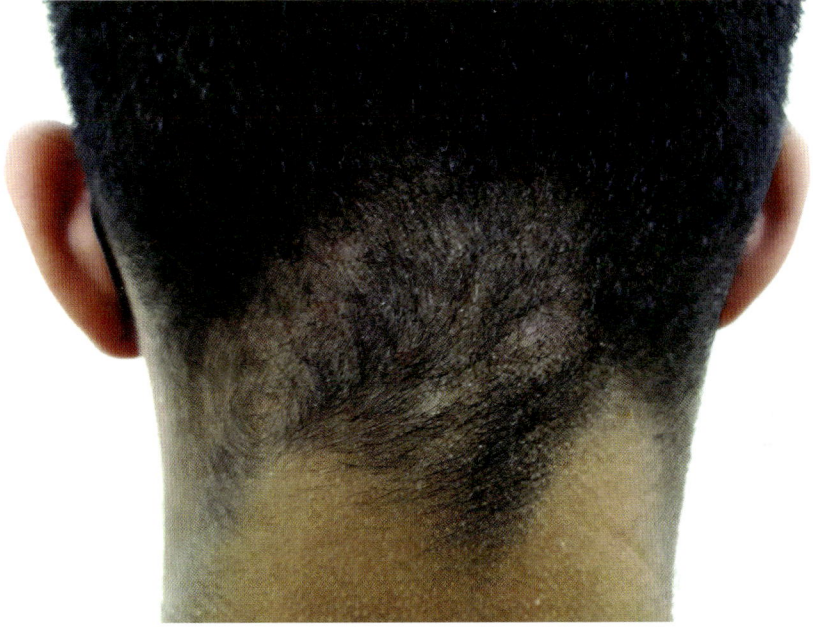

FIGURE 5–1. Asymmetrical nonscarring patches of incomplete hair loss with a bizarre-shaped pattern and irregular borders.
Source. Dr. Asmahane Souissi.

moving their own hair when they are older, switching from the automatic type to the focused type (Anwar and Jafferany 2019). In TTM, the repetitive behavior is irresistible. The patient feels an intense hair-pulling urge and is unable to control the urge. Usually, they feel pleasure and temporary relief during and immediately after pulling their hair. However, this feeling of relief quickly turns into guilt and shame. The urge to pull hair is then reinforced in a harsh cycle to cope with negative emotional states.

Clinical Features

The most common site of TTM is the scalp. Eyebrows, eyelashes, and the pubic area may be involved. Rarely, beard, chest hair, underarms, and limbs may also be affected. Clinically, patients with TTM present with asymmetrical nonscarring patches of incomplete hair loss with a bizarre-shaped pattern and irregular borders (Figure 5–1). The frontoparietal region of the scalp is more often involved, but diffuse alopecia may also be observed (Figure 5–2). The Friar Tuck sign suggestive of TTM corresponds to alopecia of the crown surrounded by a rim of normal hair at the

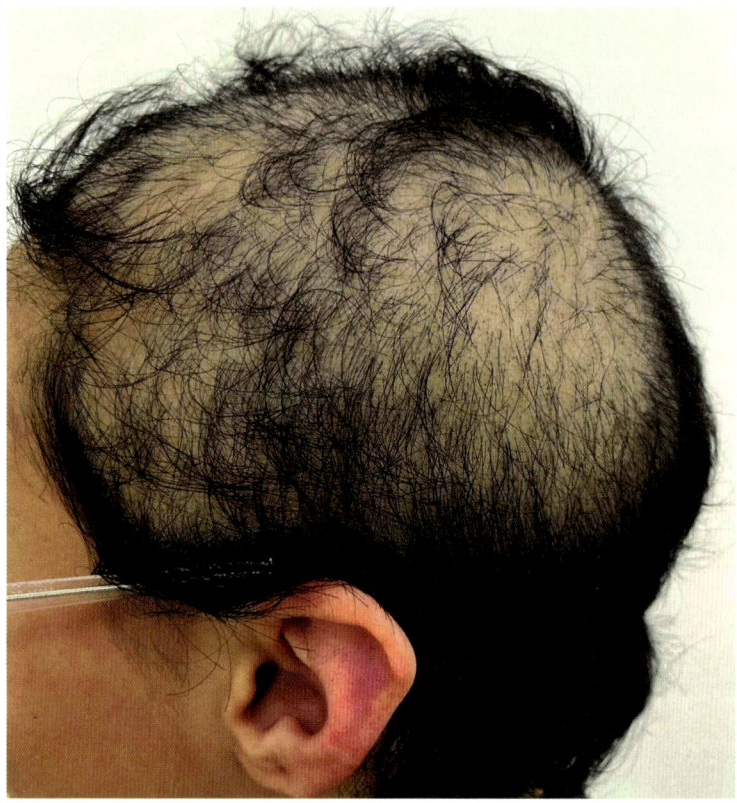

FIGURE 5–2. Diffuse alopecia secondary to trichotillomania.
Source. Dr. Asmahane Souissi.

periphery. On examination, broken hairs of various lengths may be observed depending on the fracture point of each pulled hair. Typically, there is no inflammation or scaling, and the hair-pull test is negative.

Trichoscopy

Patients with TTM usually deny the habit of deliberately pulling hair. Trichoscopy, which reveals the fractures of the hair shafts related to pulling, is the main method for diagnosing TTM. It will show broken hairs of varying lengths and shapes depending on the strength of the applied mechanical forces. Trichoscopic findings in TTM include the following:

- Coiled hairs with irregular appearance and frayed ends (Figure 5–3)
- Flame hairs: semitransparent and cone-shaped

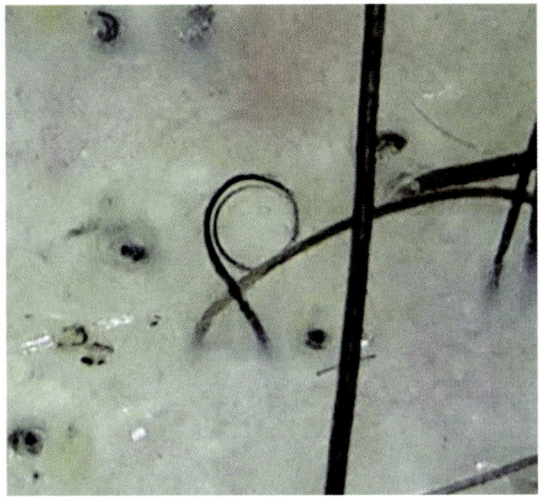

FIGURE 5–3. Coiled hair.
Source. Dr. Asmahane Souissi.

- Trichoptilosis corresponding to short hair splitting into many parts (Figure 5–4)
- Tulip hairs: the distal end is darker and has the shape of a tulip petal
- Hook hairs, the most specific finding, with a 100% positive predictive score (Kaczorowska et al. 2021): hook hairs have a distal end shaped in the form of a hook (Figure 5–5)
- In patients with TTM, trichoscopy may also show V sign (Figure 5–6), hair powder, black dots, and hemorrhages.

The association of several different signs in a single view is very characteristic of TTM and creates a chaotic trichoscopic pattern (Figure 5–7).

Histopathology

Dermatologists usually make the diagnosis of TTM based on patient history, clinical examination, and trichoscopic findings. In rare cases, a clinical diagnosis can be challenging to make; in such cases, a trichoscopy-guided biopsy may be performed. Specific histopathological features in TTM are trichomalacia and pigmented casts. In trichomalacia, the hair shaft is dysmorphic and has irregular pigmentation and incomplete cornification. Nonspecific histological findings include reversed anagen/telogen ratio,

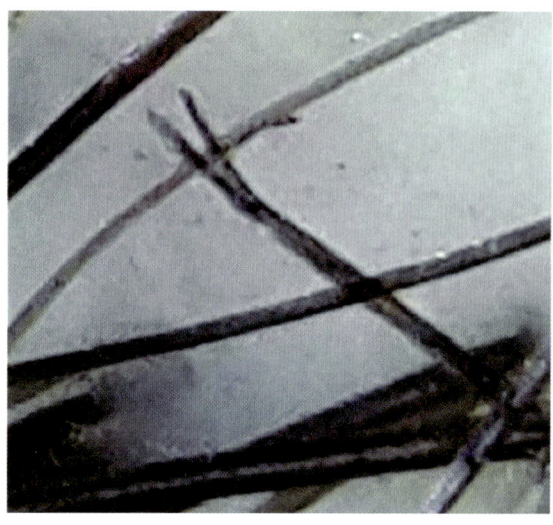

FIGURE 5–4. Trichoptilosis.
Source. Dr. Asmahane Souissi.

follicular plugging, decreased number of sebaceous glands, melanoderma, and peripilar and intrapilar hemorrhage.

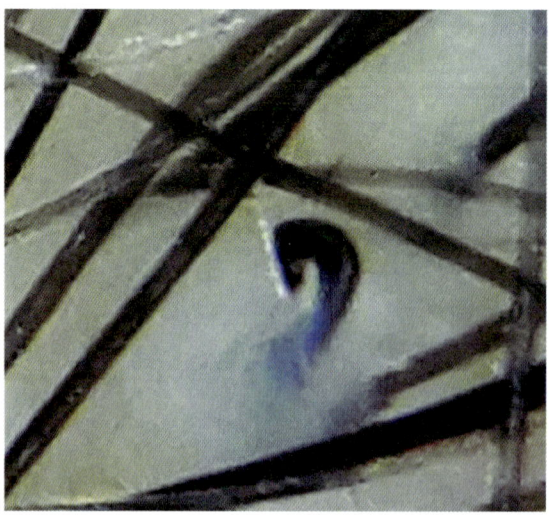

FIGURE 5–5. Hook hair.
Source. Dr. Asmahane Souissi.

Diagnosis

TTM is included in DSM-5-TR (American Psychiatric Association 2022) as a disorder related to OCD. The current diagnostic criteria are shown in Box 5–1.

Box 5–1. Diagnostic Criteria for Trichotillomania (Hair-Pulling Disorder)

A. Recurrent pulling out of one's hair, resulting in hair loss.
B. Repeated attempts to decrease or stop hair pulling.
C. The hair pulling causes clinically significant distress or impairment in social, occupational, or other important areas of functioning.
D. The hair pulling or hair loss is not attributable to another medical condition (e.g., a dermatological condition).
E. The hair pulling is not better explained by the symptoms of another mental disorder (e.g., attempts to improve a perceived defect or flaw in appearance in body dysmorphic disorder).

Source. Reprinted from American Psychiatric Association: *Diagnostic and Statistical Manual of Mental Disorders*, 5th Edition, Text Revision. Washington, DC, American Psychiatric Association, 2022. Copyright © 2022 American Psychiatric Association. Used with permission.

Although TTM is considered a psychiatric diagnosis, many patients with TTM do not meet all the psychiatric criteria. Moreover, the majority of TTM patients initially present to a dermatologist for evaluation of hair loss. The dermatologist's capacity to make the diagnosis of TTM is vital to avoid unnecessary tests and provide adequate care. The diagnosis of TTM is considered based on clinical examination. The presence of patches of incomplete hair loss with an irregular pattern, broken hairs of varying lengths, and the absence of inflammation and scaling are highly suggestive of the diagnosis. Trichoscopy is a fast, noninvasive technique that allows dermatologists to identify hair-pulling behaviors.

Assessment Tools

A variety of assessment tools and scales are used in the diagnosis and prognosis of TTM. A variety of clinician rating scales are used to measure the severity of TTM, such as the Yale-Brown Obsessive-Compulsive Scale-Trichotillomania (Y-BOCS-TM), the Psychiatric Institute Trichotillomania Scale (PITS), and NIMH's Trichotillomania Symptom Severity Scale (NIMH-TSS). Various assessment scales are shown in Table 5–1 (Jafferany 2021). Several self-report measures in use demonstrate patients'

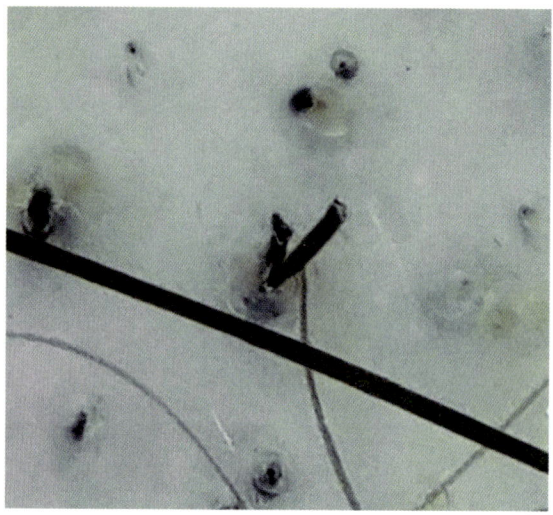

FIGURE 5–6. V sign.
Source. Dr. Asmahane Souissi.

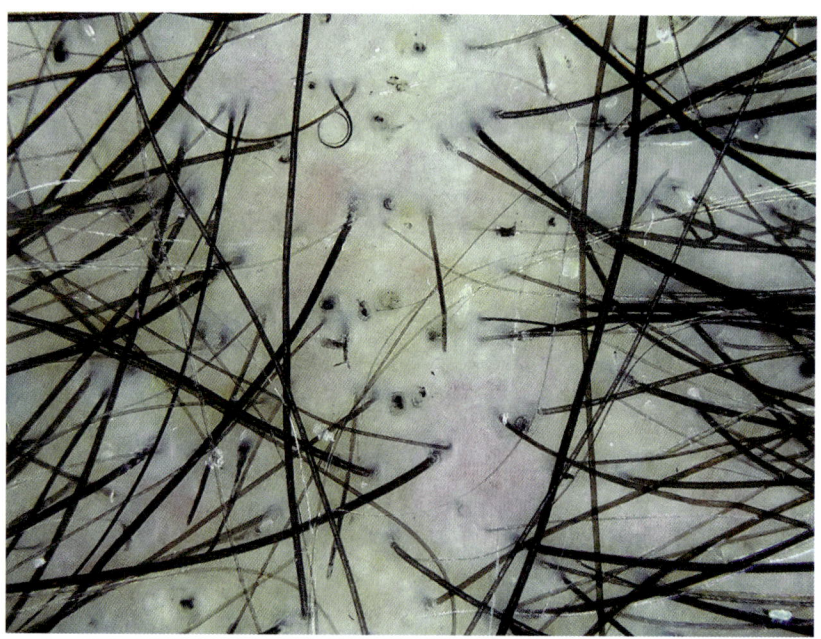

FIGURE 5–7. Broken hairs of different lengths and shapes.
Source. Dr. Asmahane Souissi.

TABLE 5–1. Assessment tools in trichotillomania

Type	Tool	Abbreviation
Clinician rating scale	Yale-Brown Obsessive-Compulsive Scale-Trichotillomania	Y-BOCS-TM
	Psychiatric Institute Trichotillomania Scale	PITS
	Trichotillomania Symptom Severity Scale	NIMH-TSS
Self-report measure	Milwaukee Inventory for Subtypes of Trichotillomania	MIST
	MGH Hair Pulling Scale	
	Hair-pulling surgery	
Self-monitoring	Saving pulled hair	
	Keeping daily record	
Collateral report	Family members	
	For children	
	For those who are cognitively impaired	
Objective measure	Pre- and posttreatment photographs	

Note. MGH=Massachusetts General Hospital; NIMH=National Institute of Mental Health.
Source. Adapted from Jafferany 2021.

pulling behavior, severity, and intensity of TTM, and the results ultimately may guide the direction of treatment. Saving pulled hair and keeping a daily record is a useful self-monitoring method by patients. Similarly, collateral reports from family members are a very important part of the history, especially for children and cognitively impaired patients. As an objective measure, pre- and posttreatment photographs may help and direct the course of the treatment.

Differential Diagnosis

Differential diagnosis of TTM mainly includes alopecia areata, traction alopecia, tinea capitis, and secondary syphilis. Diffuse TTM may mimic telogen effluvium.

Comorbidities and Complications

TTM may be associated with several disorders, such as anxiety, PTSD, depression, and substance abuse. These concomitant psychiatric conditions may be observed in 80% of cases (Woods and Houghton 2014). Patients with TTM sometimes ingest the pulled hair (trichophagia), causing trichobezoar formation and intestinal complications. In Rapunzel syndrome, the tail of the trichobezoar extends into the intestine, leading to intestinal obstruction and the need for surgical intervention.

In patients who eat their hair, evaluation should focus on these gastrointestinal symptoms, such as epigastric pain, vomiting, diarrhea, constipation, and weight loss. Appropriate interventions should include abdominal examination, blood tests to assess for anemia, and potentially a CT scan to make the diagnosis of trichobezoar (Grant and Chamberlain 2016).

The psychological impact of TTM can be significant—the act of pulling hair causes significant distress, guilt, and shame. Patients may fear being judged by others. They often avoid getting haircuts and social situations such as sporting activities or dating, leading to self-isolation and depression. Stress is a trigger factor for TTM, but TTM itself may cause stress, creating a vicious cycle that aggravates the disorder and decreases the patient's quality of life. The impact of TTM on social, academic, and professional areas is significant. Therefore, early intervention is crucial to control the disorder and its mental sequelae.

Prognosis

TTM is generally a chronic disorder with recurrent relapses interspersed with periods of remission. Although the course of TTM may vary, if untreated, it may lead to significant psychological dysfunction and, in rare cases, to life-threatening conditions.

Treatment

TTM is a chronic, relapsing disorder. It presents along a continuum from mild to severe. The aim of the treatment is to develop effective coping strategies and improve the patient's quality of life. Treatment is challenging, as patients often refuse to comply with treatment strategies. Additionally, most patients do not realize that TTM is a recognized disease. They fear health providers' reactions and do not believe that an effective treatment may exist. A patient with TTM should receive a comprehensive evaluation to determine if there is a personal history of trauma and potential comorbidities. The psychiatry-dermatology collaboration plays a crucial role in a comprehensive treatment plan and good outcomes. Parents of patients should be educated to avoid punishment and support their child to achieve remission. There are currently no FDA-approved medications for TTM; however, a variety of medications have been used with inconstant efficiency.

Comorbid disorders must also be considered, and the treatment options must be reevaluated accordingly and tailored individually.

Early-onset TTM, before the age of 5 years, is often benign and can be managed by simple interventions including reassurance and suggestion; drug therapy is rarely used at this age. Parental counseling is important to inform them about the nature of the condition, to not punish the child for pulling hair, and to not have a judgmental attitude toward the child.

Adult patients often believe that there is an underlying medical problem causing hair loss and are unwilling to accept the self-inflicted nature of TTM. In other cases, they believe that pulling hair is just a "bad habit" and avoid seeking treatment owing to shame and embarrassment. During the management of TTM, the physician should have an empathic attitude toward the patient (e.g., should not confront or blame the patient). The physician should, however, ask about other habits such as nail biting or skin picking to help the patient to gain awareness of the disorder.

Nonpharmacological Treatments

Several psychotherapeutic techniques have been used in the management of TTM, with promising results.

Habit Reversal Training

Habit reversal training (HRT) is a subtype of CBT. HRT is considered the treatment of choice for TTM. The aim of this therapy is to increase the patient's awareness of their hair-pulling behavior and help them replace it with another behavior that does not decrease their quality of life. HRT has been used successfully in combination with pharmacological drugs.

HRT consists of four steps. The first step is *awareness training*, which helps the patient monitor their awareness of their hair-pulling behavior, for example by filling out the self-monitoring form so they can identify triggering factors, vulnerable situations, and daily emotions leading to pulling hair.

The next step of HRT is called *competing response practice*, which involves avoiding stressful situations, triggers, feelings, and vulnerable places before hair pulling begins. This may consist of removing things that facilitate hair pulling or developing a competing behavior such as squeezing a stress ball or other gestures. After the successful development of a replacement behavior, *habit control motivation* techniques encourage the patient to maintain the avoidance of harmful behaviors and prevent relapse. Social support procedures involve having family members and therapists point out when the patient relapses and motivate them to avoid the unwanted behavior. Finally, *generalization training* allows the patient to imagine themselves initiating the behavior but stopping it and performing the alternative behavior instead (Rahman et al. 2023).

Acceptance and Commitment Therapy

Acceptance and commitment therapy (ACT) involves helping the patient to approach hair pulling from the perspective of commitment to personal goals instead of considering it as an urge to cope with negative emotions. A randomized trial compared 12 patients who received combined ACT/HRT (10 sessions over 12 weeks) with 13 waitlist control patients. The ACT/HRT group showed a significant reduction in TTM severity/impairment and a greater reduction in anxiety, depression, and experiential avoidance in comparison with the waitlist subjects (Woods et al. 2006). Another study evaluated ACT (10 sessions) as a stand-alone treatment for TTM versus a waitlist group in a randomized clinical trial ($N=39$). Findings suggested that ACT alone is an effective treatment; results were similar to trials that associated ACT and HRT (Lee et al. 2020).

Psychodynamic Therapy

Psychodynamic therapy has been used to treat self-mutilation and self-inflicted dermatoses, and there is increasing evidence that supports this therapy for the management of TTM. Aukerman et al. (2022) described an 11-year-old patient who was diagnosed with TTM, with a history of multiple surgeries to correct a congenital spinal imbalance. The patient and his parents underwent psychodynamic therapy weekly for 15 months. During each session, he expressed his emotions and admitted what memories caused anxiety for him. He also learned to replace the act of pulling hair by other less destructive sensory behaviors such as picking fluff off his socks. Breath work also showed efficacy to control anxiety, and he practiced this technique outside of therapy. After therapy, the patient was able to regulate his emotions and stop hair-pulling, a result that was maintained 6 months later. The authors speculated that medical trauma from the multiple surgeries acted as a trigger and that TTM served as self-regulation in an overstimulated nervous system. The psychodynamic approach proved to be a successful coping strategy to regulate the underlying psychological distress that triggered TTM in this patient (Aukerman et al. 2022).

Microneedling

Christensen et al. (2022) recently described three TTM patients who were treated with microneedling. Each patient was given a dermaroller with 0.5-mm needles and asked to use the dermaroller on their scalp whenever they felt the urge to pull hair; they also received minoxidil to stimulate hair regrowth. The microneedling was to create percutaneous wounds to stimulate hair regrowth; in addition, the sensation of needles may simulate the act of hair pulling and replace the harmful behavior. Evaluation at 6 or 12 months showed clinical and trichoscopic improvement of the involved patches (Christensen et al. 2022).

Pharmacological Treatment

Pharmacological treatments for TTM include tricyclic antidepressants, selective serotonin reuptake inhibitors (SSRIs), antipsychotics, and glutamate modulators. Their efficacy is questionable; positive effects have been shown in some case reports only.

Tricyclic Antidepressants

Clomipramine is used in the management of TTM. It blocks norepinephrine and serotonin reuptake, as well as muscarinic, cholinergic, adrenergic, H1, and 5-hydroxytryptamine receptors. Some authors reported successful treatment with clomipramine at doses of 50 mg twice a day or 125 mg/day in addition to nonpharmacological treatments (Bartley et al. 2017; Mariusso et al. 2020; Sani et al. 2019).

Selective Serotonin Reuptake Inhibitors

Because of their efficacy in the management of depression and anxiety that are commonly associated with TTM, SSRIs have been widely prescribed as a treatment for TTM. SSRIs act by inhibiting the reuptake of serotonin in synapses. A randomized controlled study examined the efficacy of fluoxetine (60 mg/day) in behavioral therapy and a waiting-list control group. Forty patients completed the trial (11 in the fluoxetine group, 14 in the behavioral therapy group, and 15 in the waiting-list group). The authors concluded that behavioral therapy was highly effective in reducing symptoms, whereas fluoxetine was not (van Minnen et al. 2003). Other studies concluded poor efficacy of SSRIs in the treatment of TTM. Nevertheless, the efficiency of these molecules in the treatment of comorbid psychiatric conditions such as depression and anxiety can make them useful in managing TTM (Everett et al. 2020).

Antipsychotics

Second-generation antipsychotics such as olanzapine or aripiprazole modulate dopamine receptors. Side effects including extrapyramidal symptoms and metabolic dysfunction must be considered when prescribing these drugs. A randomized, double-blind, placebo-controlled trial of olanzapine at a mean dosage of 10.8 mg/day showed reduced symptoms of TTM after 12 weeks of treatment (Van Ameringen et al. 2010).

N-acetylcysteine

N-acetylcysteine (NAC) is thought to work through the regulation of synaptic glutamate levels in the brain and reduction of glutamate toxicity. Özcan and Seçkin (2016) reported the efficacy and safety of NAC at 1,200 mg/day in two patients with TTM. After the treatment was initiated, there was a significant reduction in hair pulling after 2 months for the first patient and after 2 weeks for the second patient. Complete hair regrowth was noted after 4 and 6 months in the first and second patients, respectively. NAC also demonstrated efficacy at the dose of 1,200 mg twice a day for a duration of 9 weeks in a double-blind, placebo-controlled study in 50 patients with TTM (Grant et al. 2009). Because NAC is relatively safe, well tolerated, and inexpensive, it is reasonable to include this drug in a patient's regimen. However, one randomized, double-blind, placebo-controlled trial did not show any efficacy of NAC in the treatment of TTM in children. The authors concluded that it did not work because of the absence of the urge to pull hair (children are typically unaware of the pulling behavior) (Bloch et al. 2013).

Memantine

Memantine is a glutamate modulator used to treat the symptoms of Alzheimer's disease. In a recent study conducted by Grant et al. (2023), memantine resulted in a statistically significant decrease in hair-pulling and skin-picking symptoms compared with placebo and was well tolerated.

Variants of Trichotillomania

Several variants of TTM are characterized by self-inflicted hair loss. They are sustained by similar psychological distress, and their management is challenging. Trichotemnomania, trichoteiromania, and trichodaganomania are less common than TTM and often underdiagnosed. Early diagnosis and treatment are crucial to avoid mental sequelae associated with these variants.

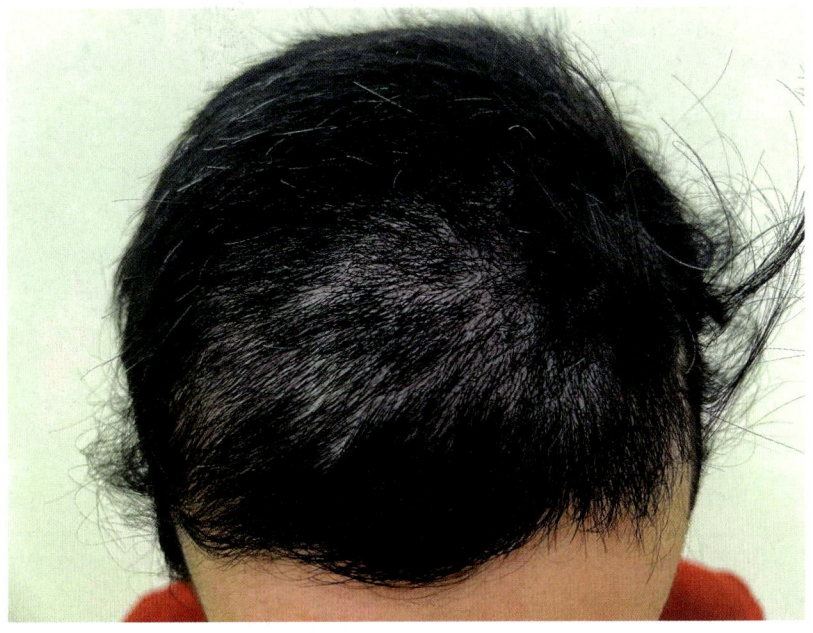

FIGURE 5–8. Decreased hair density on the frontal region related to compulsive cutting in the context of trichotemnomania.
Source. Dr. Asmahane Souissi.

Trichotemnomania

Trichotemnomania is a compulsive hair disorder characterized by hair loss due to cutting or shaving one's hair with scissors or a razor. It is less known than TTM and is mostly misdiagnosed. Few cases have been reported in the literature. Like TTM, trichotemnomania is more frequently seen in women (Patil and Dowd 2001). The main differential diagnosis includes TTM and alopecia areata.

Clinically, trichotemnomania is characterized by patches of hair loss with no signs of inflammation or scarring (Figure 5–8). Close inspection shows short hairs of equal lengths with normal morphology and sharply cut ends. The hair pull test is negative. In cases of shaving hair, examination reveals follicle openings filled with black hair shafts. Trichotemnomania may involve eyebrows, eyelashes, and axillary and pubic areas. Eyelashes and eyebrows may appear to have a trimmed appearance. Microscopic examination shows that the hair stubs have cleanly cut surfaces. Patients experience the urge to cut or to shave their hairs to relieve tension and to reduce stress. They usually deny the act out of guilt.

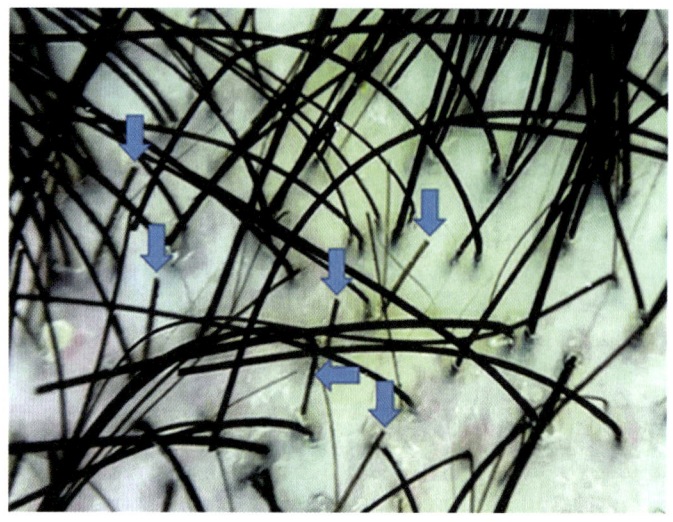

FIGURE 5–9. Short, healthy-looking hair shafts with similar length and clean-cut distal ends (blue arrows) in a patient with trichotemnomania.
Source. Dr. Asmahane Souissi.

Trichoscopy of trichotemnomania reveals follicular openings filled with black dots corresponding to hair shafts recently shaved. Patients cutting their hair with scissors or who have shaved their hair a few days before examination show short healthy-looking hair shafts with similar length and clean-cut distal ends, giving the hair a trimmed appearance (Figure 5–9).

The main differential diagnosis of trichotemnomania includes TTM and alopecia areata. TTM is characterized by broken hairs of irregular lengths and shapes. Trichoscopy reveals flame hairs, trichoptilosis, coiled hairs, and hook hairs. All these findings are lacking in trichotemnomania. On the other hand, TTM is characterized by histopathologic changes such as trichomalacia and an increased number of catagen hair follicles with pigment casts, whereas trichotemnomania reveals normal histologic structures. In alopecia areata, trichoscopy reveals yellow dots with regular distribution, exclamation mark hairs, and black dots. Trichoscopy is very useful to differentiate these diagnoses. As for TTM, the main treatment options are HRT combined with pharmacological molecules.

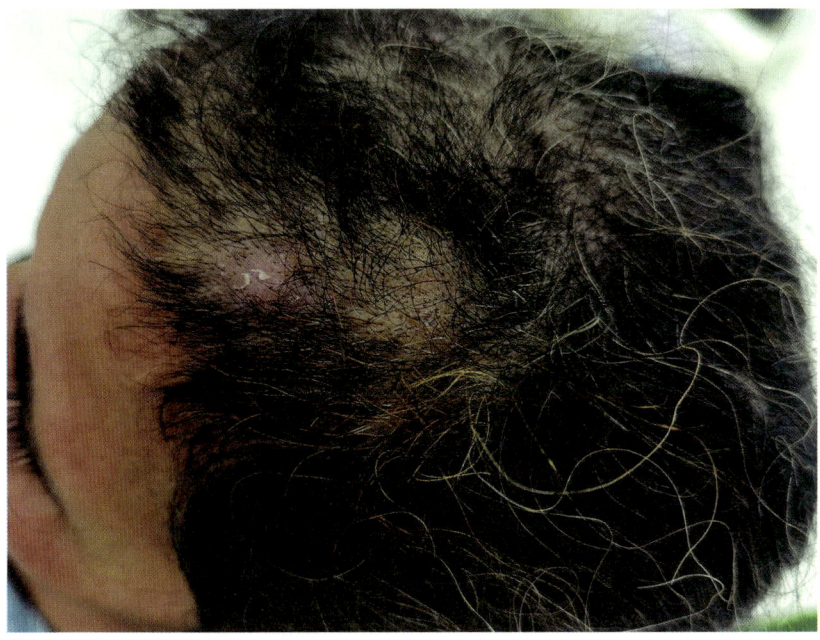

FIGURE 5–10. Irregular patches with scaling and hair loss in a patient with trichoteiromania.
Source. Dr. Asmahane Souissi.

Trichoteiromania

Trichoteiromania is defined as the compulsive habit of rubbing one's hairs, which results in fracturing of the hair shaft. Trichoteiromania is a rare cause of alopecia, often underdiagnosed.

Clinically, trichoteiromania is characterized by single or multiple irregular patches with scaling and hair loss related to fracture of hairs (Figure 5–10). The patient often gives a history of rubbing the scalp to get relief from pruritus. They may admit rubbing their scalp for many hours a day. Trichoteiromania may be confused with a scalp disorder such as eczema, psoriasis, or seborrheic dermatitis. Careful examination may reveal broken hairs at different lengths with white tips. Broken hairs emerge from thickened, rough skin with grayish-brown pigmentation (Ankad and Smitha 2022). The examination of the rest of the scalp shows normal-looking hairs. The hair pull test is negative. In some cases, erosions and hematic crusts are observed. Light microscopy also reveals brush-like splitting of the distal ends.

Under trichoscopy, the lesions show erythema, peri- and interfollicular scaling, and broom hairs corresponding to short broken hair shafts longi-

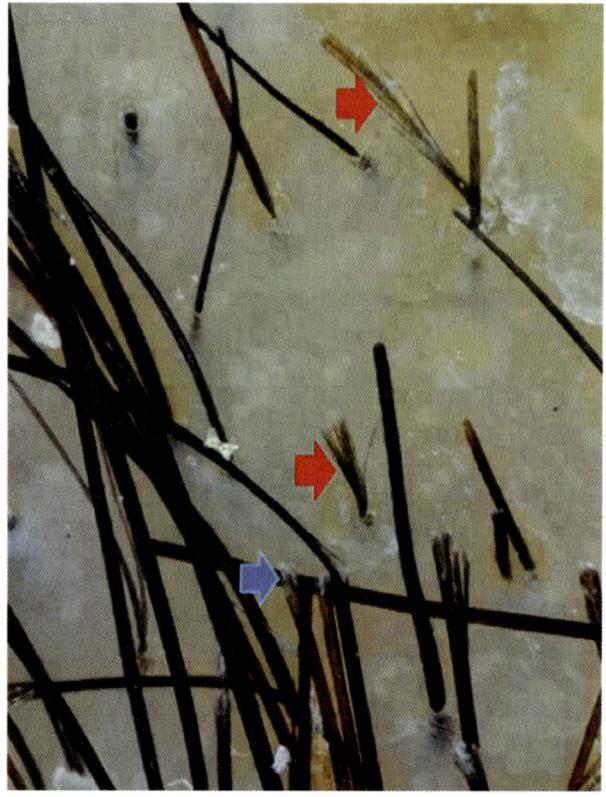

FIGURE 5–11. Trichoscopy in a patient with trichoteiromania: broom hair (red arrows) and white specks (blue arrow).
Source. Dr. Asmahane Souissi.

tudinally split into two to several parts. Broom hairs result from the continuous frictional damage of the hairs (Salas-Callo and Pirmez 2019) and have been considered to be highly suggestive of trichoteiromania (Salas-Callo and Pirmez 2019). Nevertheless, they have also been described in TTM (Kaczorowska et al. 2021). Trichoscopy also shows white specks at the distal end of the hair shaft from distal splitting (Figure 5–11) that are due to transparent hair shaft and scales at the surface (Ankad and Smitha 2022). In addition, trichoscopy may show trichorrhexis nodosa (Fowler and Tosti 2019), which results from the longitudinal splitting of the hair into small fibers that bulge out and cause the appearance of small white nodules visible along the hair shaft (Figure 5–12).

Broom hairs in TTM are associated with broken hair shafts with varying lengths and shapes, such as hook hairs, flame hairs, and tulip hairs. In

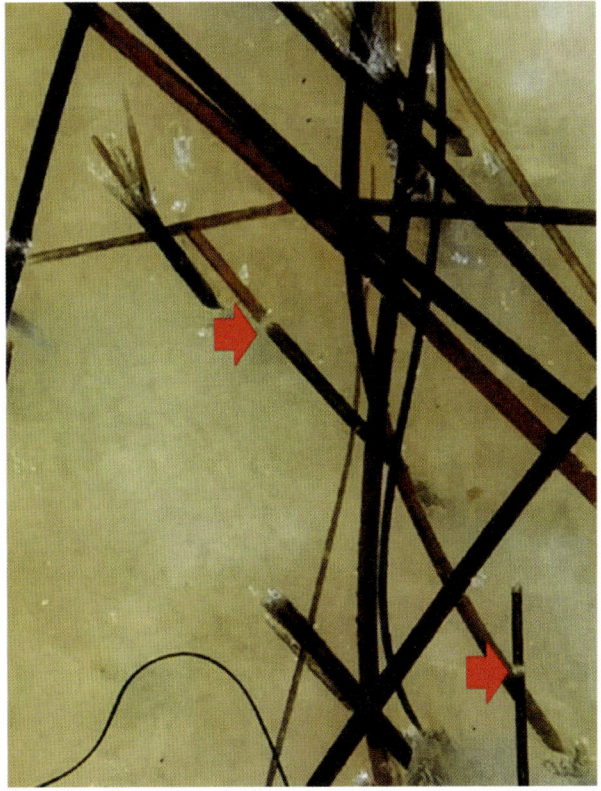

FIGURE 5–12. Trichorrhexis nodosa (red arrows) in a patient with trichoteiromania.
Source. Dr. Asmahane Souissi.

contrast, trichoscopy in trichoteiromania shows erythema, lichenification with scaling, and hyperpigmentation. The presence of clusters of broom hairs is highly suggestive of trichoteiromania (Salas-Callo and Pirmez 2019). Other differential diagnoses are psoriasis, tinea capitis, and localized hair shaft disorder. Meticulous trichoscopy examination may allow avoiding misdiagnosis.

Trichoteiromania is difficult to manage. The therapeutic options include topical and intralesional glucocorticoids with variable efficacy. The itch-rub/scratch-itch cycle may be managed by CBT to decrease the impulse to scratch. Salas-Callo and Pirmez (2019) described a case of complete hair regrowth within 16 weeks in a patient with trichoteiromania treated with NAC 1,200 mg/day. Further studies are necessary to confirm its efficacy and safety in the long term.

Trichodaganomania

Trichodaganomania is characterized by the compulsive habit of biting one's own hair on accessible sites, resulting in hair loss. As in TTM, the patient has an irresistible urge, in this case to bite the hair from easily approachable sites, triggering feelings of gratification and relief. Trichodaganomania was first described by Jafferany et al. (2009) in a 17-year-old patient who presented with patchy alopecia on both forearms with comorbid anxiety and depression. Physical examination revealed oblong areas of hair loss on both the right and the left dorsal surfaces of the forearms. The hair pull test was negative. The patient admitted to biting his hair on the affected areas during period of stress and anxiety. Microscopy of the bitten hairs showed smooth, sharply demarcated, blunted shafts secondary to being bitten.

Conclusions

TTM and its variants are complex disorders that may be sustained by genetic factors, neurobiological alterations, and social environments. Systematic and controlled epidemiological studies are required to investigate this relationship further. In all these compulsive hair disorders, psychological evaluation is necessary, and treatment of comorbid disorders is requisite. Pharmacological treatment is currently based on case reports and limited trials. Psychotherapy, particularly HRT, is the mainstay of treatment. A multidisciplinary approach involving dermatologists, psychiatrists, and pediatricians is crucial for long-term, successful treatment.

References

American Psychiatric Association: Diagnostic and Statistical Manual of Mental Disorders, 5th Edition, Text Revision. Washington, DC, American Psychiatric Association, 2022

Ankad BS, Smitha SV: Videodermoscopy of trichoteiromania: it is beyond broom hairs. Indian Dermatol Online J 13(2):268–269, 2022 35287407

Anwar S, Jafferany M: Trichotillomania: a psychopathological perspective and the psychiatric comorbidity of hair-pulling. Acta Dermatovenerol Alp Panonica Adriat 28(1):33–36, 2019 30901067

Aukerman EL, Nakell S, Jafferany M: Psychodynamic approach in the treatment of trichotillomania. Dermatol Ther 35(2):e15218, 2022 34816545

Bartley MM, Lapid MI, Grant JE: Pulling your hair out in geriatric psychiatry: a case report. Int Psychogeriatr 29(4):691–694, 2017 28143628

Bloch MH, Panza KE, Grant JE, et al: N-acetylcysteine in the treatment of pediatric trichotillomania: a randomized, double-blind, placebo-controlled add-on trial. J Am Acad Child Adolesc Psychiatry 52(3):231–240, 2013 23452680

Boughn S, Holdom JJ: The relationship of violence and trichotillomania. J Nurs Scholarsh 35(2):165–170, 2003 12854298

Chamberlain SR, Menzies LA, Fineberg NA, et al: Grey matter abnormalities in trichotillomania: morphometric magnetic resonance imaging study. Br J Psychiatry 193(3):216–221, 2008 18757980

Christensen RE, Schambach M, Jafferany M: Microneedling as an adjunctive treatment for trichotillomania. Dermatol Ther 35(11):e15824, 2022 36097871

Christenson GA, MacKenzie TB, Mitchell JE: Adult men and women with trichotillomania: a comparison of male and female characteristics. Psychosomatics 35(2):142–149, 1994 8171173

Everett GJ, Jafferany M, Skurya J: Recent advances in the treatment of trichotillomania (hair-pulling disorder). Dermatol Ther 33(6):e13818, 2020 32531098

Fernandes MRN, Melo DF, Vincenzi C, et al: Trichotillomania incognito: two case reports and literature review. Skin Appendage Disord 7(2):131–134, 2021 33796560

Fowler E, Tosti A: A case of friction alopecia in a healthy 15-year-old girl. Skin Appendage Disord 5(2):97–99, 2019 30815442

Grant JE, Chamberlain SR: Trichotillomania. Am J Psychiatry 173(9):868–874, 2016 27581696

Grant JE, Odlaug BL, Kim SW: N-acetylcysteine, a glutamate modulator, in the treatment of trichotillomania: a double-blind, placebo-controlled study. Arch Gen Psychiatry 66(7):756–763, 2009 19581567

Grant JE, Dougherty DD, Chamberlain SR: Prevalence, gender correlates, and comorbidity of trichotillomania. Psychiatry Res 288:112948, 2020 32334275

Grant JE, Chesivoir E, Valle S, et al: Double-blind placebo-controlled study of memantine in trichotillomania and skin-picking disorder. Am J Psychiatry 180(5):348–356, 2023 36856701

Greer JM, Capecchi MR: Hoxb8 is required for normal grooming behavior in mice. Neuron 33(1):23–34, 2002 11779477

Henkel ED, Jaquez SD, Diaz LZ: Pediatric trichotillomania: review of management. Pediatr Dermatol 36(6):803–807, 2019 31588617

Jafferany M: Handbook of Psychodermatology: Introduction to Psychocutaneous Disorders. Cham, Switzerland, Springer Nature, 2021

Jafferany M, Feng J, Hornung RL: Trichodaganomania: the compulsive habit of biting one's own hair. J Am Acad Dermatol 60(4):689–691, 2009 19293016

Kaczorowska A, Rudnicka L, Stefanato CM, et al: Diagnostic accuracy of trichoscopy in trichotillomania: a systematic review. Acta Derm Venereol 101(10):adv00565, 2021 34184065

Lee EB, Homan KJ, Morrison KL, et al: Acceptance and commitment therapy for trichotillomania: a randomized controlled trial of adults and adolescents. Behav Modif 44(1):70–91, 2020 30117327

Mariusso LM, Costa ACB, Canassa TC, et al: Trichotillomania: case report of pharmacological treatment outcome with clomipramine. Psychiatry Res 284:112663, 2020 31740214

Özcan D, Seçkin D: N-acetylcysteine in the treatment of trichotillomania: remarkable results in two patients. J Eur Acad Dermatol Venereol 30(9):1606–1608, 2016 27146087

Panza KE, Pittenger C, Bloch MH: Age and gender correlates of pulling in pediatric trichotillomania. J Am Acad Child Adolesc Psychiatry 52(3):241–249, 2013 23452681

Patil BB, Dowd TC: Trichotillomania. Br J Ophthalmol 85(11):1386, 2001 11702732

Rahman SM, Jafferany M, Barkauskaite R: Habit-reversal training: a psychotherapeutic approach in treating body-focused repetitive behaviour disorders. Clin Exp Dermatol 48(12):1310–1316, 2023 37470438

Salas-Callo CI, Pirmez R: Trichoteiromania: good response to treatment with N-acetylcysteine. Skin Appendage Disord 5(4):242–245, 2019 31367603

Sani G, Gualtieri I, Paolini M, et al: Drug treatment of trichotillomania (hair-pulling disorder), excoriation (skin-picking) disorder, and nail-biting (onychophagia). Curr Neuropharmacol 17(8):775–786, 2019 30892151

Shmelkov SV, Hormigo A, Jing D, et al: Slitrk5 deficiency impairs corticostriatal circuitry and leads to obsessive-compulsive-like behaviors in mice. Nat Med 16(5):598–602, 1p, 602, 2010 20418887

Van Ameringen M, Mancini C, Patterson B, et al: A randomized, double-blind, placebo-controlled trial of olanzapine in the treatment of trichotillomania. J Clin Psychiatry 71(10):1336–1343, 2010 20441724

van Minnen A, Hoogduin KA, Keijsers GP, et al: Treatment of trichotillomania with behavioral therapy or fluoxetine: a randomized, waiting-list controlled study. Arch Gen Psychiatry 60(5):517–522, 2003 12742873

Welch JM, Lu J, Rodriguiz RM, et al: Cortico-striatal synaptic defects and OCD-like behaviours in Sapap3-mutant mice. Nature 448(7156):894–900, 2007 17713528

Woods DW, Houghton DC: Diagnosis, evaluation, and management of trichotillomania. Psychiatr Clin North Am 37(3):301–317, 2014 25150564

Woods DW, Miltenberger RG, Flach AD: Habits, tics, and stuttering: prevalence and relation to anxiety and somatic awareness. Behav Modif 20(2):216–225, 1996 8934868

Woods DW, Wetterneck CT, Flessner CA: A controlled evaluation of acceptance and commitment therapy plus habit reversal for trichotillomania. Behav Res Ther 44(5):639–656, 2006 16039603

Case 5-1
Coexisting Trichotillomania and Onychotillomania in a 10-Year-Old Boy

Asmahane Souissi, M.D.
Chaima Kouki, M.D.
Rafik Mahmoudi, M.D.
Mohammad Jafferany, M.D.

Case Description

A 10-year-old boy, accompanied by his father, presented with hair loss on the frontal scalp for the past 6 months. He had no significant medical history. The father reported that the patient is brilliant and achieves excellent results at school. Dermatological examination revealed localized alopecic plaque on the frontal scalp region and thinning with short, broken hairs (Figure 5–13A). Further, the father reported that the patient avoided meeting with his friends and playing outside and preferred to stay at home. His parents also noticed that he was resistant to go to school.

Differential Diagnosis

- Trichotillomania
- Trichotemnomania
- Alopecia areata

Diagnosis

Trichoscopy was performed, and broken hairs were noted with different lengths and shapes (hook hair, flame hairs, and numerous black dots; Figure 5–13B). We observed no exclamation point hairs or yellow dots.

Cutaneous examination of the hands showed erythematous patches on the interphalangeal joints of the fingers. Plate abnormalities symmetrically affected all his fingernails. All nail plates were short, with brittleness, thinning, and onychoatrophy. The periungual skin was erythematous, with secondary crusting. The cuticle was absent, and lunulae were enlarged (Figures 5–14A and 5–14B). The toenails were not intact. There were no features suggestive of primary dermatosis on other areas of the skin, hair, or mucous membranes. No pruritus, pain, or other symptoms were reported.

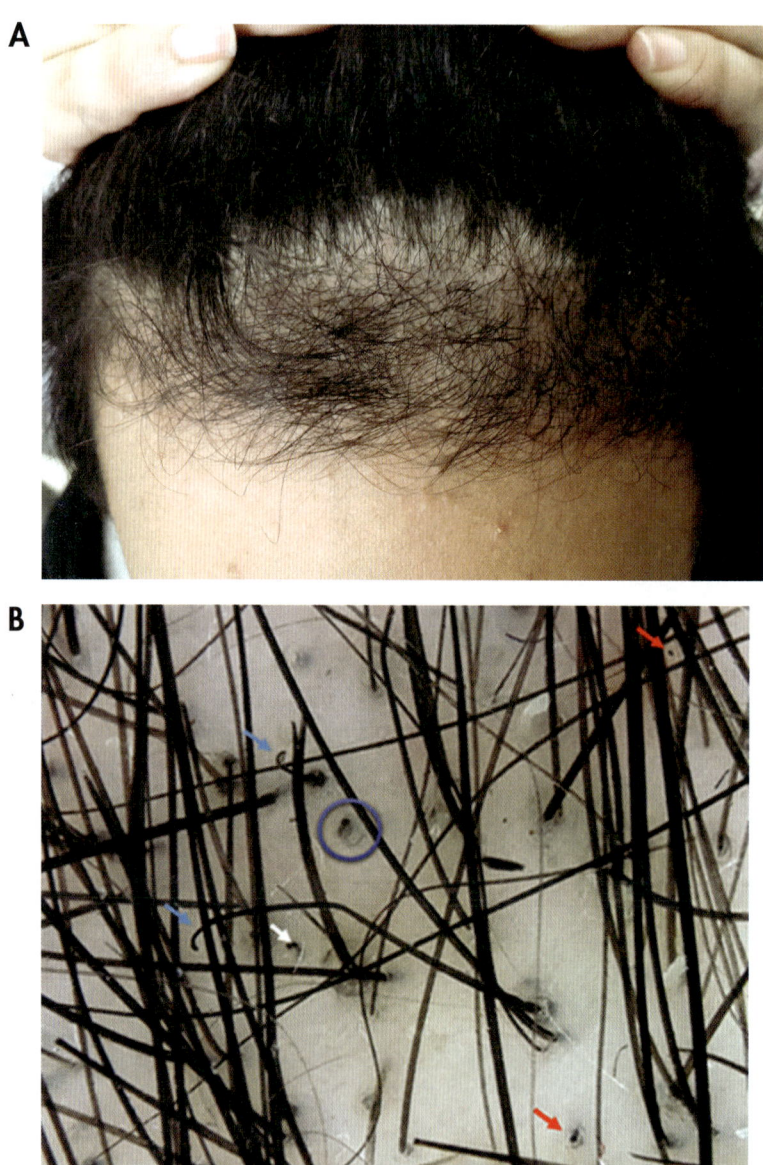

FIGURE 5–13. (A) Localized and irregular hair thinning with short hairs on the frontal region of the scalp. (B) Nonpolarized trichoscopy of scalp showing different hair lengths with hook hair (blue arrows), hair powder (blue circle), black dots (red arrows), and flame hair (white arrow).

Source. Dr. Asmahane Souissi.

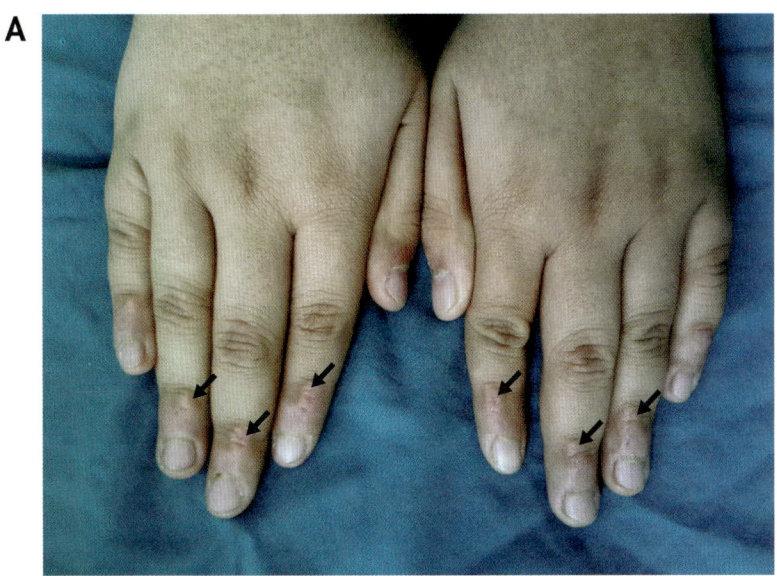

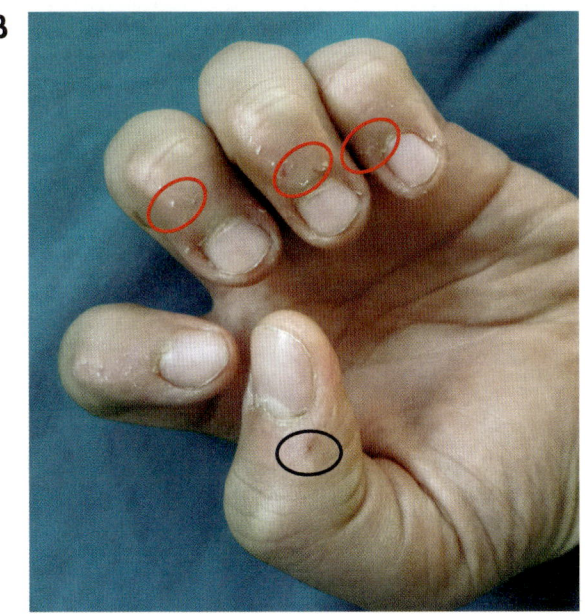

FIGURE 5–14. Erythematous patches on interphalangeal joints of the fingers (black arrows) (A). The cuticle was absent, and lunulae were enlarged. All nail plates were short with brittleness. The periungual skin was erythematous, with secondary crusting (B).
Source. Dr. Asmahane Souissi.

The patient subsequently admitted that he regularly bit the nails of his fingers and pulled his hair. He was aware of the hair pulling. In addition, he said he was going through a challenging period in his life, experiencing academic and social difficulties and striving for good grades while maintaining positive friendships. He described an uncontrollable urge to pull out his hair and a sense of relief after pulling, picking at his nails, and even biting his fingers when he felt stressed.

In light of these findings, the diagnosis of onychotillomania along with onychophagia was established.

Management

The patient was referred to a child and adolescent psychologist specializing in adolescent behavioral issues. CBT and extinction-based HRT were indicated.

After a follow-up of 4 months, significant regrowth of hair was observed. Trichoscopy showed a normal hair shaft with few interfollicular telangiectasias (Figure 5–15A and B). The patient's onychodystrophy had completely improved (Figure 5–15C), and onychotillomania remained remitted throughout the treatment.

The patient did not report any new episode of recurrence. Regular follow-up appointments with both the psychologist and dermatologist were recommended to maintain his progress.

Discussion

Body-focused repetitive behaviors (BFRBs) include hair pulling, skin picking, nail biting, teeth grinding, and other similar actions (Gupta and Gupta 2019). Patients with suspected self-induced dermatoses require both a psychiatric and a dermatological evaluation.

Diagnosis of TTM is usually based on clinical examination. Trichoscopic examination is essential for early, positive diagnosis (Elmas and Metin 2020; Grant and Chamberlain 2016; Kaczorowska et al. 2021). The most common trichoscopic findings in TTM are broken hairs and black dots. Although these features are not specific for TTM, trichoscopy remains useful in monitoring treatment efficacy, including an increase in capillary density, the presence of i-hairs, and hairs in the growth phase (Elmas and Metin 2020; Grant and Chamberlain 2016; Kaczorowska et al. 2021).

Nail-associated body-focused repetitive behaviors occur not only as a solitary obsessive-compulsive condition but also concurrently with other BFRBs of the hair and skin (Cohen 2022).

When a patient presents with a BFRB, the clinician should be cognizant of the possibility of multiple coexisting BFRBs. Even subclinical BFRBs should not be overlooked, as they can have notable dermatologic implications (Gupta and Gupta 2019). This implies the importance for an early diagnosis of a thorough clinical examination including a search for associated signs.

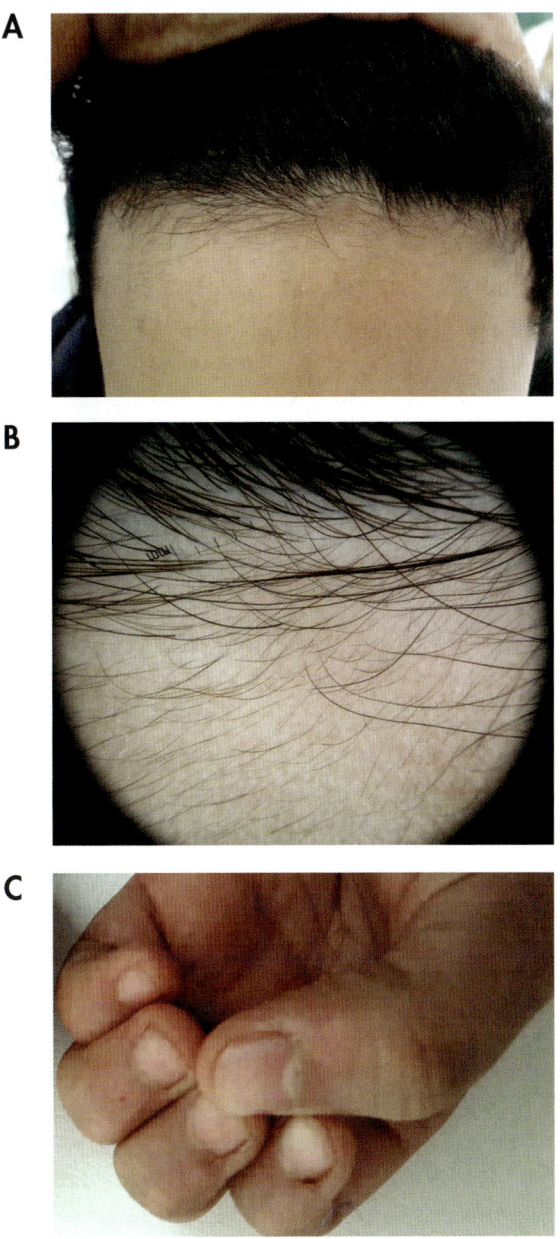

FIGURE 5–15. Complete hair regrowth with a normal appearance of terminal hair and few telangiectasia on trichoscopy (A and B). Complete healing of the onychodystrophy with regression of the periungueal signs (C).
Source. Dr. Asmahane Souissi.

HRT has a pivotal role in treating BFRBs and has emerged as a first-line psychotherapy. Additionally, therapeutic approaches may incorporate elements from ACT, dialectical behavior therapy, and traditional CBT, including cognitive restructuring techniques (Gupta and Gupta 2019).

The aspects of HRT include self-monitoring (i.e., asking the patient to track hair pulling or other behavior), awareness training, competing response training, and stimulus control procedures (i.e., modifying the environment to reduce cues for the behavior).

For HRT to be effective, the patients have to be aware of their self-injurious behavior, because HRT involves replacing the harmful urge to self-injure (Gupta and Gupta 2019). This patient was aware of the pathological nature of his behavior and was convinced of the contributing factors and triggers underlying the behavior. This represents a positive prognostic factor and may be predictive of a favorable response to standard HRT (Gupta and Gupta 2019).

TEACHING POINTS

- A range of self-induced dermatoses may simultaneously present in a single patient, and their detection may require the clinician to maintain a heightened index of suspicion and conduct a thorough examination.

- Trichoscopic examination remains essential for early, positive diagnosis and monitoring of alopecias.

- HRT, a form of CBT, is considered first-line treatment for management of BFRBs.

- It is important to identify dissociative patients who may have no recollection of having self-induced their lesions, because they tend to have greater comorbid psychopathology.

References

Cohen PR: Nail-associated body-focused repetitive behaviors: habit-tic nail deformity, onychophagia, and onychotillomania. Cureus 14(3):e22818, 2022 35382180

Elmas ÖF, Metin MS: Trichoscopic findings of trichotillomania: new observations. Postepy Dermatol Alergol 37(3):340–345, 2020 32792873

Grant JE, Chamberlain SR: Trichotillomania. Am J Psychiatry 173(9):868–874, 2016 27581696

Gupta MA, Gupta AK: Self-induced dermatoses: a great imitator. Clin Dermatol 37(3):268–277, 2019 31178108

Kaczorowska A, Rudnicka L, Stefanato CM, et al: Diagnostic accuracy of trichoscopy in trichotillomania: a systematic review. Acta Derm Venereol 101(10):adv00565, 2021 34184065

Case 5–2
A Journey of Hair Loss: From Alopecia Areata to Trichotemnomania

Asmahane Souissi, M.D.
Chaima Kouki, M.D.

Case Description

A 15-year-old healthy girl presented to the clinic with a 5-year history of hair loss and multiple alopecic patches with progressive extension. She had no personal or family history of atopy or autoimmune disease. At her initial examination, the diagnosis of alopecia areata had been made, and the patient had been treated with intralesional and oral corticosteroids, but no clinical improvement was observed 5 years later. At the current visit, the patient had a 3-year history of anxiety and depression. A psychiatrist further assessed her and found that she had clinical features of anxiety behavior related to the stress of alopecia areata.

The physical examination showed alopecic plaques on frontal and left parietal regions of the scalp, with a shaved appearance. There was preservation of normal-length hairs at the margins of the affected area, with no signs of inflammation or scarring (Figure 5–16A and B). The right region was spared. She did not have any hair loss on other body sites and had no mucosal or nail alterations. The patient denied cutting or pulling the scalp hairs.

Differential Diagnosis

- Trichotillomania
- Trichotemnomania
- Alopecia areata

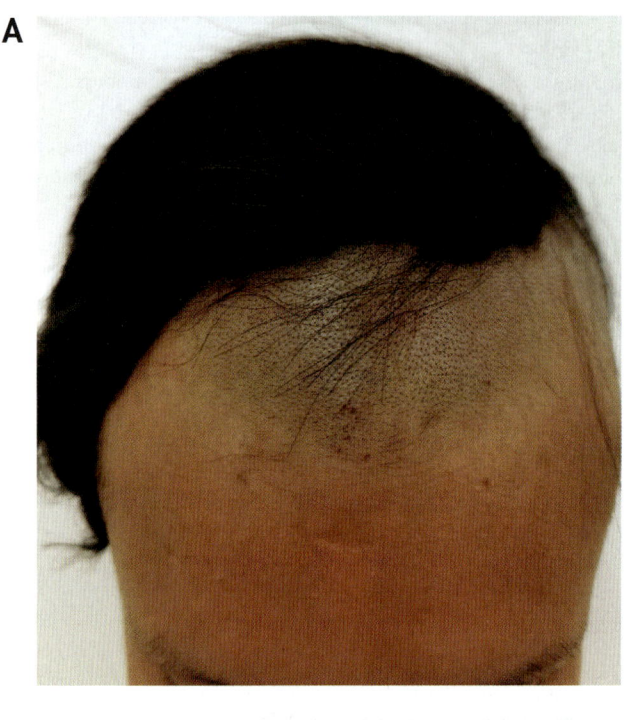

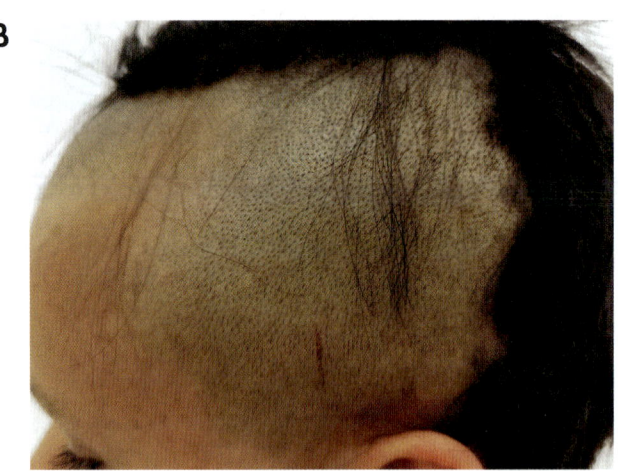

FIGURE 5–16. (A) Large alopecic plaques on frontal and left parietal regions of the scalp, with shaved appearance. (B) Normal hair length with no alopecic patches in the right region.
Source. Dr. Asmahane Souissi.

Diagnosis

On trichoscopy, there were very short broken hairs of similar length with normal morphology of the shaft (Figure 5–17A and B). There were no exclamation mark hairs, no yellow dots, no black dots, and no features of TTM. Based on these findings, a diagnosis of trichotemnomania of the scalp was established.

Management

Previously prescribed corticosteroids were stopped. The patient was referred to a child psychologist specializing in adolescent behavioral issues. Through a series of in-depth assessments, the psychologist uncovered the confirmation of trichotemnomania. A diagnosis of OCD was made, and the patient confirmed the act of shaving her hair with a razor.

After 3 months of follow-up, total regrowth of hair was observed (Figure 5–18A and B) and the patient did not report any new episode of hair loss. Regular follow-up appointments with both the psychologist and dermatologist were recommended to maintain progress.

Discussion

Alopecia areata represents a common autoimmune condition with significant psychosocial implications affecting both children and adults (Waśkiel et al. 2018). In children, nonscarred alopecia may be mistakenly identified as alopecia areata. This misdiagnosis can lead to a delay in appropriate treatment and perpetuate the progression of the underlying disease. Given the extensive use of corticosteroids in alopecia areata treatment and their substantial side effects, the diagnosis of this condition requires consideration of clinical, trichoscopic, and evolving criteria (Waśkiel et al. 2018). In this patient, the diagnosis of alopecia areata was established, and treatment with corticosteroids was maintained for an extended period. However, it was only in light of an unsatisfactory clinical progression and trichoscopic examination that the diagnosis of alopecia areata was ruled out. In fact, trichoscopy has become an essential step in alopecia examination, as it allows for the identification of both positive and negative signs, which are crucial for an accurate diagnosis (Adil et al. 2020; Porriño-Bustamante et al. 2021).

Trichotemnomania is a psychological disorder in which the act of cutting or shaving hair becomes an uncontrollable compulsion (Adil et al. 2020). It is often linked to anxiety, stress, or emotional disturbances. Alopecic patches are commonly observed on the scalp, but they can also affect other areas, such as the pubis, eyelashes, eyebrows, and axilla. Trichoscopy features are highly suggestive to diagnosis. Trichotemnomania shows hair follicles with a hair shaft in the case of shaving and terminal hair with nontapered clean-

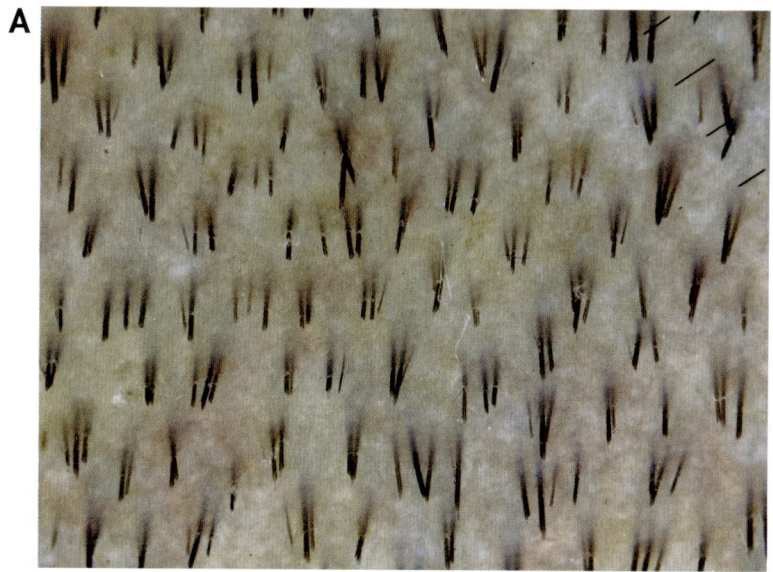

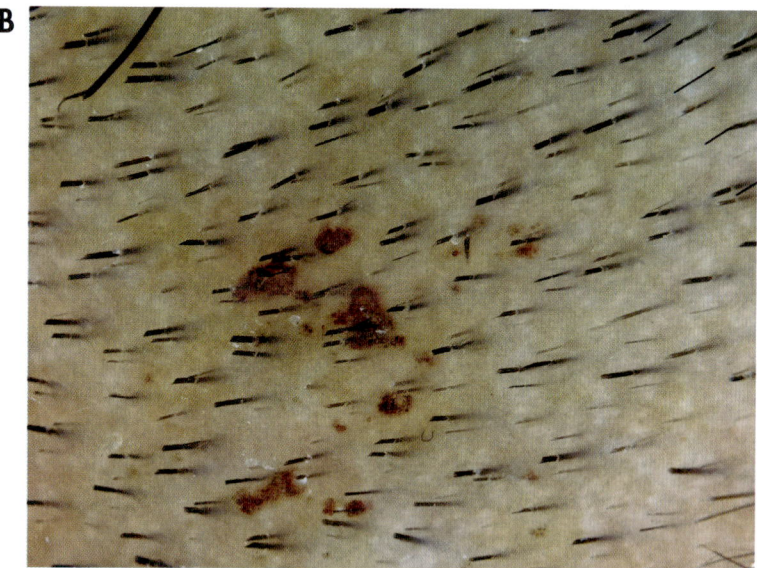

FIGURE 5–17. (A) Nonpolarized trichoscopy of scalp showing short broken hairs of similar length, with no vellus and no changes over the scalp. (B) Area of hemorrhage over the scalp.
Source. Dr. Asmahane Souissi.

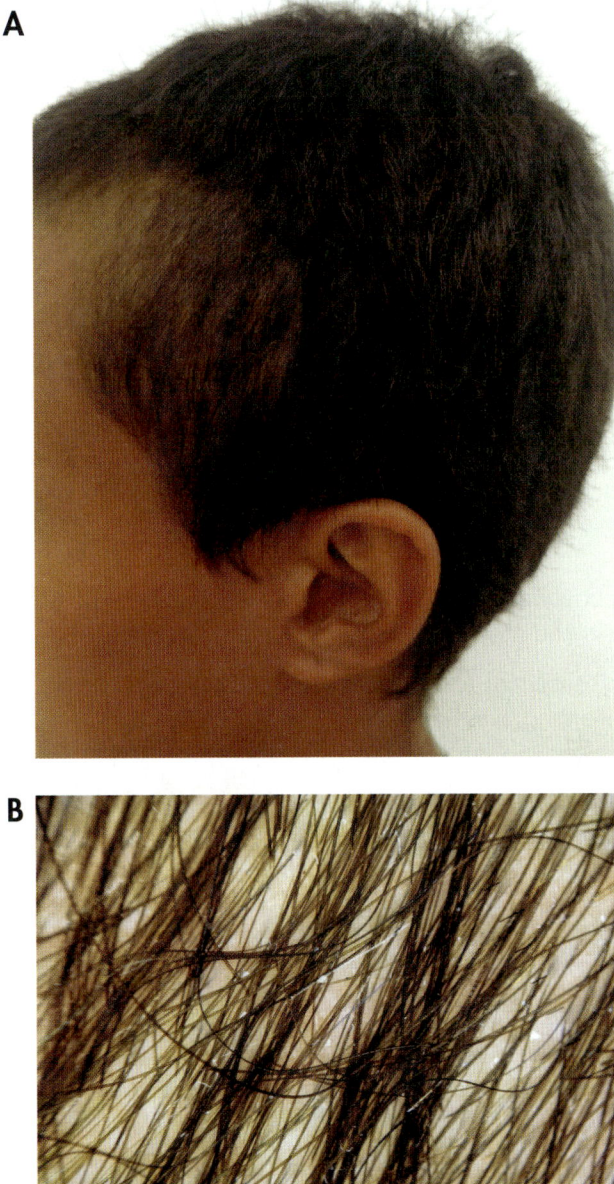

FIGURE 5–18. Complete hair regrowth (A) with normal appearance of terminal hair on trichoscopy (B).
Source. Dr. Asmahane Souissi.

cut distal ends in cases where the hair is trimmed. Alopecia areata shows yellow dots, short vellus hairs, black dots, and exclamation mark hairs (Porriño-Bustamante et al. 2021; Thadchanamoorthy et al. 2020).

TTM is characterized by alopecia patches with irregular borders. Trichoscopy in TTM shows irregular lengths of broken hair with perifollicular hemorrhage, flame hair, trichoptilosis, and black dots.

Being a causative factor or a comorbidity, trichotemnomania and alopecia areata are frequently linked to psychiatric disorders. In this case, the behavioral disturbances described by this patient were identified as a repercussion of alopecia areata. This implies the importance of collaborating with a psychiatrist in the management of these conditions to promptly identify and aid in proper diagnosis (Adil et al. 2020).

TEACHING POINTS

- Trichoscopic examination is essential for early, positive diagnosis and monitoring of alopecias.
- It is essential to consider psychological factors in patients presenting with hair loss.
- The initial diagnosis of alopecia areata, while common, may not always explain the complete picture. In cases where hair loss persists despite treatment or exhibits unusual patterns, a comprehensive evaluation, including psychological assessment, is essential.
- With the right support, care, and appropriate therapy, patients can recover from trichotemnomania and regain control over their lives, both emotionally and physically.

References

Adil M, Amin SS, Mohtashim M, et al: Concomitant trichotillomania, trichotemnomania and skin picking disorder in a woman. Indian J Dermatol Venereol Leprol 86(3):286–289, 2020 32108615

Porriño-Bustamante ML, Arias-Santiago S, Buendía-Eisman A: Concomitant occurrence of frontal fibrosing alopecia and trichotemnomania: the importance of trichoscopy. Indian J Dermatol Venereol Leprol 87(1):112–115, 2021 33580936

Thadchanamoorthy V, Thirukumar M, Dayasiri K, et al: Trichotemnomania in an adolescent girl: a case report of an Asian child and literature review. Case Rep Dermatol Med 2020:6615250, 2020 33457024

Waśkiel A, Rakowska A, Sikora M, et al: Trichoscopy of alopecia areata: an update. J Dermatol 45(6):692–700, 2018 29569271

Case 5-3
Trichoteiromania of the Beard

Asmahane Souissi, M.D.
Dorsaf Elinkichari, M.D.
Mohammad Jafferany, M.D.

Case Description

An otherwise healthy 25-year-old man presented with a symmetric patchy hair loss of the beard for 4 months. He had no history of eczema, psoriasis, or seborrheic dermatosis. Clinical examination showed well-defined, lichenified alopecic plaques, with broken hairs on the beard, and normal-appearing adjacent hair and skin (Figure 5–19). The patient acknowledged self-esteem problems and trying to cover his face with a scarf in outside gatherings. He reported that it affected his relationships and that he had a hard time being in public. His mood started feeling down, and he reported symptoms of mild depression and avoidant behavior. He denied receiving any prior treatment. The patient and his girlfriend recently broke up, and he said it has devastated him and that he is so tense that he cannot resist his hand rubbing his beard most of the time.

Differential Diagnosis

- Trichotillomania
- Trichotemnomania
- Trichoteiromania
- Psoriasis
- Tinea capitis

Diagnosis

Trichoscopy showed erythema, white scales, brown pigmentation, hematic crusts, broken hair shafts of varying lengths, and broken hair shafts longitudinally split into two to three parts, which correspond to broom hairs (Figure 5–20A and B).

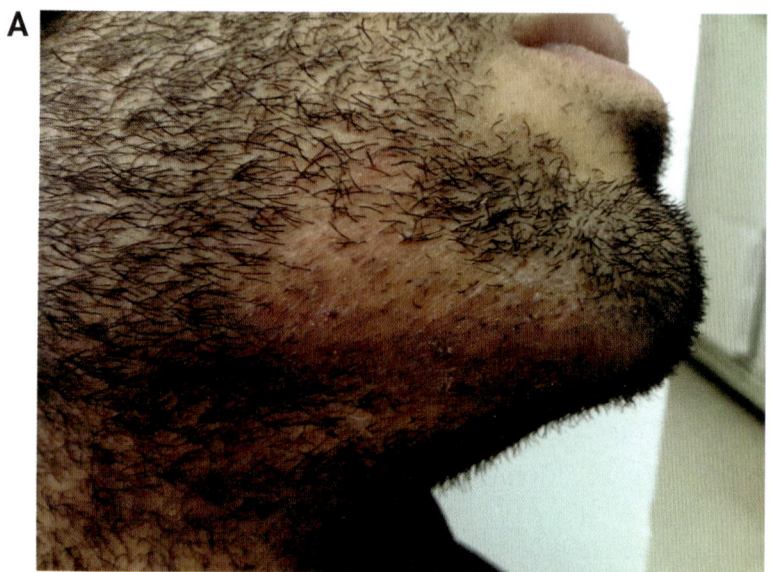

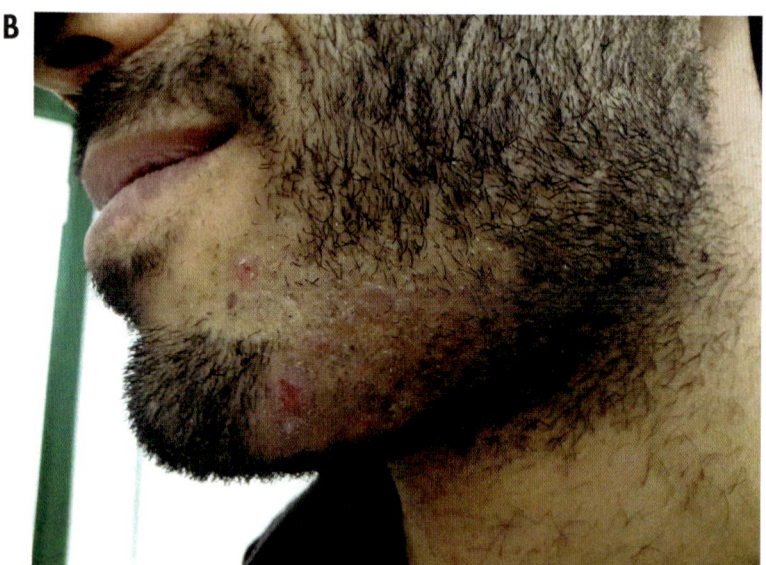

FIGURE 5–19. Symmetrical lichenified alopecic plaques of the mandibular area.
Source. Dr. Asmahane Souissi.

Trichotillomania and Its Variants

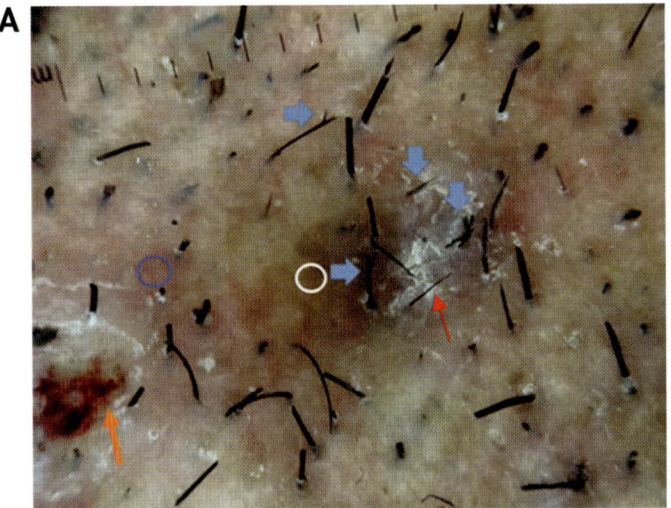

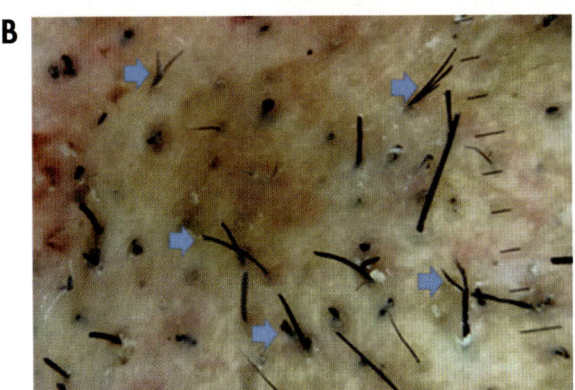

FIGURE 5–20. (A) Trichoscopy showing erythema (blue circle), white scales (red arrow), brown pigmentation (white circle), hematic crusts (orange arrow), broken hair shafts of varying lengths, and broken hair shafts longitudinally split into two to three parts (blue arrows). (B) Trichoscopy showing broken hair shafts longitudinally split into two to three parts, corresponding to broom hairs (blue arrows).
Source. Dr. Asmahane Souissi.

When questioned, the patient denied any history of hair pulling or cutting but expressed concerns about his general well-being after his recent breakup. Remarkably, during the interview, the patient was continuously rubbing his beard. He also admitted that he was inadvertently and repetitively rubbing his cheeks (at least 4 hours a day). Based on anamnesis and clinical and trichoscopic findings, the diagnosis of trichoteiromania was retained.

Management

The patient was referred to a psychiatrist for assessment and treatment. He was diagnosed with major depressive disorder, single episode moderate; unspecified anxiety disorder; and some unspecified obsessive traits. He was recommended escitalopram 10 mg daily and advised for CBT.

Discussion

Trichoteiromania is hair loss due to frequent rubbing, which leads to hair breakage at different levels and splitting at the ends. Differential diagnosis mainly includes, as in this patient, TTM and trichotemnomania, which also are self-inflicted hair disorders often seen in the context of psychiatric conditions, consisting of pulling and cutting or shaving the hair, respectively (Reich and Trüeb 2003). Trichoteiromania is characterized by the presence of thick pigmented lichenified skin underlying short shaft hairs, mimicking (as in this case) psoriasis or tinea capitis.

In trichoteiromania, trichoscopy shows longitudinal splitting of the hair shaft, called broom hairs (João et al. 2020), also termed brush hairs or trichoptilosis (Diniz et al. 2018). It is considered to be the result of traumatic splitting of the hair shafts from the constant rubbing and scratching (Quaresma et al. 2016). Although they may also be seen in other noncicatricial alopecic disorders, especially in TTM, broom hairs are by far more frequently observed in trichoteiromania. Thus, the presence of clusters of broom hairs has been considered a highly suggestive trichoscopic feature of the latter diagnosis (João et al. 2020).

Also, paying attention to the patient's gestures during the interview is very important, as they may unconsciously reproduce the gesture of rubbing, as in this patient. The diagnosis can be retained with certainty, as this patient admitted to the act of rubbing the alopecic region for hours per day (Banky et al. 2004). Similar to TTM and trichotemnomania, trichoteiromania is very likely to be an obsessive-compulsive spectrum disorder (João et al. 2020; Salas-Callo and Pirmez 2019). The onset of the disease in a young man, otherwise healthy, in a context of recent psychological and relational issues, supports this hypothesis. Collaboration between dermatologists and psychiatrists will help to clarify the psychological underpinnings of the disease.

TEACHING POINTS

- The diagnosis of trichoteiromania is challenging in the absence of specific clinical features.
- Trichotillomania is the main differential diagnosis. Clue features are the lichenified skin of the alopecic area and the patient's attitude during the anamnesis.
- Broom hairs are highly suggestive of the diagnosis but are not specific.
- Trichoscopy is very useful to establish a correct diagnosis at an early stage.
- In the clearest scenario, the patient will reveal psychological problems and the compulsive act of rubbing the alopecic area.

References

Banky JP, Sheridan AT, Dawber RPR: Weathering of hair in trichoteiromania. Australas J Dermatol 45(3):186–188, 2004 15250901

Diniz TACB, Abuawad YG, Silva FO, et al: Trichoteiromania: an atypical case associated with the Claude Bernard Horner syndrome. Skin Appendage Disord 4(4):342–344, 2018 30410912

João AL, Cunha N, Pessoa e Costa T, et al: Monotonous broom hairs: a feature of trichoteiromania. Skin Appendage Disord 6(3):168–170, 2020 32656237

Quaresma MV, Mariño Alvarez AM, Miteva M: Dermatoscopic-pathologic correlation of lichen simplex chronicus on the scalp: "broom fibres, gear wheels and hamburgers." J Eur Acad Dermatol Venereol 30(2):343–345, 2016 25308867

Reich S, Trüeb RM: [Trichoteiromania] [in German]. J Dtsch Dermatol Ges 1(1):22–28, 2003 16285289

Salas-Callo CI, Pirmez R: Trichoteiromania: good response to treatment with N-acetylcysteine. Skin Appendage Disord 5(4):242–245, 2019 31367603

Case 5-4
Trichotillomania Associated With Trichotemnomania

Tatiana Silyuk, M.D.

Case Description

A 13-year-old girl was brought in by her mother for evaluation of hair loss. She presented with a several-year history of progressive hair thinning over the crown. The patient avoided communication with classmates, skipped school, and avoided swimming lessons. After consultation with a dermatologist, she was diagnosed with alopecia areata; however, after treatment with topical steroids, there had been no improvement. Her mother was nervous about the lack of therapeutic efficacy of treatment and the emotional state and behavior of her daughter. Physical examination showed an irregular area of noncicatricial alopecia with reduced hair coverage and broken hair at different lengths (Figure 5–21). Pull test was negative. Itching, pain, burning sensations, and scales were absent. There was no inflammation of the scalp. The patient's eyebrows, eyelashes, and nails appeared normal.

Differential Diagnosis

- Alopecia areata
- Trichotillomania
- Trichotemnomania
- Traction alopecia

Diagnosis

Trichoscopy revealed broken hair shafts with various morphology: tulip hair, V-sign hairs, black dots, and flame hair. Single yellow dots were also present as well as dried drops of blood (Figures 5–22 and 5–23).

Particular attention was drawn to the ends of several hairs that appeared to be horizontally smooth, as it happens after a haircut (white arrow in Figure 5–23). Although the patient denied any manipulation with her hair, the diagnosis of TTM comorbid with trichotemnomania was considered.

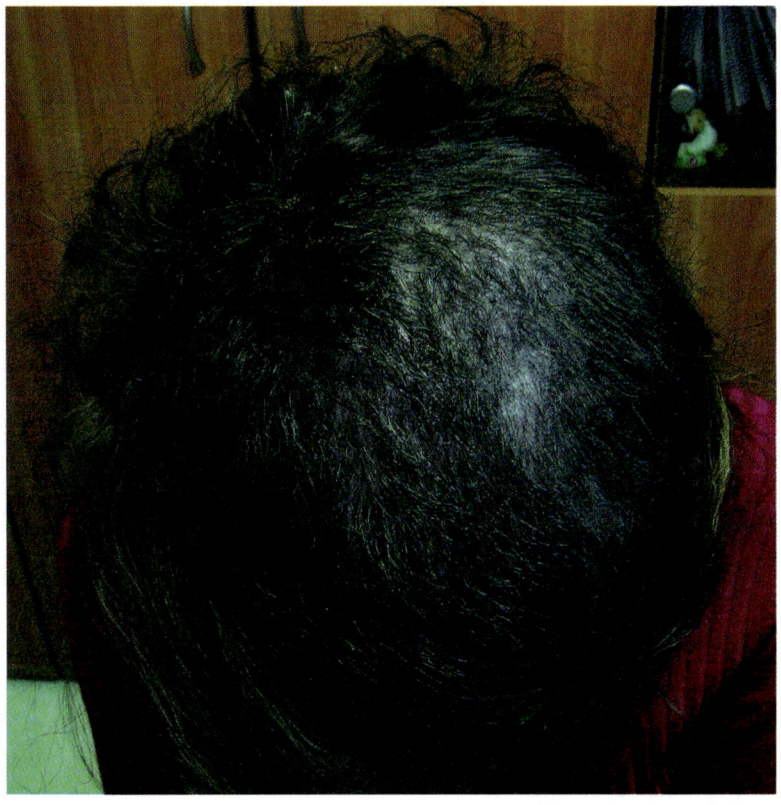

FIGURE 5–21. Irregular area with reduced hair coverage and broken hair at different lengths.
Source. Dr. Tatiana Silyuk.

Management

The patient was referred to an adolescent psychologist and received CBT, with positive behavior changes.

Discussion

The association of TTM and trichotemnomania is rarely reported in the literature (Adil et al. 2020; Gallouj et al. 2011). Trichoscopy is helpful in differentiating TTM from trichotemnomania. In this patient, trichoscopy differentiated the diagnosis of the two diseases. It showed features of both TTM (broken hairs with different shaft lengths and shapes) and trichotemnomania (hairs with horizontally smooth ends). As in this patient, hemor-

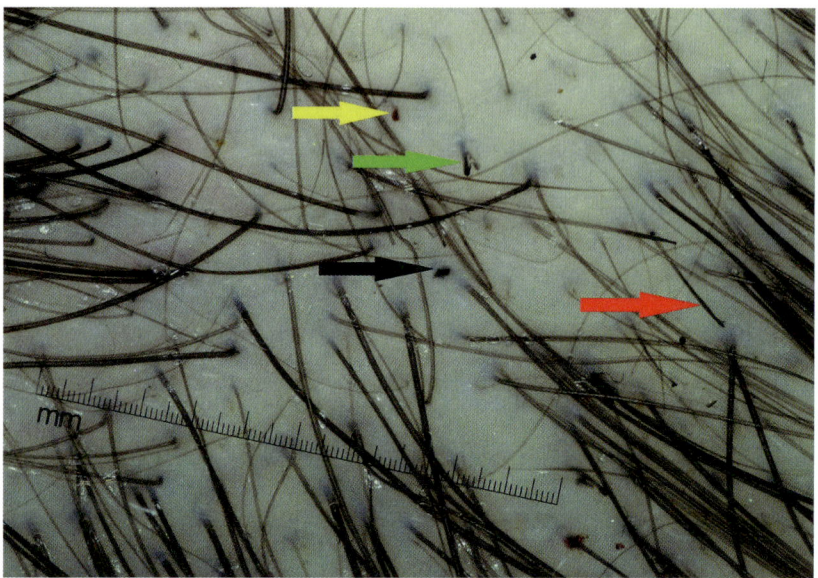

FIGURE 5-22. Tulip hair (red arrow), V-sign hairs (green arrow), black dots (black arrow), dried drops of blood (yellow arrow).
Source. Dr. Tatiana Silyuk.

rhage (extravasations) can be seen as a sign of damage to the vessels of the hair follicle during pulling.

The treatment for both disorders is the same, a combination of psychotherapy and medications targeting concomitant anxiety and depression. Making an accurate diagnosis is crucial to avoid unnecessary treatments; this patient was treated for a long time for alopecia areata.

TEACHING POINTS

- Trichotillomania and related disorders such as trichotemnomania have been classified into obsessive-compulsive spectrum disorders.
- In TTM, trichoscopy is characterized by different morphological patterns; trichotemnomania is characterized by the presence of broken hair shafts at similar lengths.
- Alopecia areata must be considered in the differential diagnosis.

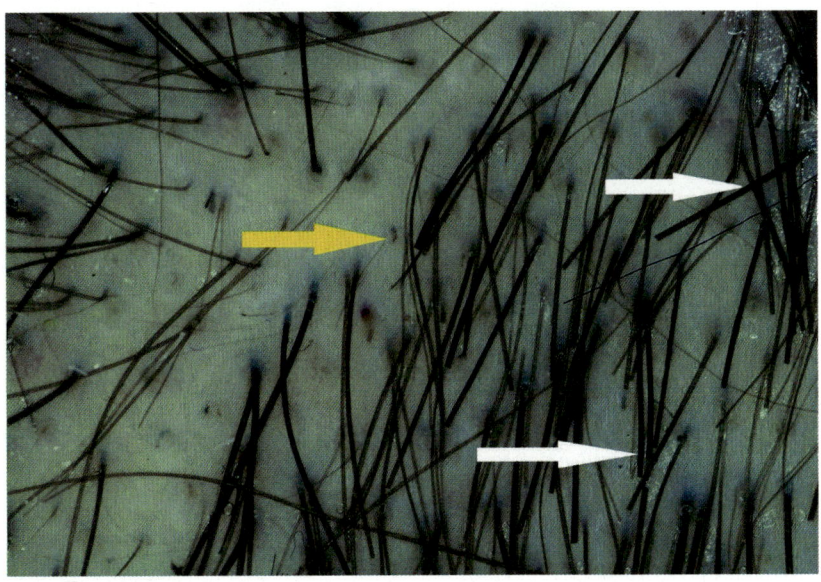

FIGURE 5-23. Flame hair (orange arrow), horizontal smooth hair ends (white arrows).
Source. Dr. Tatiana Silyuk.

References

Adil M, Amin SS, Mohtashim M, et al: Concomitant trichotillomania, trichotemnomania and skin picking disorder in a woman. Indian J Dermatol Venereol Leprol 86(3):286–289, 2020 32108615

Gallouj S, Rabhi S, Baybay H, et al: [Trichotemnomania associated to trichotillomania: a case report with emphasis on the diagnostic value of dermoscopy] [in French]. Ann Dermatol Venereol 138(2):140–141, 2011 21333827

Case 5-5

Trichotillomania: More Than Just a Hair-Pulling Disorder

Monika Fida, M.D.
Oljeda Kaçani, M.D.
Edri Stafa, M.D.
Ermira Vasili, M.D.

Case Description

A 13-year-old girl who was otherwise healthy visited our outpatient clinic with her mother and younger sister and complained about hair loss she had been experiencing for the past 6 months. The patient had been previously given a diagnosis of tinea capitis and treated empirically with systemic and topical antifungals without any success.

Physical examination revealed a clearly defined area of sparse hair on the vertex and frontoparietal region of the head, not affecting the temporal and occipital areas. These areas were covered with hair of various lengths, some with broken ends, and around the edge of the affected area was a rim of hairs that appeared to be normal (Figure 5–24). Along the margin of hair loss, the hair pull test was negative, and there was no evidence of inflammation or scaling. The patient did not express any subjective symptoms, such as pruritus or pain; instead, she appeared ashamed of her condition and felt the need to cover her hair loss with a hat all the time. Her eyebrows and eyelashes were normal, as were skin, nails, and mucosae.

Differential Diagnosis

- Alopecia areata
- Tinea capitis
- Trichotillomania
- Trichotemnomania

Diagnosis

On trichoscopic examination, reduced hair density, broken hair shafts at various lengths, short hair with trichoptilosis, V-sign, flame hairs, hook hairs, tulip hairs, black dots, broom fibers, and vellus hairs were noted (Figures 5–25 and 5–26). The physical and trichoscopy examination led to the diagnosis of TTM. When questioned about hair pulling or other attempts

Trichotillomania and Its Variants

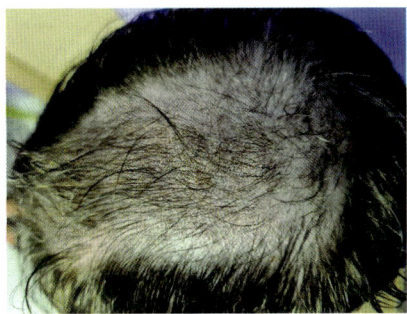

FIGURE 5-24. Tonsure pattern of alopecia (Friar Tuck sign) on the vertex and frontoparietal area, not affecting the temporal and occiput.
Source. Dr. Monika Fida.

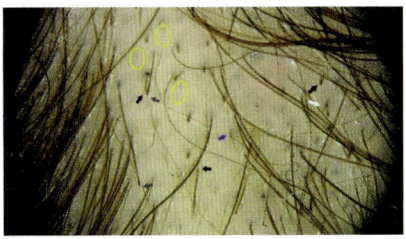

FIGURE 5-25. Trichoscopy shows tulip hair (gray arrows), broom fibers (blue arrow), V-sign (white arrow), hairs broken at different levels (black arrows), and vellus hairs (yellow circles).
Source. Dr. Monika Fida.

of self-harm, the patient denied any self-harm behavior. The younger sister said that while being engaged in activities such as studying or watching TV, she noticed the patient plucking her hair out. The parents denied that the patient was pulling her hair and insisted on the diagnosis of tinea capitis. All tests, including antinuclear antibodies, antistreptolysin O titer, serum ferritin, thyroid function, and complete blood count, were found to be normal. According to direct mycological analysis, there were no fungi present. A scalp biopsy was approved by the mother; the results showed pigmented casts and trichomalacia consistent with the clinical diagnosis of TTM.

Management

The patient underwent a complete psychiatric evaluation at the Department of Child and Adolescent Psychiatry. During her appointments with the psychiatrist, she expressed hopelessness and anxiety about the future as a result of her poor grades at school. Because of her family's financial diffi-

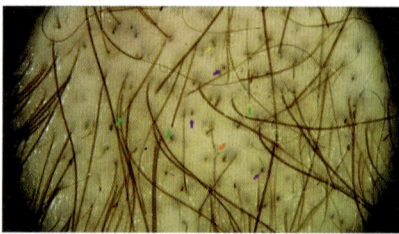

FIGURE 5–26. Trichoscopy shows reduced hair density, flame hair (yellow arrow), V-sign (purple arrows), hair with trichoptilosis (green arrows), black dots (pink arrow), and hook hair (orange arrow).
Source. Dr. Monika Fida.

culties, the girl had recently relocated to a new city and changed her school. She found it difficult to build solid relationships with her classmates, and she experienced loneliness. Although not conscious of her action while pulling out hair, she soon felt guilty and humiliated by the behavior. Therefore, she avoided many of her everyday social activities. The patient was not identified as having any other co-occurring mental disorders other than TTM. Her family's medical history was unremarkable, as was her own. She reached age-appropriate levels of development in her motor, social, and cognitive milestones.

After a multidisciplinary approach by dermatologists, psychiatrists, and psychologists and the confirmed diagnosis of TTM, the patient was started on fluoxetine 20 mg daily, N-acetylcysteine 1,800 mg daily, and CBT. A second evaluation was scheduled after 3 months of therapy.

Discussion

This patient was diagnosed with the automatic subtype of TTM, as her young sister affirmed that she was pulling hair unconsciously while studying or watching TV. Numerous onset triggers include childhood trauma, death or family illness, relocation, parental divorce, estrangement from friends, and the start of school. This patient had moved out of her city and changed school and had interpersonal isolation and difficulty making friends in a new environment.

The classic clinical appearance of alopecia is a sharply delineated incomplete patch with short and damaged hairs of various lengths. When the condition is more severe, hair pulling in and around the vertex produces the Friar Tuck sign, a common tonsure pattern of alopecia, as also seen in our patient. A rim of unaffected hair surrounds the damaged area, which is the characteristic distribution of this kind of alopecia (Yorulmaz et al. 2014).

In this case, certain distinguishing characteristics of TTM in trichoscopy, such as tulip hair, hook hair, V-sign, trichoptilosis, and flame hair, were evident. Characteristics of alopecia areata, including yellow dots and exclamation mark hair, were not present. The scalp and hair lacked scaling, comma hair, corkscrew hair, or zigzag hair as signs of tinea capitis. The mycological analysis also was negative. Histopathology was used in our case study to confirm the diagnosis, but we firmly agree that additional practice with trichoscopy interpretation and performance is essential to correctly diagnose TTM and avoid more invasive and unnecessary procedures such as scalp biopsies.

TEACHING POINTS

- Trichotillomania is a psychodermatologic condition characterized by the impulse to pluck out one's hair, causing secondary alopecia.
- Diagnosis and treatment require a multidisciplinary approach involving dermatologists, psychiatrists, and psychologists.
- Trichoscopy is a valuable tool that aids in prompt disease diagnosis and minimizes the use of invasive procedures such as biopsy.
- There is no established treatment for the disorder. Commonly used medications are SSRIs and *N*-acetylcysteine.

References

Yorulmaz A, Artuz F, Erden O: A case of trichotillomania with recently defined trichoscopic findings. Int J Trichology 6(2):77–79, 2014 25191044

Case 5-6
Trichotemnomania of the Eyebrows

Emna Chtioui, M.D.
Khadija Sallemi, M.D.
Hamida Turki, M.D.

Case Description

A 20-year-old woman presented at the emergency department, accompanied by her parents, with a 1-week history of sudden eyebrow hair loss. She did not report any hair loss on other body sites. Examination revealed symmetric hair loss of the eyebrows with no signs of inflammation or scarring. Follicle openings were filled with black hair shafts, giving a shaved appearance to the eyebrows (Figure 5–27). The scalp, eyelashes, skin, and nails did not show any abnormalities.

Upon detailed interview alone, without her parents, she acknowledged feeling stressed and anxious during the previous 3 months because of some problems with friendships and familial conflicts. She avoided social activities and experienced loneliness. When questioned, she denied any history of hair pulling or cutting. She also reported various symptoms of depression and anxiety on standard rating scales. She had experienced insomnia with frequent awakenings and unprovoked crying for the previous 2 weeks. Her appetite had also decreased. She finally admitted that she had cut the hair herself with shaver and razor to release the tension and feelings of frustration.

Differential Diagnosis

- Trichotillomania
- Trichotemnomania
- Alopecia areata

Diagnosis

Trichoscopy showed short black hairs of similar length and sharply cut ends (Figure 5–28). There were no exclamation mark hairs or yellow dots. Based on the detailed history, clinical and trichoscopic findings, and patient's confession, the diagnosis of trichotemnomania was made.

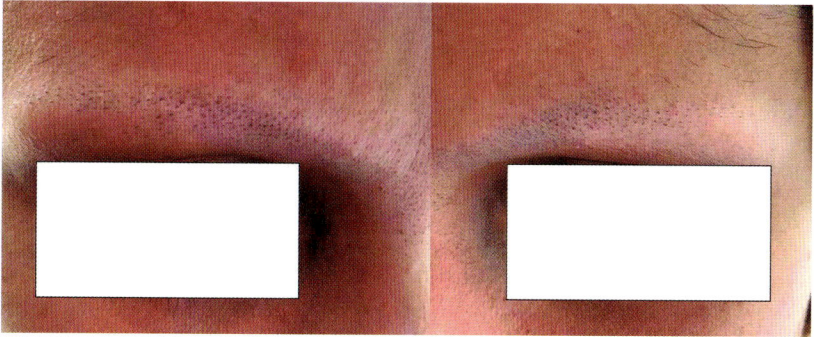

FIGURE 5–27. Symmetric hair loss of the eyebrows.
Source. Dr. Emna Chtioui.

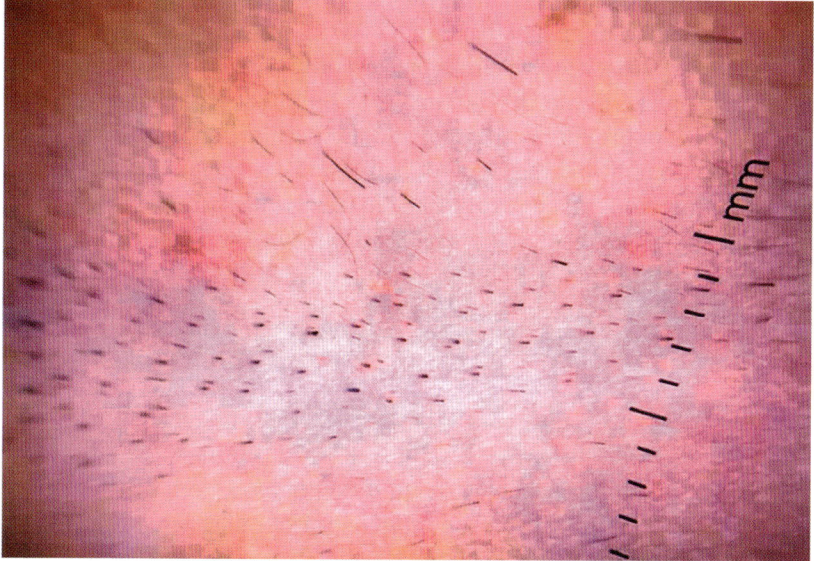

FIGURE 5–28. Nonpolarized trichoscopy of the eyebrow showing short broken hairs of similar length and sharply cut ends.
Source. Dr. Emna Chtioui.

Management

The patient was referred to a psychiatrist. The treatment strategy consisted of reinforcing parent-child relationships, along with the incorporation of CBT, and escitalopram 10 mg to address associated depression and anxiety symptoms.

Discussion

Trichotemnomania is defined as acquired, noninflammatory hair loss characterized by the patient cutting or shaving as an impulsive act. It is regarded as a variant of TTM. Clinically, trichotemnomania is characterized by the presence of broken hairs with the same length and sharply cut ends (Porriño-Bustamante et al. 2021). In this case, the main differential diagnosis included TTM and alopecia areata. In trichotemnomania, trichoscopy shows (as in this patient) broken hairs of similar length and sharply cut ends (Gallouj et al. 2011), whereas in TTM, it usually reveals broken hairs of different lengths and shapes. Alopecia areata is characterized by yellow dots, exclamation mark hairs, and vellus hairs.

Even though patients with trichotemnomania engage in cutting or shaving hairs consciously, they commonly deny it because of feelings of shame, guilt, and embarrassment. Indeed, trichotemnomania is frequently misdiagnosed as alopecia areata or TTM. In this case, the patient's acknowledgment that she shaved her own eyebrows was finally obtained in an interview alone without her parents. This highlights the importance of a trusting doctor-patient relationship and therapeutic bond.

Trichotemnomania can be debilitating, and the treatment can be challenging. Therefore, collaboration between dermatologists and psychiatrists is highly indicated. The use of behavioral therapy, sometimes in combination with SSRIs, can be helpful (Venneuguès et al. 2015).

TEACHING POINTS

- Trichotemnomania should be differentiated from other common causes of hair loss including trichotillomania and alopecia areata.
- Trichoscopy is a fast, noninvasive technique, helpful in diagnosing trichotemnomania.
- In the presence of a strong and trusting patient-doctor relationship, the patient is more likely to disclose psychological issues, including the compulsive act of shaving their own hair.

References

Gallouj S, Rabhi S, Baybay H, et al: [Trichotemnomania associated to trichotillomania: a case report with emphasis on the diagnostic value of dermoscopy] [in French]. Ann Dermatol Venereol 138(2):140–141, 2011 21333827

Porriño-Bustamante ML, Arias-Santiago S, Buendía-Eisman A: Concomitant occurrence of frontal fibrosing alopecia and trichotemnomania: the importance of trichoscopy. Indian J Dermatol Venereol Leprol 87(1):112–115, 2021 33580936

Venneuguès RV, Macbeth A, Levell NJ: Dramatic and persistent loss of eyelashes. JRSM Open 6(5):2054270415579779, 2015 26085938

6

Dermatitis Artefacta

Cemre Busra Turk, M.D.
Mohammad Jafferany, M.D.

Introduction

Factitious disorders are primary psychiatric disorders presented with the somatic expression of psychiatric stress. Patients with a factitious disorder may have various symptoms according to the targeted systems; the symptoms are produced voluntarily and consciously by the subject with subconscious motives. The primary intent of the patient is to assume the role of a sick person, without expecting other secondary gains.

Because the skin is easy to access, it is often affected in factitious disorders. To date, many different terms have been used to describe self-inflicted cutaneous lesions. Dermatitis artefacta is classified in DSM-5 as a self-imposed factitious disorder under somatic symptoms and related disorders (American Psychiatric Association 2013).

Dermatitis artefacta, also known as factitial dermatitis, is a primary psychocutaneous disorder. It is characterized by conscious, self-induced skin damage with an unconscious motive. As with all factitious disorders, the main motivation is the desire to have the role of being sick without tangible benefits for dealing with severe psychological and emotional distress.

Epidemiology

Determining the exact prevalence of dermatitis artefacta can be challenging for many reasons, including multiple caregivers involved in the process, patients disguising the deceptive behavior, and a lack of health care providers who are trained to diagnose psychocutaneous diseases. The prevalence is estimated to be 0.04%–1.5% in dermatology settings, with a female predilection of up to 20:1. Although it can occur at any age, the highest prevalence is at ~20 years old, and the mean age is ~13 years (Jafferany 2022). The patients are generally single, with low education levels and few job qualifications or skills (Rodríguez Pichardo and García Bravo 2013); remarkably, however, patients demonstrate extensive knowledge of medical specialties in producing their symptoms.

Etiology and Pathogenesis

All patients with dermatitis artefacta have an underlying psychopathology. Most patients have a history of traumatic life events, including abuse or neglect by parents, unstable care, and bullying in childhood.

Several hypotheses have been developed to understand the pathogenesis of dermatitis artefacta, including social learning, self-punishment, social signaling, implicit identification, pain-analgesia (or opiate), pragmatic, and tension regulation (Jafferany 2022). Most fundamentally, patients with dermatitis artefacta use self-harm as an emotional coping method to express their psychiatric distress. Children and adolescents may develop these symptoms to receive attention and protection from health care providers. They desire medical professionals' care as a substitution and compensation for their neglectful or abusive parents. Additionally, the act of deceiving caregivers may provide an unconscious sense of control, which helps to relieve the tension of a stressful home environment.

Patients may have additional psychiatric comorbidities that make it difficult to cope with psychological stress, such as low self-esteem, anxiety, depression, and personality disorders (Koblenzer 2000). Self-harm behaviors and painfully invasive diagnostic procedures may be seen as a punishment to deal with the guilt associated with having unstable and abusive parents, especially in patients with masochistic tendencies.

Clinical Features

Patients with dermatitis artefacta often present with various skin lesions and look anxious. Classically, they provide a "hollow history" that includes uncertain and ambiguous details about their condition. Although they tend to be secretive about their story and deny their responsibility for the lesions, they may put forward vague and exaggerated details that do not correlate with their appearance. Patients frequently report disappointment with previous caregivers, diagnostic processes, and treatments (Harth et al. 2010; Koblenzer 2000; Kuhn et al. 2017; Rodríguez Pichardo and García Bravo 2013). It is not uncommon for patients to present with additional psychiatric symptoms.

Clinically, the hallmark of dermatitis artefacta is unconscious self-harm and self-manipulation without any direct suicidal intention. Patients use various mechanical, toxic, or pharmacological techniques for self-injury. Mechanical preferences include pressure, friction, occlusion, biting, cutting, stabbing, and mutilation. They may choose to apply uric acids, alkalis, and thermal chemicals for toxic harm. Some patients, especially those educated in the medical field, may inject pharmacological agents such as insulin, heparin, warfarin, or potassium or take pills such as thyroid replacements, cortisol, or sex hormones. They may also try to exaggerate potential or preexisting infections (Jafferany 2022).

The skin lesions are generally monomorphic, cropped, and well demarcated. They have geometric shapes and sharp borders, which indicate the preferred technique. Moreover, although the lesions' morphology can imitate most dermatological pathology, characteristics and distribution of the lesions are incompatible with known dermatoses. On dermatological examination, findings may change according to the preferred self-harm technique and duration. Patients may have primary elementary lesions such as erythema, edema, papules, nodules, blisters, purpura, ecchymoses, and pigmentation alterations; they may have secondary elementary lesions such as ulcers, erosions, crusts, sclerosis, atrophy, and scars (Figures 6–1 and 6–2). The most affected sites are easy regions to reach, such as the face, arms, and legs. Hard-to-reach areas such as the middle of the back are relatively less affected. Lesions also tend to be resistant to standard dermatological treatments and to recur.

Diagnosis and Differential Diagnosis

The diagnosis of dermatitis artefacta is based on clinical suspicion and exclusion of other primary dermatological pathologies. The clinician should suspect dermatitis artefacta when the patient gives vague history and the lesions have atypical distribution, morphology, histology, or resistance to dermatological treatments. Even though clinical suspicion is essential, primary skin diseases should be ruled out before diagnosis. The most common primary dermatological conditions that may appear similar to dermatitis artefacta are summarized in Table 6–1.

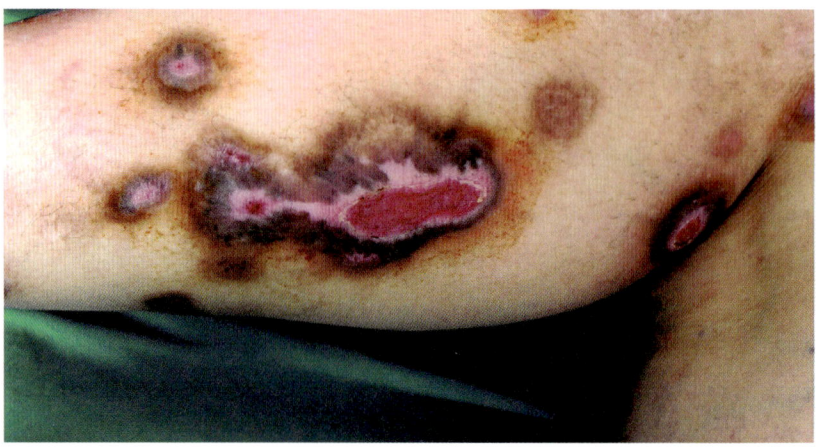

FIGURE 6–1. Ulcerative lesions with different healing stages in dermatitis artefacta.
Source. Dr. Houda Hammami.

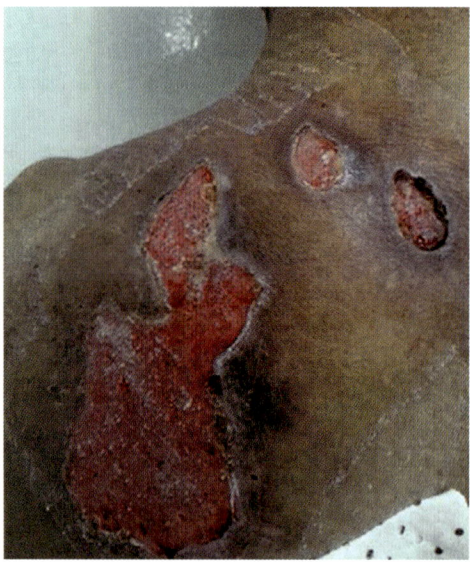

FIGURE 6–2. Ulcerative lesions in dermatitis artefacta.
Source. Dr. Asmahane Souissi.

TABLE 6–1. Differential diagnosis of dermatitis artefacta in dermatological aspect

Carcinomas
Contact dermatitis
Drug eruptions
Frostbite
Immunobullous disorders
Infections
Panniculitis
Perforating dermatoses
Phytophotodermatitis
Prurigo nodularis
Pyoderma gangrenosum
Vasculitis

TABLE 6–2. Findings that merit suspicion of dermatitis artefacta

Cultures (blood, urine, or sputum) positive for unexpected organisms
Female patient
Health care training in the patient
Lack of objective findings to support history
Multiple emergency department visits or hospitalizations (doctor shopping)
Suspicious shape and color of the lesions on examination
Vague symptoms and history

Source. Adapted from Jafferany 2022.

Routinely, a skin biopsy is not performed because there are no specific histopathological features of dermatitis artefacta (Kuhn et al. 2017). However, a specimen taken by the edge of an ulcer may help differentiate and exclude other skin pathologies. Notably, the presence of epidermal multinucleated keratinocytes (more than five nuclei) has been suggested as an important finding in dermatitis artefacta.

Several features in the clinical suspicion of dermatitis artefacta may be helpful in dermatology settings. These warning signs are listed in Table 6–2.

After initial clinical suspicion and completing the exclusion processes, patients should be directed to dermatologists who are well trained in psychocutaneous disorders or to a psychiatrist. According to DSM-5-TR (American Psychiatric Association 2022), there are four criteria for the factitious disorder diagnosis (Box 6–1).

Box 6–1. Diagnostic Criteria for Factitious Disorder

Factitious Disorder Imposed on Self

A. Falsification of physical or psychological signs or symptoms, or induction of injury or disease, associated with identified deception.
B. The individual presents himself or herself to others as ill, impaired, or injured.
C. The deceptive behavior is evident even in the absence of obvious external rewards.
D. The behavior is not better explained by another mental disorder, such as delusional disorder or another psychotic disorder.

Specify:
Single episode
Recurrent episodes (two or more events of falsification of illness and/or induction of injury)

Factitious Disorder Imposed on Another (Previously Factitious Disorder by Proxy)

A. Falsification of physical or psychological signs or symptoms, or induction of injury or disease, in another, associated with identified deception.
B. The individual presents another individual (victim) to others as ill, impaired, or injured.
C. The deceptive behavior is evident even in the absence of obvious external rewards.
D. The behavior is not better explained by another mental disorder, such as delusional disorder or another psychotic disorder.

Note: The perpetrator, not the victim, receives this diagnosis.

Specify:
Single episode
Recurrent episodes (two or more events of falsification of illness and/or induction of injury)

Source. Reprinted from American Psychiatric Association: *Diagnostic and Statistical Manual of Mental Disorders*, 5th Edition, Text Revision. Washington, DC, American Psychiatric Association, 2022, p. 367. Copyright © 2022 American Psychiatric Association. Used with permission.

Before establishing a diagnosis of factitious disorder, other possible psychiatric pathologies need to be reviewed and ruled out (Table 6–3), including skin-picking disorder (SPD), malingering, somatoform disorders, conversion disorder, and OCD. Patients with SPD accept responsibility for producing the lesions, unlike those with dermatitis artefacta. SPD patients

TABLE 6–3. Differential diagnosis of factitious disorders

Production	Motive	Disorder	Notable Feature
Conscious	Conscious	SPD	Only nails or tweezers are used
		OCD	Repetitive; provides instant relief
		Malingering	Secondary gain motive
Conscious	Unconscious	Dermatitis artefacta	Various methods of self-harm Seeks access to care providers
		Somatoform disorders	High levels of anxiety and fear from physical symptoms
Unconscious	Unconscious	Conversion	Genuine physical symptoms Acute psychological distress

damage their skin using their nails or tweezers, whereas dermatitis artefacta patients use various methods. In malingering, the subject consciously produces the signs or symptoms for secondary gain. Patients with somatoform disorders unconsciously produce their physical symptoms, causing high levels of anxiety and distress in their lives. They are not motivated to assume the sick role or get any other secondary gain. Patients with conversion disorder have genuine physical symptoms resulting from acute psychological distress. They are not conscious of their symptoms and motives.

Anxiety disorders, psychotic disorders, affective disorders with psychotic components, autism spectrum disorder, emotionally unstable personality, child abuse, and hypochondriacal delusions should also be evaluated.

Management

The management of dermatitis artefacta can be challenging. It should be led by a multidisciplinary team of dermatologist, psychiatrist, primary care physician, therapist, social worker, and family members. The aim of management should be to help the patient develop insight into their condition and continue treatment and recovery. The treatment approach is based on limiting self-harm behaviors, the risk of adverse events, and the health care costs of unnecessary treatment and diagnostic tests. The relationship between the patient and physician should be empathic and nonjudgmental. Confrontation with a dogmatic and aggressive approach may cause the patient to become defensive and drop out of the therapeutic process. If a patient refuses a psychiatry referral, the use of psychotropic drugs by the psychodermatologist can be helpful. The treatment plan should consist of

TABLE 6–4. Management guidelines for dermatitis artefacta

Basics	Nonconfrontational and neutral attitude
	Detailed clinical history and dermatological exam
	Exclusion of the differential diagnosis
	Evaluation of potential comorbid psychiatric symptoms
	Multidisciplinary approach
Dermatology	Topical products (bathing with soap-free ingredients, gentle emollients)
	Occlusive bandaging, perhaps with aluminum foil
	Topical antimicrobials (if indicated)
Psychiatry	Focus on history of childhood trauma and abuse
	Psychoeducation about the illness
	Encourage patient to understand symptoms as a request for help
	Face-saving techniques to prevent any humiliation and damage to patient reputation
	Inexact interpretation; inform the patient that the existing problem is related to psychological factors
Psychotherapy	Psychodynamic therapy to interpret unconscious conflicts
	Cognitive-behavioral therapy to modify the beliefs and behaviors
	Relaxation therapy to reduce physical and mental tension
	Family therapy to increase compliance
	Psychotropic therapy; to treat psychiatric comorbidities
Medications	Selective serotonin reuptake inhibitors
	Antipsychotics
	Mood stabilizers
	Antianxiety agents

skin repair and psychiatric therapies. Management guidelines for dermatitis artefacta are outlined in Table 6–4.

Regarding the dermatological aspects of the disease, the initial approach is topical regimens. If there is a secondary infection, topical antimicrobials should be added. Additionally, occlusive applications can contribute to clinical improvement by preventing patient manipulation. Improvement that occurs under the occlusion supports the diagnosis.

For the psychological aspect of the disease, the first-line treatment is psychotherapy. Psychodynamic therapy helps uncover underlying unconscious conflicts that may trigger the disease. There is no standard psychotropic medication, but selective serotonin reuptake inhibitors (SSRIs), antipsychotics, mood stabilizers, and antianxiety agents can be used to treat comorbid psychiatric symptoms.

Prognosis

Generally, untreated dermatitis artefacta tends to be chronic, with recurring episodes. Sometimes, a lack of communication or a lack of awareness about psychocutaneous disorders among health care professionals may worsen the prognosis. Psychiatric comorbidities and psychosocial context also affect prognosis. Better prognostic features include being young and without severe comorbidities, having a shorter disease duration, and having an understanding of social context.

An essential point for health care providers is that those with childhood dermatitis artefacta may abuse their future children when they become parents. It is known that adults who experienced abuse or neglect as children are more likely to become abusers themselves. Through this process, the offspring of adults who coped with childhood abuse through dermatitis artefacta may be at higher risk of becoming victims of dermatitis artefacta imposed on another. This condition, Munchausen syndrome by proxy, can be the reason for the intergenerational transfer of dermatitis artefacta. Health care providers should be aware of this to prophylactically provide for the children of patients with dermatitis artefacta.

References

American Psychiatric Association: Diagnostic and Statistical Manual of Mental Disorders, 5th Edition. Arlington, VA, American Psychiatric Association, 2013

American Psychiatric Association: Diagnostic and Statistical Manual of Mental Disorders, 5th Edition, Text Revision. Washington, DC, American Psychiatric Association, 2022

Harth W, Taube KM, Gieler U: Factitious disorders in dermatology. J Dtsch Dermatol Ges 8(5):361–372, quiz 373, 2010 20163503

Jafferany M: Factitious disorders (dermatitis artefacta), in Handbook of Psychodermatology: Introduction to Psychocutaneous Disorders. Cham, Switzerland, Springer, 2022, pp 103–111

Koblenzer CS: Dermatitis artefacta: clinical features and approaches to treatment. Am J Clin Dermatol 1(1):47–55, 2000 11702305

Kuhn H, Mennella C, Magid M, et al: Psychocutaneous disease: clinical perspectives. J Am Acad Dermatol 76(5):779–791, 2017 28411771

Rodríguez Pichardo A, García Bravo B: Dermatitis artefacta: a review. Actas Dermosifiliogr 104(10):854–866, 2013 23266056

Case 6-1
Dermatitis Artefacta Mimicking Palmoplantar Keratoderma

Gulhima Arora, M.D.
Sandeep Arora, M.D.

Case Description

A 20-year-old woman was brought to an outpatient dermatology department with a history of recurrent bleeding lesions on the soles of her feet, bilaterally, for the past 8 years. The lesions were spontaneous in onset, with a mild degree of burning before their appearance. She gave a history of repeatedly rubbing her feet with pumice stone to attempt to alleviate the burning sensation. There was no history of any pain, trauma, or similar lesions on the palms or elsewhere on the body. She denied any self-inflicted injury.

The patient was initially managed with traditional therapies, with no relief. A dermatology referral was sought for the first time when she was 16 years old. At the time, she was misdiagnosed with allergic contact dermatitis, psoriasis, and idiopathic palmoplantar keratoderma and treated with topical emollients and oral antihistamines, with no relief. Her routine lab work was negative.

Upon presentation to the outpatient department at age 20, her examination revealed a well-kept individual who appeared anxious but was not in obvious pain or discomfort. Dermatological examination revealed fresh, superficial, linear lacerations on both soles interspersed with similar lacerations in various stages of healing (Figure 6–3). The skin of the soles was lichenified from repeated rubbing with the pumice stone, giving an appearance of plantar keratoderma. Palms and the rest of the cutaneous integument were not involved.

Differential Diagnosis

- Allergic contact dermatitis
- Psoriasis
- Idiopathic palmoplantar keratoderma
- Dermatitis artefacta

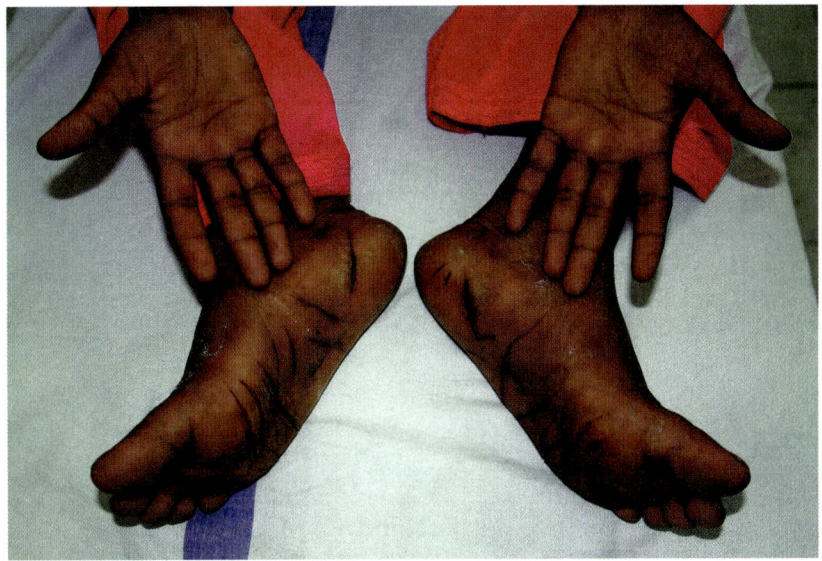

FIGURE 6–3. Fresh superficial linear cuts over both plantar surfaces of feet, with normal palms.
Source. Dr. Gulhima Arora.

Diagnosis

Because of the atypical presentation and sudden spontaneous appearance of superficial linear lacerations without trauma, in addition to the absence of obvious discomfort and lack of involvement of other body parts, the patient was suspected to have dermatitis artefacta, and she was admitted for observation.

Management

Dry dressings were placed to prevent access to the feet, with removal occurring only during bathing time. In a week, the lacerations had healed considerably (Figure 6–4), and the patient was then observed without use of the dressings. The next morning, similar fresh lacerations were observed over both soles. An alert staff member noticed the patient had a razor blade in her possession.

Psychiatric evaluation revealed multiple stressors in the patient's day-to-day life. Psychometric evaluation revealed features of anxiety during a Rorschach test and a need for nurturance and affiliation in a thematic appreciation test. In a counseling session after 6 weeks, she admitted to using

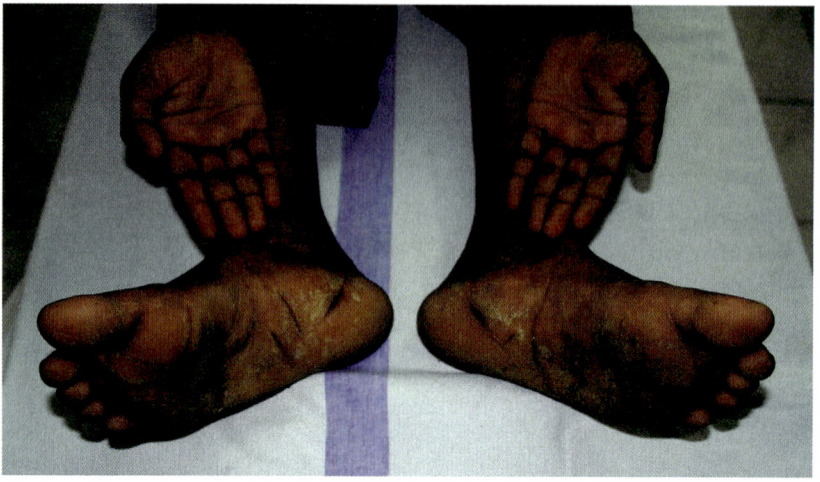

FIGURE 6–4. Partial healing of cuts after 1 week of occlusive dressing.
Source. Dr. Gulhima Arora.

the razor blade for deliberate self-harm repeatedly over the past 8 years. Active psychiatric intervention was attempted in the form of anxiolytics (buspirone 5 mg 3 times a day), relaxation measures, family therapy, and environmental interventions. She relapsed twice over a 3-month period and gradually improved. Features of dermatitis artefacta subsequently subsided, with no fresh lesions observed in the follow-up period of 1 year. She continues follow-up with psychiatry.

Discussion

Dermatitis artefacta is an uncommon disorder that is often missed in daily clinical practice. Its presentation is varied (Saha et al. 2015; Verraes-Derancourt et al. 2006), but suspicious manifestation includes geometric or linear lesions on accessible sites, with normal skin in between. An unexplained lesion distribution with unexplained chronology and sudden onset, especially around a stressful life event, should alert the physician to the possibility of dermatitis artefacta (Arora et al. 2013).

In this case, at the age of 8, the patient lost her mother to a prolonged illness, the suspected event of onset for her disease. Somatization of skin with recurrent burning sensation and repeated rubbing with a pumice stone led to lichenification of skin. Lacerations on a background of plantar lichenification gave an impression of fissuring in a case of plantar keratoderma. She was hence managed for a differential of plantar keratoderma. However, bland symptomatology, sudden onset of lesions, features of somatization, inconsistent distribution, and improvement when access to the site was limited alerted us to the possibility of dermatitis artefacta.

Identifying an underlying etiology of such lesions usually takes time, and confrontation must be avoided. Psychological support of the patient and family and gradual buildup of mutual trust and rapport between care providers and the patient are essential for management (Mohandas et al. 2013), as are early psychiatric review with objective assessment, psychotherapy, and pharmacological interventions (Shivakumar et al. 2021).

TEACHING POINTS

- The morphology of lesions in dermatitis artefacta may mimic several skin diseases, which can delay proper diagnosis.

- Patients with dermatitis artefacta tend to use tools such as knives or razors to produce the lesions. Health care providers and family members should look for these tools to help make the diagnosis.

- Dry dressing may be a useful tool for diagnosis; improvement while the area is inaccessible favors the diagnosis of dermatitis artefacta.

References

Arora S, Arora G, Gupta AK, et al: Bullous auto erythrocyte sensitization syndrome in alcohol dependence. Indian J Dermatol Venereol Leprol 79(2):269, 2013 23442486

Mohandas P, Bewley A, Taylor R: Dermatitis artefacta and artefactual skin disease: the need for a psychodermatology multidisciplinary team to treat a difficult condition. Br J Dermatol 169(3):600–606, 2013 23646995

Saha A, Seth J, Gorai S, et al: Dermatitis artefacta: a review of five cases: a diagnostic and therapeutic challenge. Indian J Dermatol 60(6):613–615, 2015 26677280

Shivakumar S, Jafferany M, Kumar SV, et al: A brief review of dermatitis artefacta and management strategies for physicians. Prim Care Companion CNS Disord 23(4):20nr02858, 2021 34228404

Verraes-Derancourt S, Derancourt C, Poot F, et al: [Dermatitis artefacta: retrospective study in 31 patients] [in French]. Ann Dermatol Venereol 133(3):235–238, 2006 16800172

Case 6–2
A Case of Dermatitis Artefacta

Pavel V. Chernyshov, M.D.

Case Description

A 53-year-old woman presented to the dermatology clinic with a 1-month history of two ulcers on her face. On examination, there were two geometric-shaped ulcers with sharp margins adjacent to normal skin on the left cheek (about 2.5 cm wide and 7 cm long) and the forehead (about 3 cm wide and 5 cm long). Multiple atrophic scars of different sizes and shapes in accessible parts of the body (predominantly on the head) were present (Figure 6–5A and B). The patient could not explain the cause of present or past lesions. Routine laboratory tests were normal. The patient denied any chronic conditions.

Differential Diagnosis

- Pyoderma gangrenosum
- Dermatitis artefacta

Diagnosis

An initial diagnosis of pyoderma gangrenosum was established. Oral prednisolone, doxycycline, and topical methylene blue were prescribed under hospitalization. After 3 days, the doctors noticed that signs of healing were present during the day (fibrin clot formation), but aggravation of lesions was prominent each morning. The patient denied any role in manipulation of the lesions. Nightly occlusive dressings were recommended, which resulted in fast healing of ulcers (Figure 6–5B). The diagnosis of dermatitis artefacta was made.

Management

After several discussions, the patient agreed to consultation with a psychiatrist after release from the hospital.

Discussion

Dermatitis artefacta falls into the category of factitious disorders. Patients usually hide responsibility for their actions from their doctors and may reject a referral to see a mental health provider (Jafferany et al. 2020). Typical

Dermatitis Artefacta

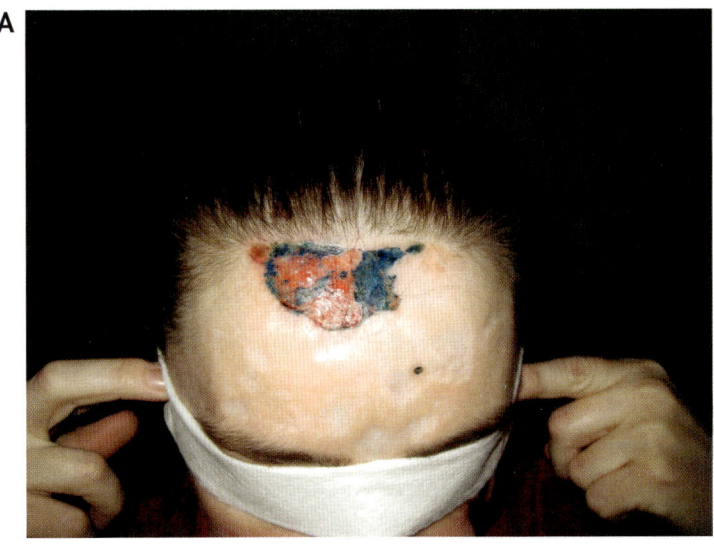

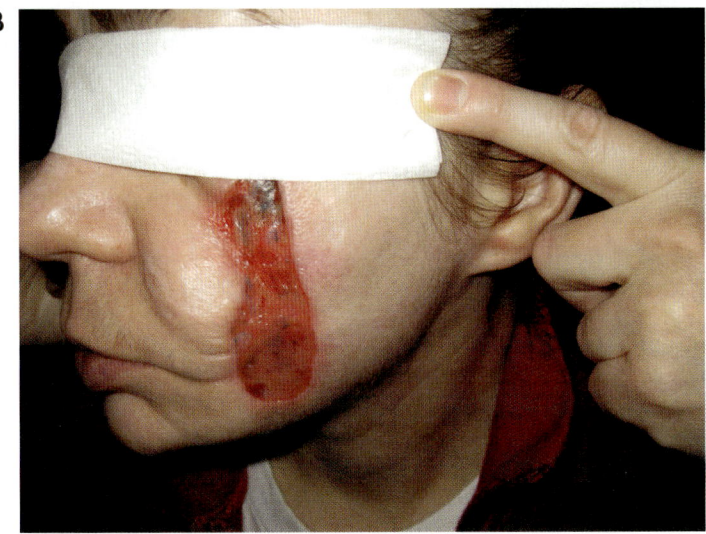

FIGURE 6–5. Geometric-shaped ulcers with sharp margins adjacent to normal skin on the forehead (A) and left cheek (B).
Source. Dr. Pavel Chernyshov.

presentation includes cutaneous lesions that are bizarre in shape and do not conform to any recognizable skin disease. Most patients have more than one skin lesion. The face is the most common site of dermatitis artefacta lesions, as in this patient (Chandran and Kurien 2023).

Patients with dermatitis artefacta often use specific tools to produce the lesions. Occlusive dressings may prevent damage (Jafferany et al. 2020). The underlying mental health disorder must be addressed and treated (Chandran and Kurien 2023).

TEACHING POINTS

- The presence of multiple lesions of different stages, varying sizes and shapes, and geometric forms is a clue for the diagnosis of dermatitis artefacta.

- Pyoderma gangrenosum is one of the main differential diagnoses of dermatitis artefacta. The absence of improvement after treatment is suggestive of the diagnosis of dermatitis artefacta. Skin biopsy may also be helpful to differentiate the two diseases by showing unspecific results in dermatitis artefacta.

References

Chandran V, Kurien G: Dermatitis Artefacta. Treasure Island, FL, StatPearls Publishing, 2023

Jafferany M, Ferreira BR, Patel A: The Essentials of Psychodermatology. Cham, Switzerland, Springer, 2020, p 128

Case 6–3
Dermatitis Artefacta in a 27-Year-Old Woman

İsa An, M.D.
Ayşe Serap Karadag, M.D.

Case Description

A 27-year-old woman was admitted to the clinic with the complaint of painful lesions on both forearms and legs. The patient stated that she had not

Dermatitis Artefacta **143**

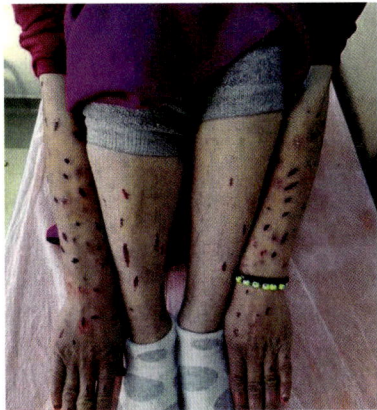

FIGURE 6–6. Multiple linear ulcerated lesions of varying sizes are observed on the back of both hands, forearms, and legs.
Source. Dr. Isa An.

had any previous skin disease and that the existing lesions occurred spontaneously at night while she was sleeping. Dermatological examination revealed multiple linear ulcerated lesions of varying sizes on the back of both hands, forearms, and legs (Figure 6–6). Collateral information from her mother revealed that the patient did not have any dermatological or psychiatric diseases previously, but she had been living an introverted life for the last 3 months as she was in the process of getting a divorce. Routine hematological and biochemical tests were within normal limits.

Differential Diagnosis

- Prurigo
- Skin-picking disorder
- Dermatitis artefacta

Diagnosis

Based on history and clinical findings, the diagnosis of dermatitis artefacta was considered. In the psychiatric evaluation, the patient was diagnosed with dermatitis artefacta and concomitant major depressive disorder.

Management

The patient was given epithelial cream for her lesions. An official psychiatry consultation was made, but she refused to comply with the psychiatric treatment and she could not be reevaluated.

Discussion

Dermatitis artefacta is a psychocutaneous disorder in which patients consciously create lesions in different forms on the skin, hair, nails, or mucous membranes to meet a psychological need, attract attention, or avoid responsibility (Gupta and Gupta 2014; Rodríguez Pichardo and García Bravo 2013). Dermatitis artefacta can accompany psychiatric diseases such as schizoaffective disorder, depression, and psychosis (Lavery et al. 2018; Nielsen et al. 2005). This patient was diagnosed with major depressive disorder accompanying dermatitis artefacta.

The lesions of dermatitis artefacta are often observed in areas where the dominant hand can easily reach. Although the lesions can be seen anywhere on the body, they are frequently seen on the face and dorsum of the hands (Mohandas et al. 2013; Saha et al. 2015). This patient had linear ulcerated lesions from scratching with fingernails, particularly on the anterior surfaces of the forearms and legs, where the hands can easily reach. Because the clinical appearance of the lesions was typical, histopathological examination was not performed. The patient was diagnosed with dermatitis artefacta based on the inconsistent history of the occurrence of lesions as well as the typical clinical appearance of the lesions due to scratching with nails.

The patient was referred to the psychiatry service to diagnose and treat the underlying mental health disorder. Because dermatitis artefacta is a disease with dermatological and psychiatric components, in which relapses are seen frequently, these patients should be followed up regularly by dermatologists and psychiatrists. In this case, the patient refused to comply with the psychiatric treatment.

TEACHING POINTS

- The diagnosis of dermatitis artefacta is mainly based on the patient's history and clinical features. Performing skin biopsy is usually unnecessary.

- Follow-up can be difficult, as patients may refuse psychiatric treatment.

References

Gupta MA, Gupta AK: Current concepts in psychodermatology. Curr Psychiatry Rep 16(6):449, 2014 24740235

Lavery MJ, Stull C, McCaw I, et al: Dermatitis artefacta. Clin Dermatol 36(6):719–722, 2018 30446194

Mohandas P, Bewley A, Taylor R: Dermatitis artefacta and artefactual skin disease: the need for a psychodermatology multidisciplinary team to treat a difficult condition. Br J Dermatol 169(3):600–606, 2013 23646995

Nielsen K, Jeppesen M, Simmelsgaard L, et al: Self-inflicted skin diseases: a retrospective analysis of 57 patients with dermatitis artefacta seen in a dermatology department. Acta Derm Venereol 85(6):512–515, 2005 16396799

Rodríguez Pichardo A, García Bravo B: Dermatitis artefacta: a review. Actas Dermosifiliogr 104(10):854–866, 2013 23266056

Saha A, Seth J, Gorai S, et al: Dermatitis artefacta: a review of five cases: a diagnostic and therapeutic challenge. Indian J Dermatol 60(6):613–615, 2015 26677280

Case 6–4
Dermatitis Artefacta in a 51-Year-Old Woman

Dimitry V. Romanov, M.D.
Anna V. Michenko, M.D.
Andrey N. Lvov, M.D.

Case Description

A 51-year-old woman presented with pseudosomatic complaints that appeared after childbirth when she was 24. At that time, she had unusual sensations of twitching and contractions in the veins and muscles of the shins. Over the years, the discomfort in the shins became more frequent. Starting at the age of 40, there were sensations of twitching and "swarming" in the shins, numbness of the little fingers and forearms of both hands, and headaches that were tight in nature in the occipital region of the head. Neurological examinations were insignificant, and functional (conversional) neurological complaints were considered. Regarding these complaints, she had been self-medicating since the age of 43; she visited a sanatorium annually where she received hirudotherapy (medicinal leeches) and drank mineral waters.

At the age of 46, she took orlistat to lose weight for 3 months and lost 15 kg. After discontinuing the medication, the feeling of twitching veins on her legs increased. Simultaneously, she noticed a "pimple" around the right nasolabial fold that was accompanied by a feeling of itching and bursting from the inside, "as if something foreign was growing." The skin sensations were accompanied by ulcers that spread over both cheeks and chin.

The patient was anxious about her condition and consulted with various medical specialists, mainly dermatologists and parasitologists. Various diagnoses were considered (e.g., pyoderma, dermatitis, larva migrans, actinomycosis), none of which was confirmed. Eventually, she was sent for a consultation with a psychiatrist. At the psychiatric examination, she complained of painful rashes on the facial skin that differed from the "usual pimple" in density and were accompanied by a feeling of the presence of foreign bodies in the skin. She described two types of unpleasant sensations. First, she described itching and swarming from the inside of her skin. Second, she described the feeling of sharp "tugs" inside the skin and the feeling of "something quickening" under the skin. However, she denied the presence of parasites or other infesting objects.

She complained that when a pimple appeared, she also felt an irresistible desire to remove it from under the skin. After removing the subcutaneous contents with a needle, she noted temporary relief of the itching and other skin sensations. Within 3 days, however, the sensations would resume in the same place, and she would think that "something was not completely squeezed out" and resume her skin mutilation. In addition to pimples, she described the presence of "pouches in the cheek" that reached a maximum size of 1.5×0.5 cm. She admitted that she opened them with a needle and physically squeezed to extract their contents: "bright-yellow fluid with black fine hairs, threads and balls looking like bunches of grapes."

The patient's skin presented with artificial lesions localized on the face, including the skin of the chin and cheeks bilaterally. The skin eruptions presented with localized deep ulcers and hemorrhagic crusts, sharply delineated from normal skin, surrounded by erythematous and white scars with irregular borders on the right cheek; atrophic superficial scars with irregular borders and few excoriations partly covered with hemorrhagic crusts on the left cheek; and a linear scar with central linear ulcer on the chin (Figure 6–7A, B, and C).

Differential Diagnosis

Dermatitis artefacta should be distinguished from primary dermatoses or systemic disease with skin presentations (e.g., pyoderma gangrenosum, syphilitic gumma) and other primary psychiatric disorders causing secondary self-inflicted skin symptoms (e.g., skin-picking disorder, factitious disorder, delusional parasitosis, Morgellons syndrome, schizophrenic psychosis).

Diagnosis

The patient was diagnosed with dermatitis artefacta or factitial dermatitis (L98.1 according to ICD-10) or artefactual skin disorder (ED00 according to ICD-11) and comorbid somatoform disorder (F45.1 according to ICD-10) or bodily distress disorder (6C20 according to ICD-11).

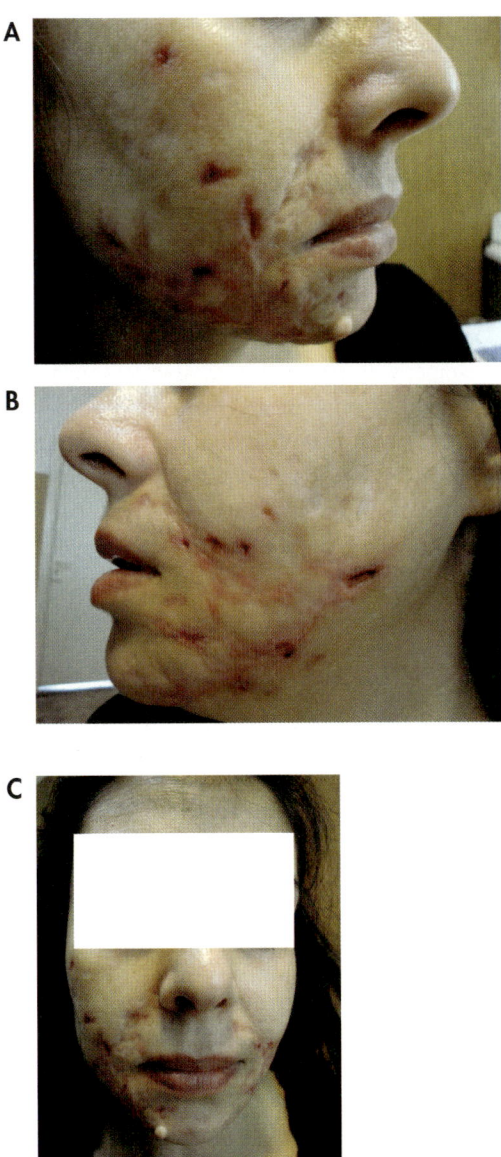

FIGURE 6–7. Artificial skin lesions (ulcers and scars) of the right cheek, left cheek and chin.
Source. Dr. Dimitry Romanov.

Management

The patient was prescribed olanzapine 10 mg daily and given occlusive dressings with mupirocin cream three times a day for a week, then switched to cream with sulfathiazole silver. Before cream application, wound irrigation was performed with 0.1% water solution of chlorhexidine. The long-lasting (6-month) treatment course resulted in elimination of pathological skin and other body sensations as well as self-mutilation. Skin ulcers receded, and residual scars remained.

Discussion

The dermatological diagnosis of dermatitis artefacta or artefactual skin disorder in this case meets ICD-11 criteria (code ED00) (World Health Organization 2022). It encompasses the self-inflicted skin injuries that are provoked by mechanical means. The patient's skin presentations share characteristics of most dermatological descriptions of the disorder: distinctive and geometric, with sharp borders, and cannot be otherwise explained. For a long time, there was also denial of a conscious or deliberate producing of the lesions, a course considered typical for dermatitis artefacta (Conde Montero et al. 2016; Laughter et al. 2020). The patient also fulfilled criteria for somatoform disorder that she suffered since her 20s: recurrent distressing physical symptoms with negative medical findings. Treatment requires dermatological medications, psychotherapy, and psychopharmacology. The latter includes anxiolytics, antidepressants, and low-dose antipsychotics.

TEACHING POINTS

- Dermatitis artefacta is considered a rare condition; however, dermatologists should be aware of it, particularly in cases of localized, persistent ulcers that are sharply delineated from normal skin margins and feature a purulent center surrounded by scar tissue.

- Precise psychiatric examination is required to bring to light underlying psychopathology and other comorbid psychiatric conditions.

- Treatment of dermatitis artefacta requires cooperation of a dermatologist and a psychiatrist, as a combined management with skin medications and psychopharmacotherapy and psychotherapy is required.

References

Conde Montero E, Sánchez-Albisua B, Guisado S, et al: Factitious ulcer misdiagnosed as pyoderma gangrenosum. Wounds 28(2):63–67, 2016 26891139

Laughter MR, Florek AG, Wisell J, et al: Dermatitis artefacta, a form of factitial disorder imposed on self, misdiagnosed as pyoderma gangrenosum for eight years. Cureus 12(7):e9054, 2020 32782873

World Health Organization: International Statistical Classification of Diseases and Related Health Problems, 11th Revision. Geneva, World Health Organization, 2022

Case 6-5
A Case of Dermatitis Artefacta in a 54-Year-Old Man

Brunilda Bardhi, M.D.
Monika Fida, M.D.
Arbnore Tafica, M.D.

Case Description

A 54-year-old man visited the dermatology outpatient clinic complaining about sudden onset of nodular lesions on his forearms bilaterally. He was concerned about his condition because the lesions were increasing in size and now had hemorrhagic secretions. The lesions continued for almost 8 months. He stated that at the time of onset he started misusing alcohol because of family problems. Even though he then stopped drinking in excess, the lesions did not improve. The patient denied self-inducing the lesions. When asked about stress, he refused to answer.

Dermatological examination revealed multiple circular erosions with hemorrhagic crusts in the center, excoriations, and some nodular lesions that were in different stages of appearance in the form of postinflammatory hyper-/hypopigmentation. They were clearly demarcated from surrounding normal skin (Figure 6–8). Routine lab work was within normal limits. A biopsy of the edge of the lesion was performed, which showed the presence of epidermal multinucleated keratinocytes and epidermal necrosis.

Differential Diagnosis

- Pyoderma gangrenosum
- Insect bite
- Dermatitis artefacta

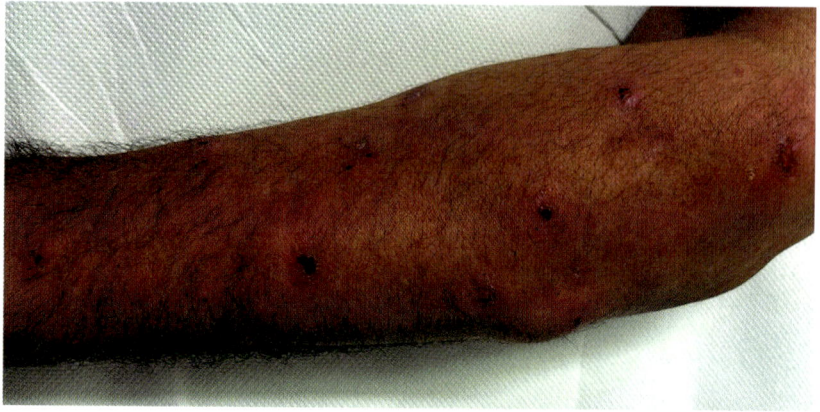

FIGURE 6–8. Circular red erosions with ulcers and hemorrhagic crusts in the center and nodular subcutaneous lesions.
Source. Dr. Brunilda Bardhi.

Diagnosis

Based on the patient's medical history, physical examination, and biopsy, the diagnosis of dermatitis artefacta was suspected, and the patient was referred to a psychiatrist.

Management

The erosive lesions were treated with fusidic acid cream locally and occlusive zinc-medicated dressings. Fortunately, the patient accepted the referral to a psychiatrist and reported that he couldn't control himself and kept touching the lesions all the time. Sometimes it felt like he had something under his skin, and he wanted to pull it out. His actions were motivated by his divorce from his wife, and he tried to draw attention to himself by self-inducing the skin lesions. After the detailed psychiatric evaluation, the psychiatrist suggested CBT without any medication. The patient showed improvement after therapy.

Discussion

In dermatitis artefacta, the patient develops skin lesions due to a psychological demand, frequently a need for attention. Patients typically deny that they intentionally caused their skin damage and typically give a vague history (Jafferany 2022). In this case, the patient referred to scratching his skin with the purpose of drawing his wife's attention. The lesions, which had no recognizable characteristics of primary skin disease, were found on physically reachable areas of the body such as the face, upper trunk, and extremities. Additionally, normal lab results and nonspecific histopathological findings in this case pointed to the diagnosis of dermatitis artefacta.

In the treatment of dermatitis artefacta, it is important to determine whether the patient has ever received a psychiatric diagnosis or whether they have a personal or familial history of mental illness.

TEACHING POINTS

- Patients with dermatitis artefacta can induce their lesions to draw the attention of other people.
- The role of biopsy is controversial, but it may be performed in selected and individualized cases to rule out other skin conditions.

References

Jafferany M: Primary psychiatric disorders, in Handbook of Psychodermatology: Introduction to Psychocutaneous Disorders. Cham, Switzerland, Springer, 2022, p 30

Case 6–6
Dermatitis Artefacta in a 26-Year-Old Woman

Rozana Cela, M.D.
Etleva Jorgaqi, M.D.

Case Description

A 26-year-old woman presented with multiple painful erosions and scarring on the lower extremities (Figure 6–9). There was no evidence of an insect bite or contact dermatitis. She denied any self-inflicted nature of her injury such as scratching or rubbing with any object. The lesions were bizarre, with tapering, and were in various stages of healing. The lesion pattern was not compatible with any known dermatological disorder.

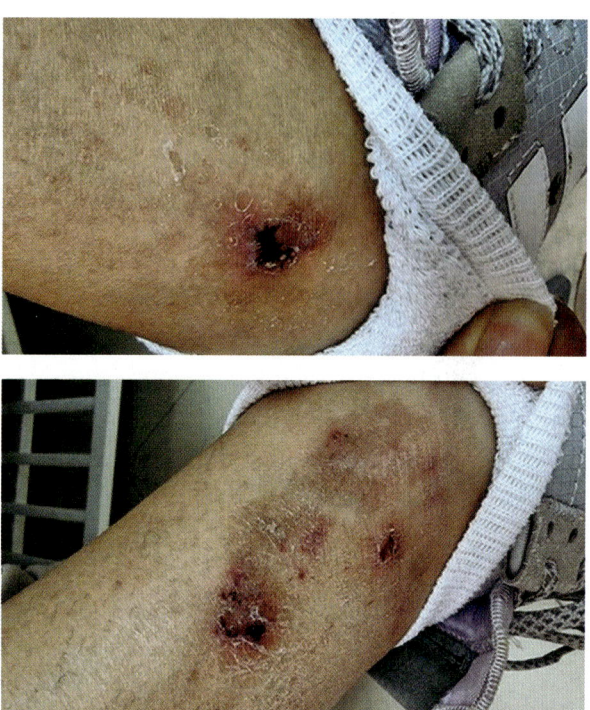

FIGURE 6–9. (A) Erosions and scarring in a linear distribution on the lower extremities. (B) Close-up view showing scarring and erosion.
Source. Dr. Rozana Cela.

Histopathological findings were nonspecific. Her psychiatric evaluation revealed emotional and physical abuse. She acknowledged feeling moody, depressed, and stressed out.

Differential Diagnosis

Dermatitis artefacta has no specific clinical appearance, and the lesions may vary as vastly as the patient's imagination. Dermatitis artefacta may resemble almost any dermatologic condition, such as vasculitis, pyogenic granuloma, or cutaneous T-cell lymphoma. Sometimes, histopathology analysis of a biopsy specimen can be used to rule out other dermatologic conditions. Once a diagnosis of self-induced dermatosis is made, the main challenge is to rule out malingering, deliberate self-harm, Munchausen syndrome, delusions, and neurotic excoriations.

Diagnosis

In this case, clinical history with no previous history of skin disease, physical examination, the presence of physical and emotional abuse, and nonspecific biopsy findings led to the diagnosis of dermatitis artefacta.

Management

Treatment with occlusive therapy completely healed the lesions within 2 weeks. The patient did not return for follow-up.

Discussion

Dermatitis artefacta is a type of factitious disorder produced by deliberate action of the patient to satisfy some deep-seated, psychiatric need (Jafferany 2022). Denial regarding the self-inflicted nature of the injuries is a common finding, consistent with this case. Therefore, confrontation to explore the underlying psychosocial conflicts should be strongly discouraged. Rather, a gentle, nonjudgmental, and empathetic approach often works. A sense of hesitancy and difficulty in making eye contact are useful clues to such strange behavior. External incentives (whether economic, legal, or related to body image) are typically absent.

The pathophysiology of dermatitis artefacta is still an enigma. Factors such as delayed developmental milestones, marital disputes, loss of loved ones in the recent past, self-guilt, disturbed parent-child relationships, bipolar personality disorder, and sexual and substance abuse are implicated as precipitating factors, as in this case.

Dermatological care with a bland emollient, topical antibiotics, and occlusive dressing should not be underestimated, as the patients tend to be emotionally attached to their skin. This patient showed significant improvement with this approach.

TEACHING POINTS

- Laboratory investigations, including histopathological examination, are usually nonspecific and do not give a correct clue to diagnosis.

- Lack of proper identification of underlying psychiatric disturbances may be the major cause of the loss of follow-up.

References

Jafferany M: Primary psychiatric disorders, in Handbook of Psychodermatology: Introduction to Psychocutaneous Disorders. Cham, Switzerland, Springer, 2022, p 30

Case 6-7
Dermatitis Artefacta: A Diagnostic and Therapeutic Challenge

Ilirjana Zekja, M.D.
Malbora Xhelili, M.D.
Monika Fida, M.D.

Case Description

A 15-year-old girl presented to the dermatology department with multiple painful, well-demarcated skin lesions and erosions with some scarring over her face for the past 3 months (Figure 6–10). Each lesion measured about 2 cm in length and 1 cm in width. There was no evidence of insect bite, drug or food allergy, or inflammatory skin condition. The main complaint was the pain of the lesions, as well as headache. The patient denied any self-inflicted nature of her injury, such as scratching or rubbing with any object. The lesions seemed bizarre and were not compatible with any known dermatological disorder. Blood test results were normal. Histopathological findings were nonspecific for any inflammatory or infectious disease. MRI of the head was performed to rule out any pathology and produced a normal result. The patient was referred to the neuropsychiatric department for an evaluation of her psychological state.

Differential Diagnosis

- Impetigo
- Leishmaniasis
- Discoid lupus erythematosus
- Dermatitis artefacta

Diagnosis

During the examination, the patient appeared sad and depressed after repeated interviews with the neurologist and psychiatrist. The patient's birth

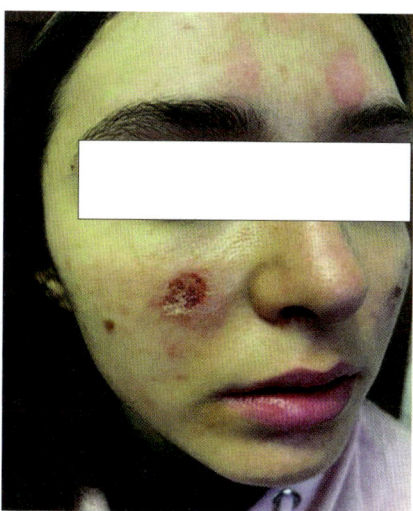

FIGURE 6–10. Well-demarcated patches and erosions on the face.
Source. Dr. Monika Fida.

history was uneventful, and she had no major medical illness. Her motor, social, and cognitive milestones developed at age-appropriate levels.

It was discovered that she dropped out of school for a short period because of poor academic performance and underwent constant criticism by her family and friends. Family history revealed that her father had remained away from the home for economic reasons starting when the patient was 3 years old. She lived with her mother, whom she described as authoritative, with overinvolvement and overprotection. The entire family believed her to be a physically and mentally weak person, from childhood. She had frequent conflicts with her friends at school.

The patient's personality was assessed with psychological tests. She had feelings of inadequacy and was hypersensitive to negative evaluation, which was apparent by her avoidance of occupational activities. She manifested instability of her interpersonal relationships and affect and had a disturbed self-image. She had constant emotions of worry and concern regarding her health and future. She met the criteria of borderline personality disorder. The diagnosis of dermatitis artefacta was made.

Management

The patient was prescribed 20 mg fluoxetine and anxiolytics, along with supportive and insight-oriented psychotherapy and family counseling. For the skin lesions on the face, a local antibiotic cream (mupirocin 2%) and an epithelial cream were prescribed. She continued under the care of a dermatologist. Within 4–5 months, she showed improvement. The skin lesions had resolved, and she reported feeling emotionally better.

Discussion

Physicians must rely on clinical presentation, careful observation, and detailed careful history from the patient and family members. A careful systematic approach to diagnosis includes taking a detailed history and ruling out other potential pathologies. Lesions may be circular blisters or erosions, burns, cryodamage, excoriations, hemorrhages, indurations, or necrosis. Traces or evidence of these are noticeable on close examination of crude dermatitis (Pradhan et al. 2019). Any part of the body can be affected, but the most common site in all age groups is the face, followed by dorsum of the hands and forearm of the nondominant limb. Direct confrontation should be avoided, and medical staff should try to create an accepting, empathetic, and nonjudgmental environment.

The types of lesions seen in dermatitis artefacta may mimic other dermatitis or inflammatory skin diseases. This patient presented with erosions, crusted lesions, discolored macules, and erythematous papules. The differential diagnosis included impetigo, leishmaniasis, and discoid lupus erythematosus. In some cases, a skin biopsy to exclude other dermatoses is worth considering.

Treatment of dermatitis artefacta sometimes is a challenge and requires involving a multidisciplinary team of a dermatologist, family physician, psychiatrist, and psychologist (Jafferany 2007). Strong and trusted relationships between the health care providers and the patient are key for success. Some specific psychopharmacologic medication may be prescribed by specialists, and the patient should be monitored closely during this treatment.

TEACHING POINTS

- Dermatitis artefacta can develop in patients during childhood as a desire to receive attention or obtain protection from health care providers to compensate for an abusive home environment.
- Treatment aims to limit the patient's self-injurious behavior and avoid unnecessary diagnostic tests.

References

Jafferany M: Psychodermatology: a guide to understanding common psychocutaneous disorders. Prim Care Companion J Clin Psychiatry 9(3):203–213, 2007 17632653

Pradhan S, Sirka CS, Dash G, et al: Dermatitis artefacta in a child: an interesting morphological presentation. Indian Dermatol Online J 10(1):72, 2019 30775305

Case 6–8
Dermatitis Artefacta as a Complication of Posttraumatic Stress Disorder

Adem Cemerlic, M.D.
Asja Prohić, M.D., Ph.D.

Case Description

A 58-year-old woman presented to the department of dermatology with a large number of varying skin lesions on her abdomen and extremities. She stated that her skin lesions first appeared in 1992, shortly after the start of the Bosnian war, and attributed them to sleeping in the prone position on an uncomfortable basement floor. The patient claimed that the lesions occur sporadically and were not constantly present. Despite the war having resolved >20 years ago, she stated she still slept in the same location, which resulted in her dermatologic condition.

The patient appeared unkempt, was slightly irritable but cooperative, and stated she was sent to the dermatology clinic by her primary care physician. When questioned whether these lesions gave her discomfort, she stated that she was most troubled by the death of her husband in the Bosnian war, the economic migration of her eldest son to Germany, and the fact that her daughter could not find work here in Sarajevo; her attitude toward her lesions seemed indifferent.

On examination, numerous erosions, hyperpigmentations, and scars, bizarrely shaped in a linear distribution, were noted on her trunk, arms, and legs (Figures 6–11 and 6–12). Histopathological findings were nonspecific and unremarkable.

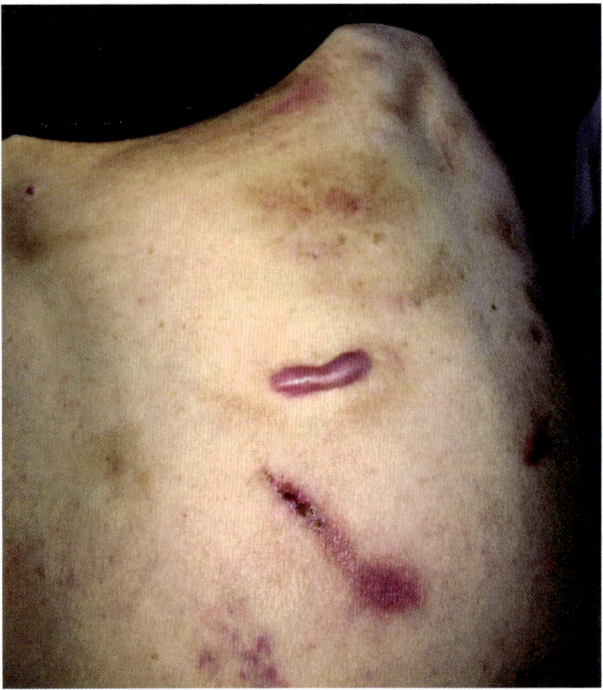

FIGURE 6–11. Bizarrely shaped hyperpigmentation, crusts, and hypertrophic scars on the trunk.
Source. Dr. Adem Cemerlic.

Differential Diagnosis

Dermatitis artefacta mimics any dermatologic condition, such as vasculitis, pyoderma gangrenosum, necrotizing vasculitis, cutaneous T-cell lymphoma, malingering, deliberate self-harm, Munchausen syndrome, delusional infestation, and neurotic excoriations.

Diagnosis

In this case, the clinical history and physical examination with no previous history of skin disease, the presence of physical and emotional trauma, and nonspecific biopsy findings led to the diagnosis of dermatitis artefacta. The psychiatric exam concluded that the patient suffered from PTSD, which was untreated and likely resulted in her case of dermatitis artefacta. Upon further questioning, she admitted to using her long, unkempt nails to induce the lesions. Conservative symptomatic care of the lesions was conducted, and the patient was enrolled in the outpatient psychiatric program.

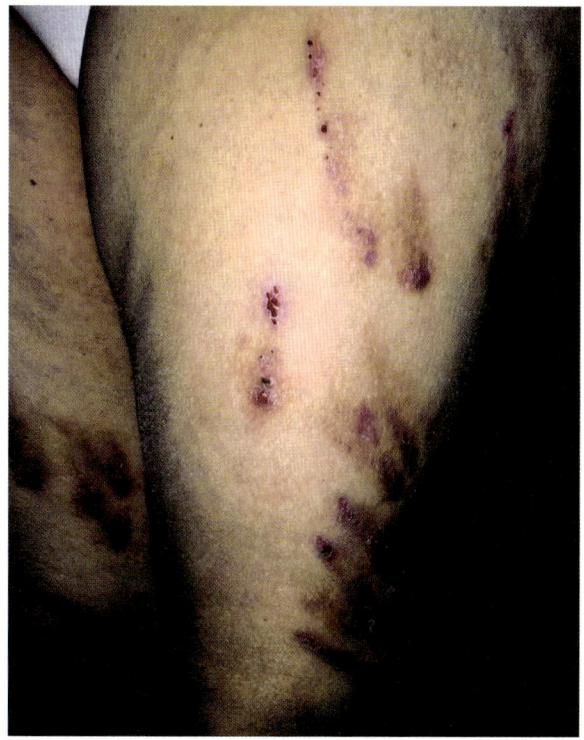

FIGURE 6–12. Erosions, hyperpigmentation, crusts, and scars in linear distribution on the lower extremities.
Source. Dr. Adem Cemerlic.

Discussion

The dermatologic manifestations of dermatitis artefacta are wide ranging but typically stem from unresolved psychological and psychiatric qualms (Shivakumar et al. 2021). When assessing patients with dermatitis artefacta, a thorough history should be taken. Often, the interview may produce clues as to a troubling psychiatric background, which eventually results in the lesions of dermatitis artefacta. Despite thorough questioning, patients often provide vague and misleading answers, readily denying having caused the lesions. It should be noted that patients with dermatitis artefacta are not motivated by financial gain (malingering).

Diagnosing dermatitis artefacta is often challenging, as lesions and the mechanisms causing them may be various in appearance. Pathognomonic signs include lesions on areas of the body that are easily accessible, such as the face, extremities, and anterior trunk. The lesions are usually bizarre and geometrical and do not conform to any recognizable skin disease. In addition, the lesions may exhibit varying temporal presentations in regard to their onset and timely resolution, with different stages of healing present among the lesions. Healthy-looking adjacent skin regions, unremarkable or inconclusive histopathological examinations, normal laboratory studies, and resolution of the presenting lesions following occlusion therapy are all characteristics associated with dermatitis artefacta (Saha et al. 2015).

Physicians should consider the various approaches that may be undertaken to induce the lesions of dermatitis artefacta, including thermally (hot/cold), chemically, and often mechanically induced injury (Lavery et al. 2018). Pyoderma gangrenosum, necrotizing vasculitis, and cutaneous T-cell lymphoma should also be considered as potential diagnoses. These should be ruled out before proceeding with dermatitis artefacta, a diagnosis of exclusion.

Dermatitis artefacta is very likely more prevalent than has been documented, because of low levels of physician recognition, patient reluctance to admit self-inflicted lesions, and lack of clinical follow-up. Typically (but not necessarily), patients are single, female, and of lower socioeconomic backgrounds. However, patients may come from all walks of life. A noteworthy association is a history of psychiatric illness (Cotterill 1992).

Although the lesions of dermatitis artefacta may resolve quickly, the long-term nature of psychiatric treatment in these patients should be recognized. Treating these patients may be tricky, but certain attitudes and approaches are likely to be fruitful. Initially, frank confrontation of the self-injurious behavior should be avoided, as this is likely to weaken the therapeutic alliance between patient and physician. Physicians should be understanding, nonjudgmental, and empathetic to patients with dermatitis artefacta, as a delicate and harmonious collaboration is likely to optimize treatment outcomes. Of integral importance is CBT, helping patients to slowly gain insight into their state and confer more positive and healthy responses to their impulses. Family therapy is likely helpful as well. Although clear consensus regarding pharmacologic approaches is still lacking, it is postulated that SSRIs may aid these patients (Koparde et al. 2018).

This case is interesting for several reasons; chiefly, it exemplifies the strong association between psychiatric illness and dermatitis artefacta. Moreover, it highlights the poor recognition and treatment of dermatitis artefacta on the primary levels of health care and beyond. Profound levels of clinical judgment are needed to recognize and treat dermatitis artefacta.

TEACHING POINTS

- Dermatitis artefacta is often the dermatologic manifestation of a deeply rooted psychiatric illness.

- Patients with dermatitis artefacta often go untreated or undertreated because of poor identification by health care providers, unclear clinical presentations, and poor patient compliance.

- Compassionate, patient, and nonconfrontational approaches should be used in addressing and treating patients with dermatitis artefacta.

References

Cotterill JA: Self-stigmatization: artefact dermatitis. Br J Hosp Med 47(2):115–119, 1992 1543958

Koparde V, Patil S, Patil S: Dermatitis artefacta (factitious dermatitis) responding to high-dose sertraline. Journal of Ment Health and Human Behavior 23(1):67–68, 2018

Lavery MJ, Stull C, McCaw I, et al: Dermatitis artefacta. Clin Dermatol 36(6):719–722, 2018 30446194

Saha A, Seth J, Gorai S, et al: Dermatitis artefacta: a review of five cases: a diagnostic and therapeutic challenge. Indian J Dermatol 60(6):613–615, 2015 26677280

Shivakumar S, Jafferany M, Kumar SV, et al: A brief review of dermatitis artefacta and management strategies for physicians. Prim Care Companion CNS Disord 23(4):20nr02858, 2021 34228404

Case 6-9
Giant Facial Ulcer as a Clinical Manifestation of Dermatitis Artefacta

Marta Szepietowska, M.D.
Barbara Białynicka-Birula, M.D.
Jacek C. Szepietowski, M.D.

Case Description

A 32-year-old man presented with pruritic ulcerative skin lesions on his face. He reported that the first skin lesion appeared about 18 months earlier, and within a few weeks, new lesions appeared and spread, affecting the face, chest, and upper extremities. The lesions started as pruritic papules and erythematous plaques. Constant scratching resulted in excoriations with subsequent ulcers. The patient denied any triggering factors or stress. On examination, the patient presented with an ulcer (4 cm×2 cm) localized on the left cheek (Figure 6–13). Several scars were found on the face, chest, and both arms. Detailed history revealed family discord and marital difficulties. Routine lab work was negative.

Differential Diagnosis

- Dermatitis artefacta
- Basal cell carcinoma
- Squamous cell carcinoma

Diagnosis

The patient was seen by a psychiatrist, who documented increased anxiety accompanied by high tendency to manipulation. The patient was diagnosed with dermatitis artefacta associated with anxiety disorder.

Management

Based on the psychiatric consultation, the patient was prescribed pregabalin 75 mg twice a day, subsequently increased to 300 mg per day. He was offered supportive therapy and CBT, which he declined. He was prescribed doxycycline 100 mg twice a day to address the bacterial infection. The patient's

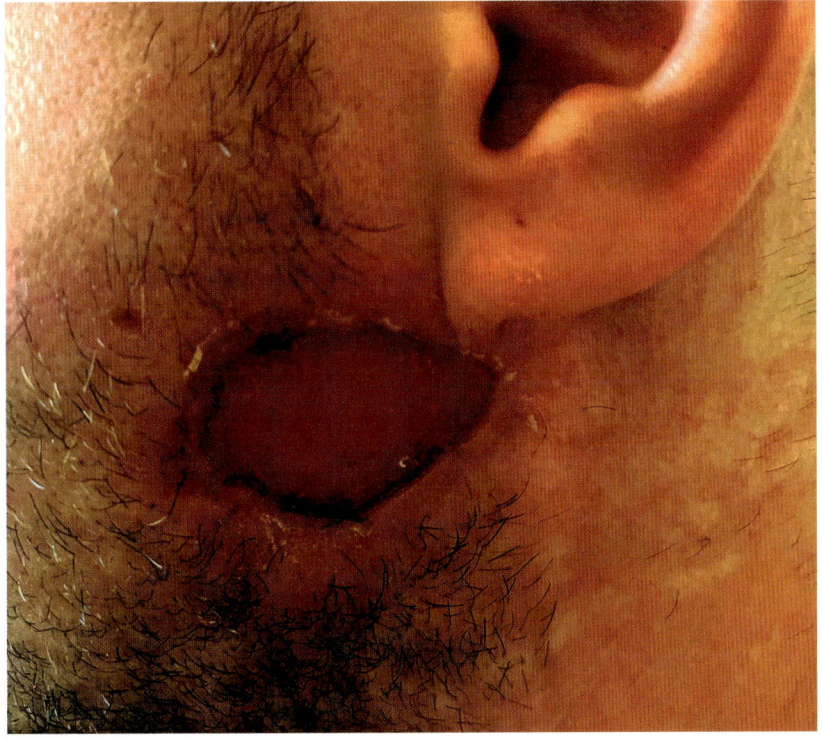

FIGURE 6–13. Giant ulcer on the left cheek.
Source. Dr. Marta Szepietowska.

lesions showed some improvement, and he was referred to a dermatologist for further treatment. The patient was lost to follow-up.

Discussion

Dermatitis artefacta is a psychodermatological condition in which patients self-inflict skin lesions owing to underlying undiagnosed psychological stress (Gieler et al. 2013). Dermatitis artefacta is a primary psychiatric condition. It is often associated with disorders such as borderline personality disorder and PTSD. Traumatic childhood experience, including abuse and neglect, or any challenging situation at the formative stage of life, is often part of the history. Patients are mentally unstable and translate their internal struggles through self-harm (Shivakumar et al. 2021).

Clinical manifestation varies. Usually, lesions are present on easily accessible parts of the body, as in this patient. The lesions may have different shapes, and shape and size can be related to the methods used for self-harm

(Shivakumar et al. 2021). A negative laboratory workup should be a hint for the physician to look closer at psychiatric aspects. Another relevant signal is that the lesions heal well when occluded during hospitalization (Nayak et al. 2013).

The management of dermatitis artefacta is difficult and requires a multidisciplinary approach among dermatologists, psychiatrists, and psychologists. Dermatological treatment, including antiseptics and occlusive dressings, should be continued. Very often occlusion helps the lesions to heal quickly, which may give additional confirmation of the diagnosis. SSRIs to address anxiety and depression are frequently prescribed. Some patients, especially those not responding to SSRIs, may benefit from antipsychotics. Some authors have documented positive outcomes with the use of gabapentinoids (Hong et al. 2022).

TEACHING POINTS

- Dermatitis artefacta presents with bizarre lesions that do not conform to any recognized skin condition.
- Lesions of dermatitis artefacta vary between patients and may show different morphological patterns and stages of healing.
- A holistic and multidisciplinary approach among dermatologists, psychiatrists, and psychologists is mandatory for good management.

References

Gieler U, Consoli SG, Tomás-Aragones L, et al: Self-inflicted lesions in dermatology: terminology and classification: a position paper from the European Society for Dermatology and Psychiatry (ESDaP). Acta Derm Venereol 93(1):4–12, 2013 23303467

Hong JSW, Atkinson LZ, Al-Juffali N, et al: Gabapentin and pregabalin in bipolar disorder, anxiety states, and insomnia: systematic review, meta-analysis, and rationale. Mol Psychiatry 27(3):1339–1349, 2022 34819636

Nayak S, Acharjya B, Debi B, et al: Dermatitis artefacta. Indian J Psychiatry 55(2):189–191, 2013 23825858

Shivakumar S, Jafferany M, Kumar SV, et al: A brief review of dermatitis artefacta and management strategies for physicians. Prim Care Companion CNS Disord 23(4):20nr02858, 2021 34228404

Case 6-10
Factitious Hand Lymphedema in a 19-Year-Old Female

Maha Lahouel, M.D.
Nour El Imene Ouni, M.D.
Mohamed Denguezli, M.D.

Case Description

A 19-year-old woman presented to the dermatology outpatient clinic with recurrent, painless swelling of the left hand developing over the previous 3 years. No trauma or infection was reported. Clinical examination revealed swelling on the back of the left hand extending to the forearm. Numerous scars of previous surgical procedures were present on the dorsum of the hand (Figure 6–14). The right hand was unaffected. Sensation, mobility, and arterial measurement of the upper limbs were normal. No underlying pathology was demonstrated on x-ray, MRI, vascular Doppler ultrasonography, lymphoscintigraphy, or laboratory studies.

The patient was a student living alone. Further inquiry revealed that during one of the acute episodes, she underwent a surgical procedure. The diagnosis of abscess was ruled out. As the condition worsened, the patient received below-elbow cast immobilization, and the swelling reduced significantly. However, the patient returned 2 weeks later with developing edema on the contralateral hand (Figure 16–15). Physical examination identified a constrictive band in the wrist with signs of strangulation (Figure 16–16). The patient was unable to give any explanation for the elastic wrist band, and it appeared she was trying to hide something. She was referred to a psychiatrist for evaluation.

Differential Diagnosis

- Lymphatic obstruction
- Hand algodystrophia
- Cellulitis/cutaneous abscess
- Drug extravasation
- Factitious lymphedema

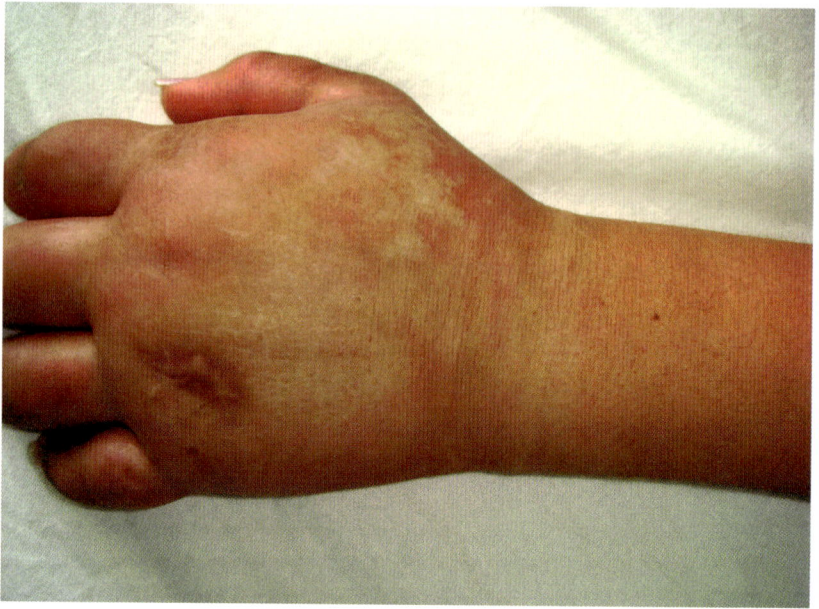

FIGURE 6–14. Swelling on the back of the left hand.
Source. Dr. Mohamed Denguezli.

Diagnosis

Based on the presence of the elastic band, the diagnosis of factitious lymphedema was suspected.

Management

Compression with limb elevation was applied, leading to rapid regression of lymphedema. During follow-up, the recurrence of edema in the left hand was observed. Subsequently, the patient was referred to the psychiatry department for assessment and appropriate management. During the psychiatric evaluation, she continued to deny self-infliction of the edema; however, she reported familial conflicts and stressful relationships in her school. Standardized rating scales and assessments revealed symptoms of depression, anxiety, and borderline personality disorder. She was prescribed SSRIs to address her anxiety and depression symptoms, but she declined.

Discussion

Lymphedema is characterized by an abnormal accumulation of fluids in the tissues caused by failure of the lymph drainage system (De Fátima Guerreiro Godoy and Pereira De Godoy 2015). Factitious lymphedema is a rare form of factitious disorder in which the patient applies a tourniquet around

Dermatitis Artefacta

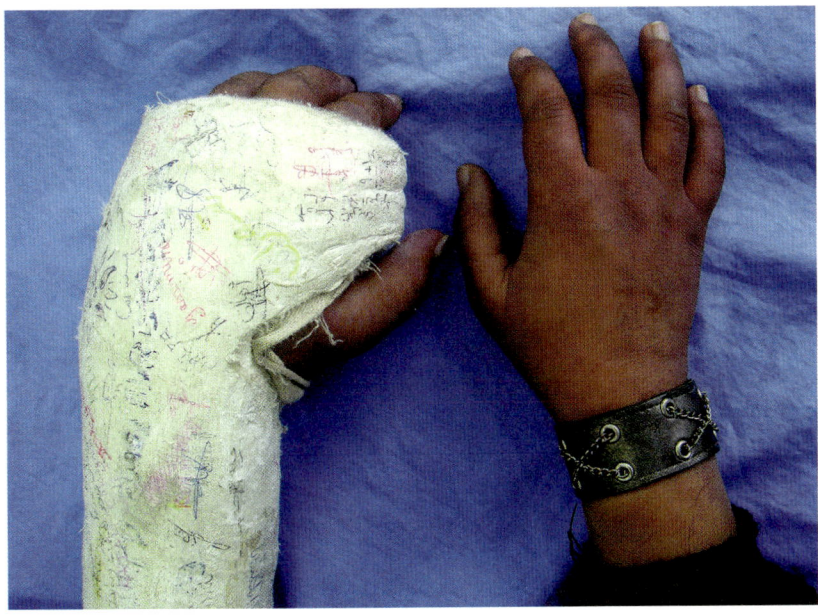

FIGURE 6-15. Edema on the contralateral hand.
Source. Dr. Mohamed Denguezli.

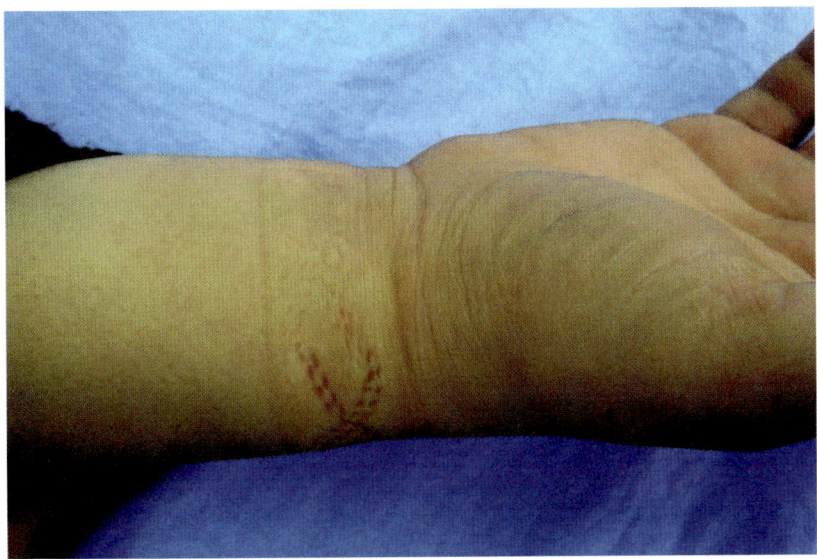

FIGURE 6-16. Constrictive band in the wrist with signs of strangulation.
Source. Dr. Mohamed Denguezli.

the limb, causing edema (Birman and Lee 2012). The diagnosis of factitious lymphedema is challenging. As in this case, it may lead to a delay in diagnosis or to unnecessary investigations or surgical procedures. Patients usually deny any role in causing the lymphedema. The physician should look for clues that suggest the diagnosis of factitious lymphedema. Clinically, a noticeable demarcation line or bands of redness, discoloration, or bruises often separate the unaffected and lymphedematous regions of the limb (Birman and Lee 2012).

Treatment consists of a combination of nonsurgical management and appropriate psychiatric counseling. Elevating the extremity with a spica cast is recommended. The patient should be referred to psychiatry to address the underlying psychiatric illness (Birman and Lee 2012).

TEACHING POINTS

- The self-induced nature of lymphedema should be considered in patients presenting with psychological symptoms, vague history, and no apparent cause on investigation.
- Early diagnosis of factitious lymphedema is crucial to avoid unnecessary surgical procedures.
- Treatment of factitious lymphedema requires a multidisciplinary approach including dermatologists, psychiatrists, and orthopedists.

References

Birman MV, Lee DH: Factitious disorders of the upper extremity. J Am Acad Orthop Surg 20(2):78–85, 2012 22302445

De Fátima Guerreiro Godoy M, Pereira De Godoy JM: Factitious lymphedema of the arm: case report and review of publications. Eur J Phys Rehabil Med 51(3):337–339, 2015 25692686

Case 6-11
Occupational Dermatitis Artefacta in a Soldier

Malek Ben Slimane, M.D.
Wafa Kabtni, M.D.
Abdel Aziz Oumaya, M.D.
Mohamed Raouf Dhaoui, M.D.

Case Description

A 29-year-old man serving in the military was referred to the dermatology department for pruritic plaques of the nipple, left ear, and pubic region developing over 2 weeks. He denied any history of trauma or recent new medications. Physical examination revealed erythematous crusted plaques with excoriations localized on the nipple, auricle, and pubic region (Figures 6–17 and 6–18). The patient was prescribed topical steroid ointment. As symptoms worsened under treatment, a skin biopsy of the affected area was performed. It revealed parakeratosis, acanthosis, spongiosis, exocytosis of lymphocytes, and the presence of eosinophils in the upper dermis. Blood tests were unremarkable.

Differential Diagnosis

- Allergic contact dermatitis
- Psoriasis
- Discoid lupus erythematous
- Occupational dermatitis artefacta

Diagnosis

Clinical and histological findings were consistent with the diagnosis of allergic contact dermatitis. Because the patient did not respond to standard treatment and his symptoms were worsening, he was referred to the psychiatry department for further consultation. During the psychiatric evaluation, the patient admitted that he was deliberately applying the substances to his skin to resemble eczema and obtain sick leave. The diagnosis of occupational dermatitis artefacta was made.

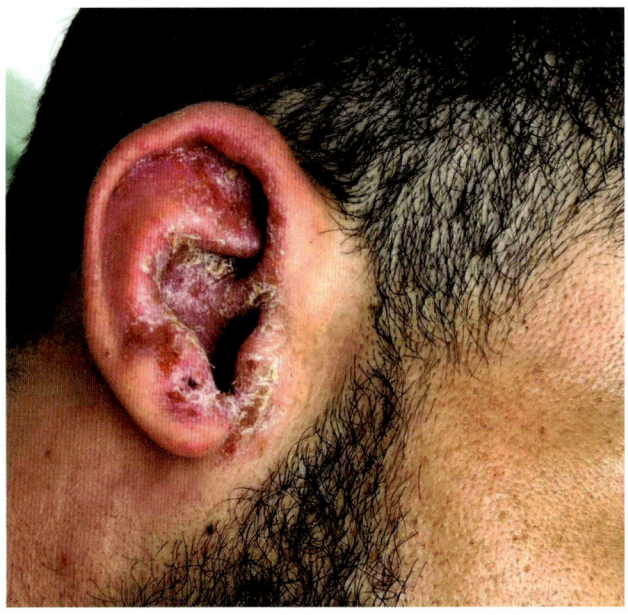

FIGURE 6–17. Erythematous crusted plaque with excoriations on the left ear.
Source. Dr. Malek Ben Slimane.

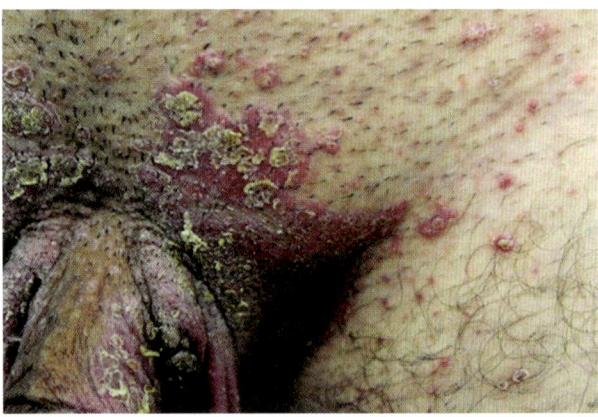

FIGURE 6–18. Erythematous, crusted plaque in the pubic region.
Source. Dr. Malek Ben Slimane.

Management

The patient was put on daily topical steroids. A nurse applied the ointment under occlusive bandaging. Skin lesions gradually improved. The patient was advised for CBT.

Discussion

Malingering in dermatology is the deliberate imitation or production of skin lesions with an intent of secondary gain. Occupational dermatitis artefacta is an infrequent subtype of malingering. In this context, the intentional production of skin lesions is motivated by its recognition as an occupational affliction, attaining a higher class of disability pension, or obtaining continuation of a prior disease (Bonamonte et al. 2022). Through the infliction of dermatitis artefacta, malingering soldiers try to gain sick leave and reduce their duties (Cohen and Vardy 2006). Occupational dermatitis artefacta is characterized by bizarre morphological features and repeated negative findings of all clinical consultations and tests. These patients always have some workplace conflicts and stressful situation with their superiors.

Causal agents are highly varied and strange (Bonamonte et al. 2022). Several methods of malingering among soldiers have been reported, including rubbing freshly ground garlic on various areas of the skin or applying a potato or an onion to the skin with an occlusive dressing overnight (Wolf et al. 2002). The diagnosis of occupational dermatitis artefacta might be confirmed by confessions obtained from the patient after repeated confidential discussions during the interview process (Bonamonte et al. 2022). CBT and psychoanalytic psychotherapy, alone or in combination with psychotropic drugs, seem to achieve the best results in the most challenging cases (Tomas-Aragones et al. 2017).

TEACHING POINTS

- Occupational dermatitis artefacta is motivated by the gain of sick leave, reduced duties, or financial compensation.
- Treatment consists of cognitive-behavioral therapy and psychoanalytic psychotherapy, alone or in combination with psychotropic drugs.

References

Bonamonte D, Foti C, DE Marco A, et al: Self-inflicted pathological cutaneous disorders: part II. Ital J Dermatol Venereol 157(6):480–488, 2022 36177780

Cohen AD, Vardy DA: Dermatitis artefacta in soldiers. Mil Med 171(6):497–499, 2006 16808128

Tomas-Aragones L, Consoli SM, Consoli SG, et al: Self-inflicted lesions in dermatology: a management and therapeutic approach: a position paper from the European Society for Dermatology and Psychiatry. Acta Derm Venereol 97(2):159–172, 2017 27563702

Wolf R, Orion E, Matz H: Contact dermatitis in military personnel. Clin Dermatol 20(4):439–444, 2002 12208633

Case 6-12
Dermatitis Artefacta: A Case Report

Imen Baati, M.D.
Madiha Mseddi, M.D.
Rim Sellami, M.D.
Hamida Turki, M.D.

Case Description

A 27-year-old single woman who was right-handed and worked in the clothing manufacturing industry presented to the dermatology department with bulla on the limbs evolving for 12 hours. The patient reported that similar lesions had appeared 2 years earlier and then spontaneously disappeared.

She had an appendectomy 4 years earlier and no history of other medical or psychiatric disorders or consumption of psychoactive substances. On clinical examination, she was afebrile, with good general condition. Dermatological examination revealed bullous lesions on an erythematous background, located on the external surface of the right thigh and knee (Figure 6–19). Anamnesis showed no medication taken or exposure to a caustic or thermal harming agent. The patient reported professional conflicts and job abandonment 2 months before.

Differential Diagnosis

- Bullous fixed drug eruption
- Dermatitis artefacta

Dermatitis Artefacta

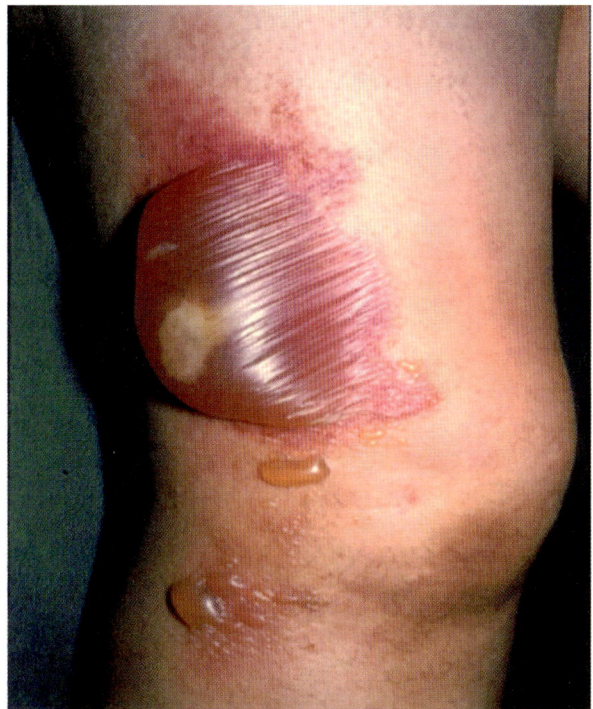

FIGURE 6-19. Vesicles and bulla on the right thigh and knee.
Source. Dr. Madiha Mseddi.

Diagnosis

Results of blood tests including complete blood count, sedimentation rate, glycemia, urea, and ionogram were normal. On psychiatric examination, the patient did not show depressive or psychotic symptoms. Her speech focused on workplace conflicts. She reported that she lost her temper at the slightest annoyance and was intolerant of frustrations. No obvious external incentives were suspected at the first psychiatric evaluation.

The diagnosis of dermatitis artefacta was retained.

Management

The patient was admitted in the dermatology department and received bubble puncture and dressing. After 6 days, blistered lesions dried up. She was referred for psychiatric outpatient consultation but was lost to follow-up.

Discussion

The patient profile of a single young female is in accordance with data in the literature about dermatitis artefacta (Bonamonte et al. 2022; Mohandas et al. 2013). Skin lesions are often polymorphic, with a sudden onset and without a prodromal stage (Bonamonte et al. 2022). The most common lesions are excoriations and ulcerated lesions (Shivakumar et al. 2021). Vesicular and bullous lesions, as in this patient, are less frequent (Bonamonte et al. 2022). The main clinical differential diagnosis includes immunobullous diseases (Mahon et al. 2019).

Young women more frequently produce lesions in uncovered accessible regions; older or perimenopausal women tend to produce lesions in hidden regions, particularly the breasts (Gregurek-Novak et al. 2005). In this patient, it was difficult to identify the mechanism causing the lesions. In fact, secrecy about the origin of the lesions favors of the diagnosis of dermatitis artefacta (Rodríguez-Pichardo et al. 2010). In the literature, self-inflicted bullous lesions can be caused using vegetable extracts or other chemical agents (Bonamonte et al. 2022), such as deodorant spray (Mahon et al. 2019).

Most patients deny having induced their skin lesions themselves. They may end up confessing to their act when an appropriate relationship has been established with the caregiver (Tomas-Aragones et al. 2017). However, they fail to explain why. For those who persist in their denial, they probably dissociate while they self-inflict. These patients would not remember how the lesions occurred and would appear emotionally uninvolved when describing the history of the illness (Shivakumar et al. 2021).

Classically, subjects with dermatitis artefacta are emotionally and socially isolated, with frequent professional instability and precarious family ties that can go back to childhood (Bonamonte et al. 2022). Some patients have experienced loss of family members and loved ones early in life (Mohandas et al. 2013). Dermatitis artefacta is likened to an emotional safety valve in vulnerable patients. Thus, it is essential to explore psychosocial stressors, rather than determining how the patient created the lesions (Mohandas et al. 2013).

The onset of this disorder often coincides with a triggering life event, such as professional conflicts in this patient's case. Life events vary according to age: school exams, harassment, and family discord in children (Mohandas et al. 2013); widowhood, estrangement from children, recent appearance of a somatic pathology in older adults (Gregurek-Novak et al. 2005).

Patients with dermatitis artefacta tend to communicate very poorly and, when upset or angry, hurt their skin to draw attention to themselves (Anwar et al. 2004) or to look for a fixed and secure relationship with a doctor (Bonamonte et al. 2022). Dermatitis artefacta remains a diagnosis of exclusion (Kuhn et al. 2017), oriented by the context in which the lesions appeared. Additional investigations and histological study, although not specific, make it possible to rule out other skin conditions that could be life-threatening, such as bullous dermatoses, autoimmune disease, and cancer.

Regarding treatment, the main benefit of hospitalization is separation from home surroundings and the isolation of lesions using occlusive dressings. These dressings have a dual interest: to obtain healing of the lesions and to confirm their provoked nature (Kuhn et al. 2017).

Self-induced lesions are the expression of psychological suffering, hence the importance of patient-dermatologist communication helping to make an earlier diagnosis of dermatitis artefacta (Tomas-Aragones et al. 2017). Skin lesions could be understood as an indirect cry for help (Bonamonte et al. 2022). Thus, each patient suspected of having dermatitis artefacta requires a psychiatric evaluation in search of the motivations for the behavior (predictive and triggering factors) and a possible underlying psychiatric disorder.

Dermatitis artefacta does not necessarily indicate a particular personality disorder, but it can be accompanied by certain traits, such as intolerance of frustration, poor self-esteem, impulsivity and emotional dependence, and "behavior of sickness" observed among major consumers of care (Lemogne et al. 2006).

The psychiatric evaluation is easier to carry out in the hospital, during the dermatology stay. Furthermore, patients referred to psychiatry are often lost to follow-up, as with this patient. One in two patients openly express their refusal to be examined by a psychiatrist (Rodríguez-Pichardo et al. 2010). This reluctance to have psychiatric follow-up results from the pejorative image and stigma of psychiatry. To focus on stress as the probable mediator of dermatitis artefacta could be a rationale for the introduction of psychotherapy or a psychiatric consultation (Tomas-Aragones et al. 2017).

TEACHING POINTS

- Given a reduced number of bullous lesions, monomorphic appearance, and absence of medication, self-induced dermatosis must be considered.
- The presence of a state of stress, conflict, or annoyance could be an additional element in favor of the diagnosis of self-induced dermatosis.

References

Anwar W, Murphy N, Powell FC: Learning the cost of dermatitis artefacta. Clin Exp Dermatol 29(5):576–578, 2004 15347361

Bonamonte D, Foti C, DE Marco A, et al: Self-inflicted pathological cutaneous disorders: part I. Ital J Dermatol Venereol 157(5):389–401, 2022 36062949

Gregurek-Novak T, Novak-Bilić G, Vucić M: Dermatitis artefacta: unusual appearance in an older woman. J Eur Acad Dermatol Venereol 19(2):223–225, 2005 15752297

Kuhn H, Mennella C, Magid M, et al: Psychocutaneous disease: clinical perspectives. J Am Acad Dermatol 76(5):779–791, 2017 28411771

Lemogne C, Fossati P, Allilaire JF: From pathomimesis to medical addiction: a dimensional approach and therapeutic perspectives. Ann Med Psychol (Paris) 164:676–681, 2006

Mahon C, Webber L, Bisson N, et al: Aerosolised deodorant-induced bullous dermatitis artefacta: a clinicopathological correlation. Australas J Dermatol 60(4):331–333, 2019 31158918

Mohandas P, Bewley A, Taylor R: Dermatitis artefacta and artefactual skin disease: the need for a psychodermatology multidisciplinary team to treat a difficult condition. Br J Dermatol 169(3):600–606, 2013 23646995

Rodríguez-Pichardo A, Hoffner MV, García-Bravo B, et al: Dermatitis artefacta of the breast: a retrospective analysis of 27 patients (1976–2006). J Eur Acad Dermatol Venereol 24(3):270–274, 2010 19694893

Shivakumar S, Jafferany M, Kumar SV, et al: A brief review of dermatitis artefacta and management strategies for physicians. Prim Care Companion CNS Disord 23(4):20nr02858, 2021 34228404

Tomas-Aragones L, Consoli SM, Consoli SG, et al: Self-inflicted lesions in dermatology: a management and therapeutic approach: a position paper from the European society for dermatology and psychiatry. Acta Derm Venereol 97(2):159–172, 2017 27563702

7

Prurigo Nodularis

Sara Al Janahi, M.D., M.Sc.
Dimitre Dimitrov, M.D., Ph.D.

Introduction

Prurigo nodularis, also termed chronic nodular prurigo or prurigo nodularis of Hyde, is a chronic inflammatory, pruritic condition that classically presents with dome-shaped papules and nodules, symmetrically distributed on the extensor extremities and trunk (Frølunde et al. 2022). The etiology of prurigo nodularis remains unclear, but the underlying mechanism is thought to be secondary to chronic pruritus, which can be of cutaneous, systemic, infectious, or neuropsychiatric origin (Iking et al. 2013). The most reported cutaneous association is atopic dermatitis, but prurigo nodularis can also be associated with plaque psoriasis, lichen planus, or dermatitis herpetiformis (Bewley et al. 2022; Iking et al. 2013). Localized disease may be secondary to venous stasis, postherpetic neuralgia, or brachioradial pruritus (Pereira et al. 2018).

Pathophysiology

The main factors theorized to be involved in the pathogenesis of prurigo nodularis are neuronal sensitization, inflammation, and pruritus (Bewley et al. 2022; Williams et al. 2021). Prurigo nodularis likely results from a multifactorial process involving T-helper 2 cytokines, specifically interleukin (IL)-4, IL-5, and IL-13 playing a crucial role (Fukushi et al. 2011; Williams et al. 2021).

Neuronal alteration is visible in prurigo nodularis lesions, with an increased number of Merkel cells in the epidermis and an increase in papillary dermal nerves (Williams et al. 2021). There is also noted to be an increased density of mast cells, neutrophils, and eosinophil-derived neurotoxins; however, there is no increase in eosinophils (Mullins et al. 2022). The pruritus is mediated by neuropeptides such as substance P, calcitonin gene-related peptide (CGRP), and vanilloid receptor subtype 1 (Mullins et al. 2022). In addition, IL-31 levels are elevated (Mullins et al. 2022). A recent study reported that increased plasma levels of eight circulating inflammatory biomarkers were ascertained in prurigo nodularis patients in comparison with control subjects (Parthasarathy et al. 2023).

Epidemiology

The estimated prevalence of prurigo nodularis in the United States is 72 per 100,000 people (Huang et al. 2020a); the prevalence in England was recently reported as 3.27 per 10,000 people (Morgan et al. 2022). Middle-aged individuals in the fifth and sixth decades of life, especially women, are most affected by prurigo nodularis (Amer and Fischer 2009). An epidemiological study reported the mean age as 50.9 years and the median age as 54; however, prurigo nodularis has also been reported in children (Boozalis et al. 2018).

Increased risk has been reported in patients of color, with Black individuals being 3.4 times more likely to develop prurigo nodularis and having higher morbidity compared with White or Hispanic individuals (Boozalis et al. 2018; Huang et al. 2020b; Sutaria et al. 2022).

Comorbidities

The impact of the systemic comorbidities of prurigo nodularis frequently outweighs that of atopic dermatitis or psoriasis (Huang et al. 2020b). Systemic associations include endocrine disorders, particularly diabetes mellitus types 1 and 2, and increased risk of hypertension, hyperlipidemia, and obesity (Boozalis et al. 2018; Huang et al. 2020a, 2020b; Mullins et al. 2022; Sutaria et al. 2022; Zeidler et al. 2021). There is also increased risk of autoimmune diseases, such as celiac disease, Hashimoto thyroiditis, ulcerative colitis, and Crohn disease (Francesco Stefanini et al. 1999; Huang et al. 2020a, 2020b). The association between prurigo nodularis and renal disease, especially end-stage renal disease, is well established (Huang et al.

2020b; Kim et al. 2022; Kowalski et al. 2019). There may be hematologic, pulmonary, and cardiovascular involvement in patients with prurigo nodularis, as well (Huang et al. 2020b).

Infectious associations include HIV and hepatitis C. In regions where HIV is endemic, such as French Guiana, prurigo nodularis has been shown to have a high positive predictive value (72%) for poorly managed HIV and advanced immunosuppression (Huang et al. 2020b; Magand et al. 2011). There have been reports of prurigo nodularis lesions responding to raltegravir, an antiretroviral agent used to treat HIV (Motegi et al. 2014; Unemori et al. 2010).

There is evidence that prurigo nodularis may arise with cutaneous lymphoma or mycosis fungoides, hematologic malignancies such as non-Hodgkin and Hodgkin lymphoma, and malignancies of the gastrointestinal tract (Funaki et al. 1996; Jerković Gulin et al. 2015; Larson et al. 2019; Rubenstein and Duvic 2006; Shelnitz and Paller 1990). Therefore, it is important to rule out those diagnoses before making the diagnosis of prurigo nodularis (Dazzi et al. 2011). Chronic pruritic dermatoses often demonstrate an association with psychiatric comorbidities, including anxiety and depression (Jafferany and Davari 2019).

Complications

Prurigo nodularis has a significant effect on quality of life, often leading to psychological distress, sleep disturbances, anxiety, and depression (Kowalski et al. 2019). Jørgensen et al. (2017) reported that the depression and anxiety experienced are often severe enough to warrant pharmacological intervention. However, there was no significant difference in the rate of completed suicides in patients with prurigo nodularis compared with control subjects (Funaki et al. 1996; Huang et al. 2020b).

Huang et al. (2020a) reported increased odds of eating disorders, self-harm, ADHD, and schizophrenia in patients with prurigo nodularis compared with age- and sex-matched control subjects. Delusional infestation has also been reported as a complication of prurigo nodularis (Dervout et al. 2020). Prurigo nodularis lesions may become infected if not properly treated.

Clinical Features

Clinical presentation includes the appearance of firm, dome-shaped, pruritic nodules, which can range in number from a few to >100 lesions and may vary from pink to brown-black in color (Figures 7–1 and 7–2). The lesions often occur in a symmetrical pattern, affecting the trunk and extensor

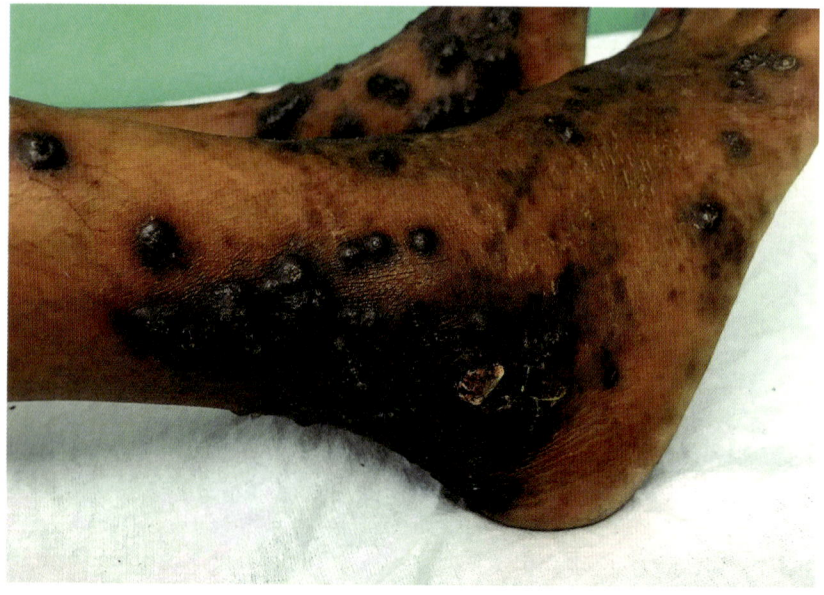

FIGURE 7–1. Nodular hyperpigmented lesions of prurigo nodularis.
Source. Dr. Prajwal Pudasaini.

extremities, but spare the face and hard-to-reach areas such as the upper mid-back (Mullins et al. 2022). This distribution is referred to as the butterfly sign (Huang et al. 2020b; Mullins et al. 2022). Pruritus is the main clinical feature, which can be exacerbated by sweating, clothing irritation, or heat. However, burning, stinging, and alterations in the temperature of the lesions have also been reported in some patients (Iking et al. 2013). Any excoriated lesions pose a risk of secondary infection (Mullins et al. 2022).

Dermoscopy

Prurigo nodularis is a clinical diagnosis, but dermoscopy can aid in distinguishing it from hypertrophic lichen planus (HLP). Nair and Patel (2019) reported red dots, globules, and pearly white areas with peripheral striations in prurigo nodularis; pearly white areas and peripheral striations, gray-blue globules, comedo-like openings, red dots and globules, brownish-black globules, and yellowish structures were observed in HLP.

Prurigo Nodularis

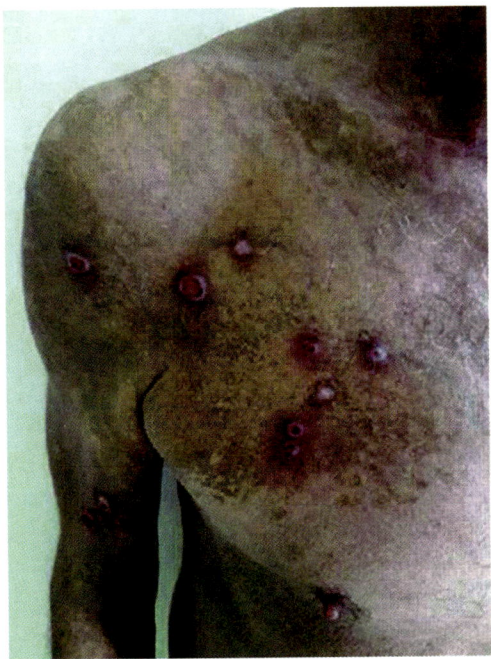

FIGURE 7–2. Ulcerated nodules on the trunk and right arm in a patient with prurigo nodularis.
Source. Dr. Asmahane Souissi.

Histopathology

A skin biopsy may be warranted for lesions that are bleeding, have formed ulcers, or are resistant to first-line therapies (Mullins et al. 2022). Biopsies of prurigo nodularis nodules show thickened, hyperplastic dermal nerve fibers with decreased density of intraepidermal nerve fibers (Huang et al. 2020b; Zeidler et al. 2021). Lesional skin may also demonstrate thickened, hyperplastic dermal nerve fibers with decreased density of intraepidermal nerve fibers (Huang et al. 2020b).

Management

Management of prurigo nodularis is multifaceted and consists of individually tailored treatment processes. General care consists of encouraging patients to keep their fingernails short, wear long sleeve clothing or gloves, and keep nodules covered with bandages. Patients should also be encouraged to maintain the skin barrier by using gentle cleansers and keeping the skin moisturized (Mullins et al. 2022).

Potent topical steroids under occlusion are suggested as a first-line therapy (Mullins et al. 2022). Intralesional triamcinolone acetonide in concentrations of 10–20 mg/mL were found to be effective in flattening lesions and providing relief from pruritus (Mullins et al. 2022).

Alternative topical agents include pimecrolimus 1%, which was as effective as hydrocortisone for non-atopic prurigo nodularis (Siepmann et al. 2013). Calcipotriol ointment showed greater efficacy than betamethasone valerate 0.1% or menthol in concentrations <5% (Patel et al. 2007; Wong and Goh 2000). Other effective therapeutic agents for prurigo nodularis include antihistamines, the Janus kinase (JAK) inhibitor tofacitinib, apremilast, azathioprine, cyclosporine, methotrexate, oral alitretinoin, oral tacrolimus, naltrexone, cyclophosphamide, thalidomide, and lenalidomide (Chen et al. 2010; Chung et al. 2020; Gupta 2016; Halvorsen and Aasebø 2015; Kanavy et al. 2012; Klejtman et al. 2018; Lear et al. 1996; Mullins et al. 2022; Peng et al. 2022; Todberg et al. 2020; Wiznia et al. 2018).

Alternative options for treatment include phototherapy (ultraviolet B [UVB], UVA, and UVA plus psoralen), excimer laser (308 nm), or acupuncture (Brenninkmeijer et al. 2010; Williams et al. 2020; Wu and Dong 2021). Cannabinoids, selective serotonin reuptake inhibitors (SSRIs), and tricyclic antidepressants (TCAs) can be considered for chronic pruritus (Khanna et al. 2021; Mullins et al. 2022). Neurokinin-1 receptor antagonists, such as aprepitant or serlopitant, reduce itch by blocking substance P and may be helpful for chronic pruritus associated with prurigo nodularis (He et al. 2017; Ständer et al. 2019).

Dupilumab is a human monoclonal IgG4 antibody that inhibits the signaling of IL-4 and IL-13 by binding to the IL-4 Ra subunit shared by the IL-4 and IL-13 receptor complexes. It is approved for use in atopic dermatitis and asthma and has shown great benefit in prurigo nodularis (Cao et al. 2023; Wieser et al. 2020). Additionally, dupilumab has been noted to significantly reduce pruritus, improve health-related quality of life, and lessen depressive symptoms in patients with prurigo nodularis (Lönndahl et al. 2022). In September 2022, dupilumab was approved by the FDA for adults with prurigo nodularis. Nemolizumab, a humanized monoclonal antibody that blocks the α subunit of the IL-31 receptor, rapidly alleviates pruritus. It also restores epithelial function and promotes skin barrier integrity, thus reducing inflammation and severity of lesions in atopic dermatitis and prurigo nodularis, making it a promising option for prurigo nodularis (Serra-Baldrich et al. 2022; Ständer et al. 2022). Another treatment option on the horizon includes KPL-716, an OSM β receptor activated by monocytes and T lymphocytes, which has been studied in atopic dermatitis and is currently being investigated for prurigo nodularis (Williams et al. 2020).

In prurigo nodularis management, it is important to appreciate the role of psychological distress in the etiopathogenesis of this difficult-to-treat chronic condition. As with other psychodermatological disorders, psychological factors are thought to play an important role in triggering and maintaining prurigo nodularis. Therefore, the best result might be expected from adding various psychopharmacological and psychotherapeutic approaches to the treatment plan. Antidepressants from various groups (SSRIs, TCAs), as well as anxiolytic drugs, may be helpful. The danger of dependence should be kept in mind with anxiolytic medications.

SSRIs may require a higher-than-usual dose to reduce the patient's compulsion to scratch, as SSRIs have independent anti-itching properties (Bewley and Barlow 2021). TCAs, such as amitriptyline or doxepin, are usually used in lower doses and can be helpful as an antipruritic agent; however, they also have significant sedative properties that may not be desirable in the long term (Bewley and Barlow 2021). Other psychotropic agents, such as antipsychotics, may be considered if a practitioner is well experienced in prescription and patient monitoring (Bewley and Barlow 2021). Control of pruritus with oral ketotifen and topical antibiotics has been reported as well (Sharma 2013).

Applying various forms of psychological therapy in prurigo nodularis may be helpful in allowing patients to understand the psychological distress that is causing and maintaining the disease. Psychoeducation is very important, as the patient will benefit from understanding the nature of the disease and the role of stress in the disease. CBT and its subtype, habit reversal training, have been used with success in many cases where compulsive scratching is prominent. Other psychotherapeutic treatments that can be used for the management of prurigo nodularis are acceptance and commitment therapy, neurolinguistic programming, and eye movement desensitization and reprocessing (Bewley and Barlow 2021). A study reported that hypnosis and acupuncture were beneficial in prurigo nodularis (Samuels et al. 2011).

Prurigo nodularis is a chronic pruritic disorder that until recently had no approved treatments. However, novel therapeutic options are promising in improving symptoms, clinical lesions, and quality of life.

References

Amer A, Fischer H: Prurigo nodularis in a 9-year-old girl. Clin Pediatr (Phila) 48(1):93–95, 2009 18648078

Bewley A, Barlow R: Nodular prurigo, in Psychodermatology in Clinical Practice. Edited by Bewley A, Lepping P, Taylor R. Cham, Switzerland, Springer, 2021, pp 185–197

Bewley A, Homey B, Pink A: Prurigo nodularis: a review of IL-31RA blockade and other potential treatments. Dermatol Ther (Heidelb) 12(9):2039–2048, 2022 35986886

Boozalis E, Tang O, Patel S, et al: Ethnic differences and comorbidities of 909 prurigo nodularis patients. J Am Acad Dermatol 79(4):714.e3–719.e3, 2018 29733939

Brenninkmeijer EE, Spuls PI, Lindeboom R, et al: Excimer laser vs. clobetasol propionate 0·05% ointment in prurigo form of atopic dermatitis: a randomized controlled trial, a pilot. Br J Dermatol 163(4):823–831, 2010 20491772

Cao P, Xu W, Jiang S, Zhang L: Dupilumab for the treatment of prurigo nodularis: a systematic review. Front Immunol 14:1092685, 2023 36742321

Chen M, Doherty SD, Hsu S: Innovative uses of thalidomide. Dermatol Clin 28(3):577–586, 2010 20510766

Chung BY, Um JY, Kang SY, et al: Oral alitretinoin for patients with refractory prurigo. Medicina (Kaunas) 56(11):599, 2020 33182351

Dazzi C, Erma D, Piccinno R, et al: Psychological factors involved in prurigo nodularis: a pilot study. J Dermatolog Treat 22(4):211–214, 2011 20666670

Dervout C, Stephan F, Misery L: Delusional infestation can be a complication of prurigo nodularis with underlying neuropathies. Acta Derm Venereol 100(14):adv00217, 2020 32556345

Francesco Stefanini G, Resta F, Marsigli L, et al: Prurigo nodularis (Hyde's prurigo) disclosing celiac disease. Hepatogastroenterology 46(28):2281–2284, 1999 10521982

Frølunde AS, Wiis MAK, Ben Abdallah H, et al: Non-atopic chronic nodular prurigo (prurigo nodularis hyde): a systematic review of best-evidenced treatment options. Dermatology 238(5):950–960, 2022 35417906

Fukushi S, Yamasaki K, Aiba S: Nuclear localization of activated STAT6 and STAT3 in epidermis of prurigo nodularis. Br J Dermatol 165(5):990–996, 2011 21711341

Funaki M, Ohno T, Dekio S, et al: Prurigo nodularis associated with advanced gastric cancer: report of a case. J Dermatol 23(10):703–707, 1996 8973036

Gupta R: Treatment of prurigo nodularis with dexamethasone-cyclophosphamide pulse therapy. Indian J Dermatol Venereol Leprol 82(2):239, 2016 26924412

Halvorsen JA, Aasebø W: Oral tacrolimus treatment of pruritus in prurigo nodularis. Acta Derm Venereol 95(7):866–867, 2015 25804254

He A, Alhariri JM, Sweren RJ, et al: Aprepitant for the treatment of chronic refractory pruritus. BioMed Res Int 2017:4790810, 2017 29057261

Huang AH, Canner JK, Khanna R, et al: Real-world prevalence of prurigo nodularis and burden of associated diseases. J Invest Dermatol 140(2):480–483.e4, 2020a 31421126

Huang AH, Williams KA, Kwatra SG: Prurigo nodularis: epidemiology and clinical features. J Am Acad Dermatol 83(6):1559–1565, 2020b 32454098

Iking A, Grundmann S, Chatzigeorgakidis E, et al: Prurigo as a symptom of atopic and non-atopic diseases: aetiological survey in a consecutive cohort of 108 patients. J Eur Acad Dermatol Venereol 27(5):550–557, 2013 22364653

Jafferany M, Davari ME: Itch and psyche: psychiatric aspects of pruritus. Int J Dermatol 58(1):3–23, 2019 29917231

Jerković Gulin S, Čeović R, Lončarić D, et al: Nodular prurigo associated with mycosis fungoides: case report. Acta Dermatovenerol Croat 23(3):203–207, 2015 26476905

Jørgensen KM, Egeberg A, Gislason GH, et al: Anxiety, depression and suicide in patients with prurigo nodularis. J Eur Acad Dermatol Venereol 31(2):e106–e107, 2017 27505149

Kanavy H, Bahner J, Korman NJ: Treatment of refractory prurigo nodularis with lenalidomide. Arch Dermatol 148(7):794–796, 2012 22801610

Khanna R, Khanna R, Denny G, et al: Cannabinoids for the treatment of chronic refractory pruritus. J Dermatolog Treat 32(2):266–267, 2021 31264498

Kim HS, Kim HJ, Ahn HS: Impact of chronic kidney disease severity on the risk of prurigo nodularis: a population-based cohort study. Acta Derm Venereol 102:adv00781, 2022 35971831

Klejtman T, Beylot-Barry M, Joly P, et al: Treatment of prurigo with methotrexate: a multicentre retrospective study of 39 cases. J Eur Acad Dermatol Venereol 32(3):437–440, 2018 29055135

Kowalski EH, Kneiber D, Valdebran M, et al: Treatment-resistant prurigo nodularis: challenges and solutions. Clin Cosmet Investig Dermatol 12:163–172, 2019 30881076

Larson VA, Tang O, Stander S, et al: Association between prurigo nodularis and malignancy in middle-aged adults. J Am Acad Dermatol 81(5):1198–1201, 2019 30954580

Lear JT, English JS, Smith AG: Nodular prurigo responsive to azathioprine. Br J Dermatol 134(6):1151, 1996 8763446

Lönndahl L, Lundqvist M, Bradley M, et al: Dupilumab significantly reduces symptoms of prurigo nodularis and depression: a case series. Acta Derm Venereol 102:adv00754, 2022 35670328

Magand F, Nacher M, Cazorla C, et al: Predictive values of prurigo nodularis and herpes zoster for HIV infection and immunosuppression requiring HAART in French Guiana. Trans R Soc Trop Med Hyg 105(7):401–404, 2011 21621233

Morgan CL, Thomas M, Ständer S, et al: Epidemiology of prurigo nodularis in England: a retrospective database analysis. Br J Dermatol 187(2):188–195, 2022 35083742

Motegi S, Kato M, Uchiyama A, et al: Persistent prurigo nodularis in HIV-infected patient responsive to antiretroviral therapy with raltegravir. J Dermatol 41(3):272–273, 2014 24479440

Mullins TB, Sharma P, Riley CA, et al: Prurigo Nodularis. Treasure Island, FL, StatPearls Publishing, 2022

Nair PA, Patel T: Dermatoscopic features of prurigo nodularis. Indian Dermatol Online J 10(2):187–189, 2019 30984602

Parthasarathy V, Cravero K, Xu L, et al: The blood proteomic signature of prurigo nodularis reveals distinct inflammatory and neuropathic endotypes: a cluster analysis. J Am Acad Dermatol 88(5):1101–1109, 2023 36806647

Patel T, Ishiuji Y, Yosipovitch G: Menthol: a refreshing look at this ancient compound. J Am Acad Dermatol 57(5):873–878, 2007 17498839

Peng C, Li C, Zhou Y, et al: Tofacitinib for prurigo nodularis: a case report. Clin Cosmet Investig Dermatol 15:503–506, 2022 35340735

Pereira MP, Basta S, Moore J, et al: Prurigo nodularis: a physician survey to evaluate current perceptions of its classification, clinical experience and unmet need. J Eur Acad Dermatol Venereol 32(12):2224–2229, 2018 29869425

Rubenstein M, Duvic M: Cutaneous manifestations of Hodgkin's disease. Int J Dermatol 45(3):251–256, 2006 16533224

Samuels N, Sagi E, Singer SR, et al: Hypnosis and acupuncture (hypnopuncture) for prurigo nodularis: a case report. Am J Clin Hypn 53(4):283–292, 2011 21598842

Serra-Baldrich E, Santamaría-Babí LF, Francisco Silvestre J: Nemolizumab: an innovative biologic treatment to control interleukin 31, a key mediator in atopic dermatitis and prurigo nodularis. Actas Dermosifiliogr 113(7):674–684, 2022 35842249

Sharma AD: Oral ketotifen and topical antibiotic therapy in the management of pruritus in prurigo nodularis: a randomized, controlled, single-blind, parallel study. Indian J Dermatol 58(5):355–359, 2013 24082179

Shelnitz LS, Paller AS: Hodgkin's disease manifesting as prurigo nodularis. Pediatr Dermatol 7(2):136–139, 1990 2359730

Siepmann D, Lotts T, Blome C, et al: Evaluation of the antipruritic effects of topical pimecrolimus in non-atopic prurigo nodularis: results of a randomized, hydrocortisone-controlled, double-blind phase II trial. Dermatology 227(4):353–360, 2013 24281309

Ständer S, Kwon P, Hirman J, et al: Serlopitant reduced pruritus in patients with prurigo nodularis in a phase 2, randomized, placebo-controlled trial. J Am Acad Dermatol 80(5):1395–1402, 2019 30894279

Ständer S, Yosipovitch G, Lacour JP, et al: Nemolizumab efficacy in prurigo nodularis: onset of action on itch and sleep disturbances. J Eur Acad Dermatol Venereol 36(10):1820–1825, 2022 35766128

Sutaria N, Semenov YR, Kwatra SG: Understanding racial disparities in prurigo nodularis. J Am Acad Dermatol 87(3):e111–e112, 2022 35577228

Todberg T, Skov L, Simonsen S, et al: Efficacy of apremilast in patients with prurigo nodularis: a proof-of-concept study. Acta Derm Venereol 100(8):adv00118, 2020 32189005

Unemori P, Leslie KS, Maurer T: Persistent prurigo nodularis responsive to initiation of combination therapy with raltegravir. Arch Dermatol 146(6):682–683, 2010 20566941

Wieser JK, Mercurio MG, Somers K: Resolution of treatment-refractory prurigo nodularis with dupilumab: a case series. Cureus 12(6):e8737, 2020 32714676

Williams KA, Huang AH, Belzberg M, et al: Prurigo nodularis: pathogenesis and management. J Am Acad Dermatol 83(6):1567–1575, 2020 32461078

Williams KA, Roh YS, Brown I, et al: Pathophysiology, diagnosis, and pharmacological treatment of prurigo nodularis. Expert Rev Clin Pharmacol 14(1):67–77, 2021 33191806

Wiznia LE, Callahan SW, Cohen DE, et al: Rapid improvement of prurigo nodularis with cyclosporine treatment. J Am Acad Dermatol 78(6):1209–1211, 2018 29438756

Wong SS, Goh CL: Double-blind, right/left comparison of calcipotriol ointment and betamethasone ointment in the treatment of prurigo nodularis. Arch Dermatol 136(6):807–808, 2000 10871962

Wu D, Dong G: A case of prurigo nodularis treating by acupuncture. Clin Cosmet Investig Dermatol 14:1815–1818, 2021 34880640

Zeidler C, Pereira MP, Augustin M, et al: Investigator's global assessment of chronic prurigo: a new instrument for use in clinical trials. Acta Derm Venereol 101(2):adv00401, 2021 33236125

Case 7-1
Prurigo Nodularis in a 45-Year-Old Woman

Prajwal Pudasaini, M.D.
Sushil Paudel, M.D.
Sadiksha Adhikari, M.D.

Case Description

A 45-year-old woman presented with nodular, pigmented lesions over her bilateral upper and lower limbs for the past 2 years. The patient is a farmer who works predominantly in the fields and gave a history of evanescent urticarial wheals, on and off, for many years, with seasonal exacerbation. She had dry skin with chronic pruritus, which interfered with her daily activities and work productivity. Her itch was exacerbated whenever she was physically and mentally stressed, affecting her quality of life.

The skin lesions started as a single, pinhead-sized, soft, raised lesion. The lesions were red in color, and they presented initially over the upper right arm and increased in both size and number along with crust formation. The lesions progressed to form nodules with surrounding brown-black pigmentation.

On examination, symmetrically distributed multiple discrete nodules and plaques were present over the bilateral upper and lower limbs, the largest one measuring 1.5 cm and oval in shape over the left upper arm (Figure 7–3). The surrounding skin was thickened and pigmented with prominent

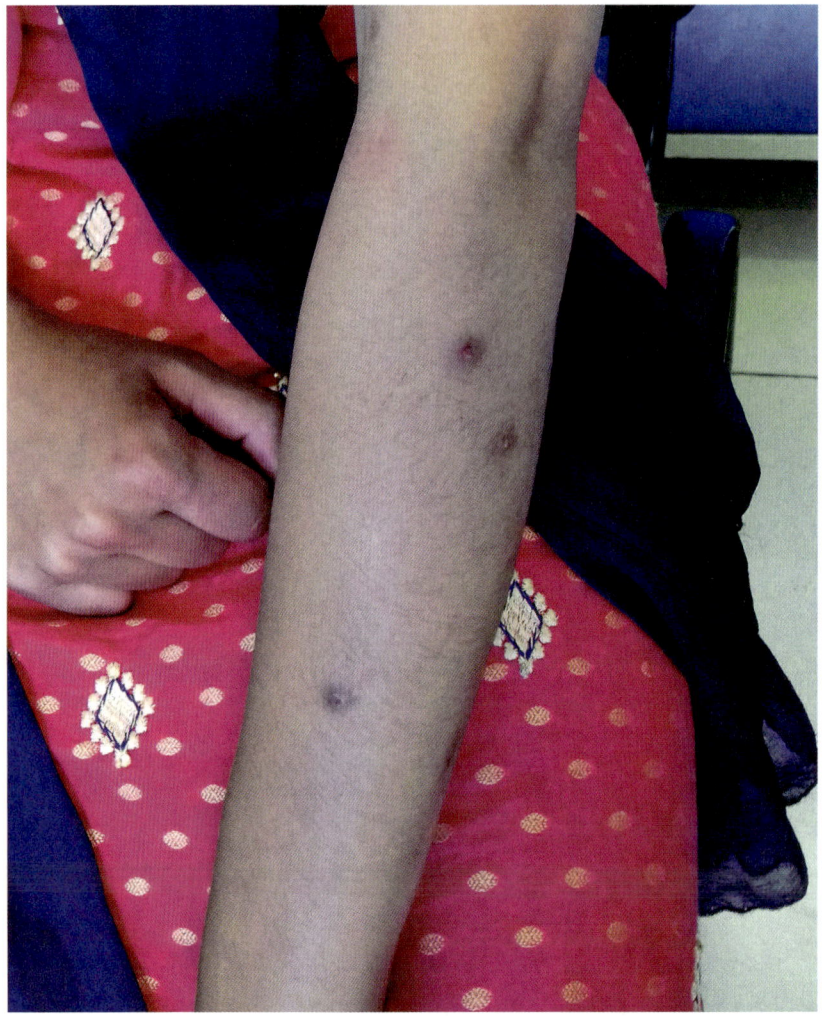

FIGURE 7–3. Typical prurigo nodularis lesion: multiple discrete nodules over the extensor aspect of the left upper arm and forearm, with crusted surface and surrounding brownish black hyperpigmentation.
Source. Dr. Prajwal Pudasaini.

margins (lichenification) (Figure 7–4). A biopsy was performed, which displayed a thick and compact keratinized layer, like volar skin, with folliculosebaceous units in nonvolar skin, pseudoepitheliomatous hyperplasia, hypergranulosis, focal parakeratosis, and increased numbers of fibroblasts and inflammatory infiltrates. These findings were suggestive of prurigo nodularis (Figure 7–5).

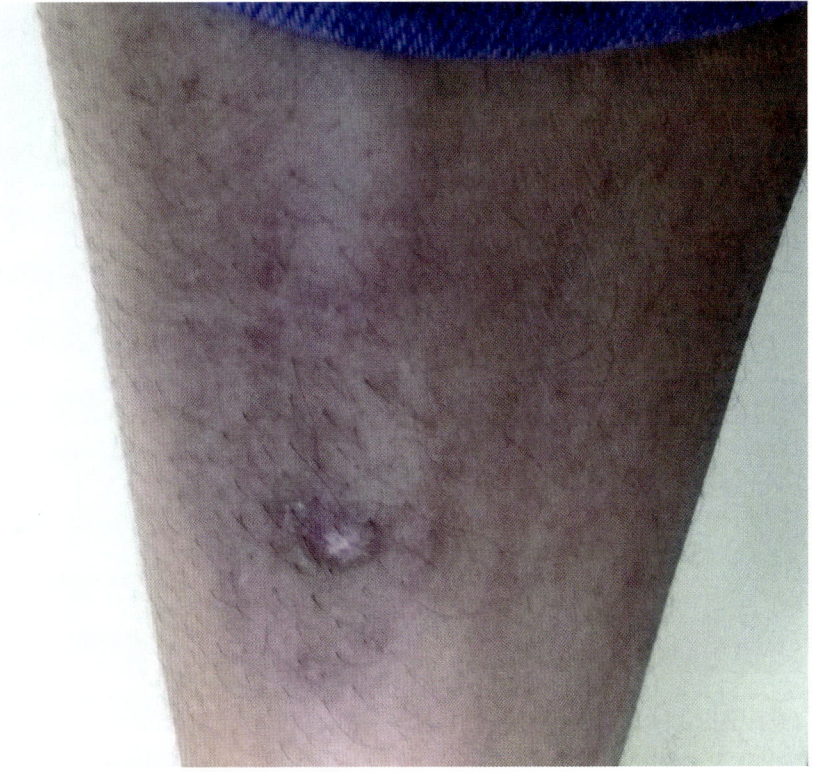

FIGURE 7–4. A solitary papulonodular lesion and central crust surrounding hyperpigmentation, with impending lichen simplex chronicus over the periphery of the right shin of the lower leg.
Source. Dr. Prajwal Pudasaini.

Differential Diagnosis

- Hypertrophic lichen planus
- Linear IgA disease
- Nodular scabies
- Actinic prurigo

Diagnosis

The clinical pictures and histopathological findings were suggestive of prurigo nodularis.

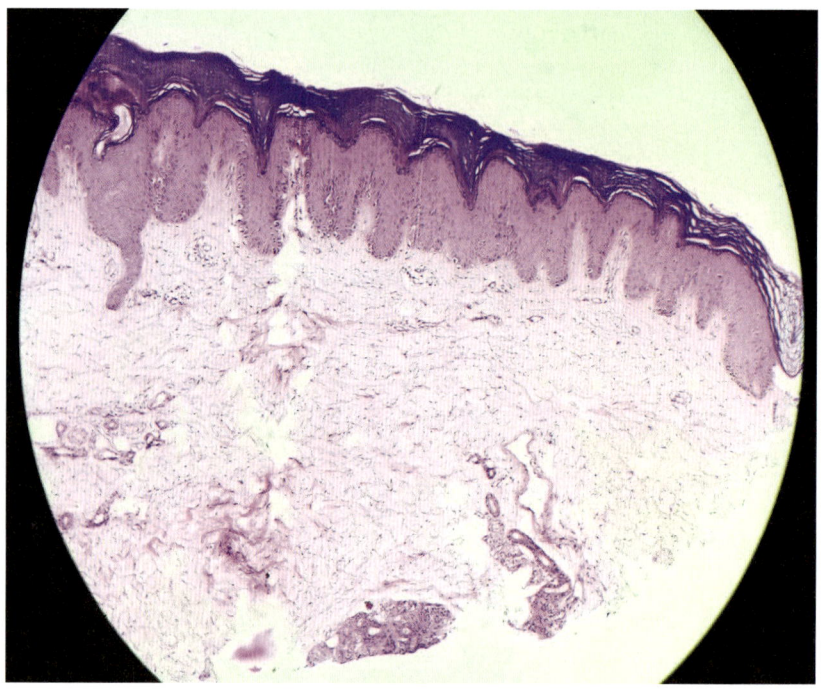

FIGURE 7–5. Biopsy shows epidermis lined by keratinized squamous epithelium with orthokeratosis, parakeratosis, and irregular acanthosis along with mild to moderate perivascular mononuclear inflammatory cell infiltrate and mild fibrosis of papillary dermis.
Source. Dr. Prajwal Pudasaini.

Management

General precautions to avoid skin irritation and excessive dryness were given to the patient. The patient was advised to avoid field work for some time and was treated for her dry skin with frequent and liberal use of petrolatum-based moisturizers along with liquid paraffin. Use of nonalkaline soaps, lukewarm showers of short duration, and application of moisturizer after showering were advised. Psychosocial counseling and educational training were provided. A menthol-based ointment was applied twice a day along with weekly pulsed topical potent steroid cream for 6 weeks, followed by tacrolimus 0.1% twice a day as maintenance therapy for 3 months. Hydroxyzine 25 mg at nighttime was given for 1 month along with oral pregabalin 75 mg for 3 months. Significant improvement in pruritus and lesion morphology was seen after 3 months. The patient has remained symptom free with only occasional exacerbations during field work.

Discussion

Prurigo nodularis is a recalcitrant, often treatment-resistant psychodermatological entity, occurring on the background of chronic pruritus of varied etiology. Clinically, it manifests with pruritic excoriated papules, nodules, or plaques localized predominantly over the extensor aspects of limbs and extremities (Mullins et al. 2019). However, the occurrence of prurigo nodularis over acral sites is not uncommon (Albinhamad et al. 2022). Treatment of prurigo nodularis comprises correct assessment and treatment of underlying causal factors of chronic pruritus, such as dermatological, systemic, neuropathic, or psychogenic diseases (Mullins et al. 2019). Among multiple etiological causal factors, patients with atopic dermatitis are more likely to have prurigo nodularis as the cutaneous complication of their disease, due to the vicious itch-pick-scratch cycle (Iking et al. 2013).

This patient, a farmer by occupation, had prurigo nodularis as a sequela of her underlying atopic diathesis, with frequent exacerbation of pruritus while she was performing field work or when she got stressed. The onset of urticarial eruptions with evanescent wheals on dry skin with exacerbation of skin lesions on exposure to dust was also suggestive of her atopic predilection (Iking et al. 2013). All these factors led to occurrence of prurigo nodularis due to intractable pruritus, with subsequent picking and scratching behavior. As prurigo nodularis occurs on the background of underlying etiologies, its diagnosis depends on histopathological corroboration of clinical findings with underlying primary dermatological conditions.

A holistic treatment approach of prurigo nodularis should incorporate objective assessment of chronic pruritus and quality of life (Janmohamed et al. 2021). Most patients with prurigo nodularis are long-term sufferers of their chronic pruritus, with significantly reduced quality of life as assessed by the Dermatology Life Quality Index, in which multiple subdomains are affected (Ruppenstein et al. 2021). As in this case, patients with prurigo nodularis have reduced quality of life due to chronic pruritus, urticarial eruptions, and effects on daily activities and work productivity; hence psychological counseling was provided. Additionally, prurigo nodularis can be caused by a psychogenic itch caused by delusional disorders, stress, or mood disorders such as major depression or anxiety (Iking et al. 2013). Patients of lower socioeconomic status are more likely to manifest with at least one of these psychological comorbidities; however, a vast majority of patients do not go for psychiatric consultation. Hence, psychotherapy along with oral antidepressants and mood stabilizers may be needed for the holistic treatment of this recalcitrant condition (Mullins et al. 2019).

TEACHING POINTS

- Prurigo nodularis is a persistent, recurrent condition occurring on a background of chronic intractable pruritus.

- Female patients of low socioeconomic status are more likely to have anxiety, depression, or mood disorder, and these patients are also less likely to seek psychiatric counseling.

- A holistic approach to treatment of any chronic skin condition should address not only physical disease, but also the mental health component with psychotherapy or psychotropic medications when needed.

References

Albinhamad A, Almazied M, Alharithy R, et al: Acral prurigo nodularis: a case report. Cureus 14(9):e29405, 2022 36304386

Iking A, Grundmann S, Chatzigeorgakidis E, et al: Prurigo as a symptom of atopic and non-atopic diseases: aetiological survey in a consecutive cohort of 108 patients. J Eur Acad Dermatol Venereol 27(5):550–557, 2013 22364653

Janmohamed SR, Gwillim EC, Yousaf M, et al: The impact of prurigo nodularis on quality of life: a systematic review and meta-analysis. Arch Dermatol Res 313(8):669–677, 2021 33108524

Mullins TB, Sharma P, Riley CA, et al: Prurigo nodularis: vulvar disease. In Vulvar Disease: Breaking the Myths. Edited by Bornstein J. Cham, Switzerland, Springer International, 2019, pp. 227–228

Ruppenstein A, Limberg MM, Loser K, et al: Involvement of neuro-immune interactions in pruritus with special focus on receptor expressions. Front Med (Lausanne) 8:627985, 2021 33681256

Case 7-2
Prurigo Nodularis in a 55-Year-Old Woman

Atiya Rahman, M.D.
Saadia Tabassum, M.D.
Tazein Amber, M.D.

Case Description

A 55-year-old woman presented to the outpatient dermatology department with a 4-year history of skin lesions all over the body, along with persistent and intractable itching. The pruritus was so intense that it hampered her daily functional activities and interfered with sleep. She would scratch the lesions relentlessly until they bled. Despite the bleeding, the patient found solace in the scratching. There was no history of any preceding redness or blisters appearing spontaneously on the skin. The patient had known hypertension, which was well controlled on amlodipine. She was married and had three children. She lived with her spouse in a rural area and had traveled to the city for management of her skin condition. She had taken various topical and oral medications with minimal benefit. Her social life had been affected significantly, as she couldn't stop itching in front of people and had noticed people avoiding her. Many mistook her skin condition as being contagious and avoided physical contact with her. Hence, she had started staying home.

On dermatological examination, there was xerosis cutis, along with multiple, firm, eroded, and crusted papules and nodules ranging from 0.5 to 1.5 cm in size, surrounded by areas of hyperpigmentation. The lesions were scattered symmetrically on the limbs and trunk as shown in Figures 7–6 and 7–7A and B. The head and neck region, mucosae, palms, and soles were spared. General physical and systemic examination was unremarkable.

Differential Diagnosis

Based on her history and examination, differential diagnosis of prurigo nodularis, HLP, and cutaneous transepithelial elimination disorder was considered. As the patient did not give history of any preceding blister formation, nor were any blisters seen during clinical examination, pemphigoid nodularis was ruled out.

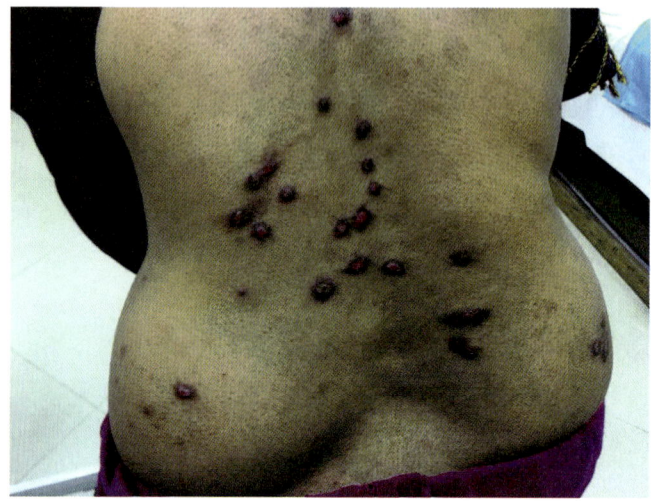

FIGURE 7–6. Excoriated papulonodular lesions with surrounding hyperpigmentation on the lower back.
Source. Dr. Atiya Rahman.

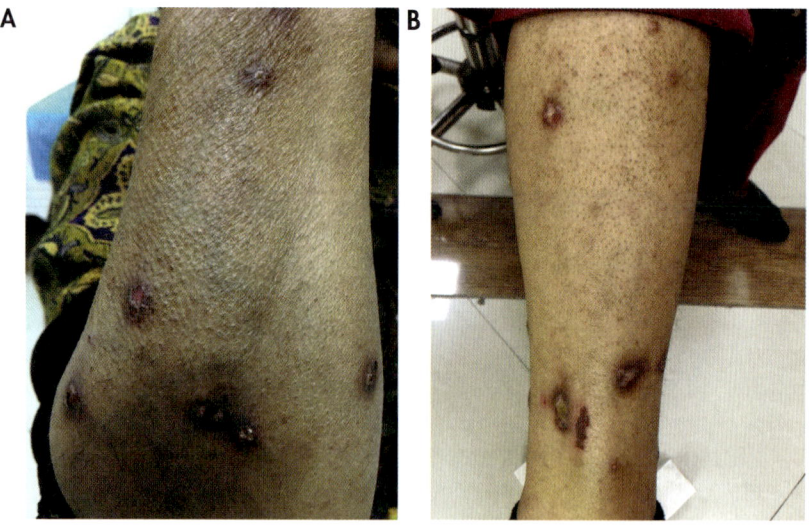

FIGURE 7–7. Prurigo nodular lesions on the extensors of limbs, with surrounding xerotic, hyperpigmented, and lichenified skin.
Source. Dr. Atiya Rahman.

Diagnosis

Laboratory investigations of complete blood count, liver function tests, renal profile, serology for hepatitis B virus and hepatitis C virus, thyroid profile, and serum immunoglobulin E levels were within normal limits. A skin biopsy for histopathology revealed epidermal hyperplasia. There was hyperkeratosis with focal parakeratosis and acanthosis. The basement membrane was intact. The dermis showed moderately dense scattered lymphohistiocytic infiltrate, with few eosinophils and neutrophils. There was accentuation of infiltrate in the perivascular region. Based on clinicopathological findings, a diagnosis of prurigo nodularis was made. Lichen planus was excluded because of the absence of interface dermatitis. Similarly, there was no evidence of transepithelial elimination.

Management

The patient was counseled about her disease and the itch-scratch-itch cycle, which was worsening the condition. On being recommended phototherapy (narrow band ultraviolet B therapy), she was reluctant, as coming to the hospital two to three times per week would be difficult. She was advised to start oral loratadine 20 mg/day, topical steroid fluocinonide 0.05% ointment twice a day, and oral gabapentin 300 mg at nighttime, along with regular use of emollients. The gabapentin was gradually increased to 1,800 mg/day.

After 6 weeks of treatment, the patient reported minimal improvement. She admitted an inability to stop herself from scratching the lesions, even though she knew that scratching would be a self-perpetuating phenomenon worsening her lesions. She was not willing to take oral methotrexate or cyclosporine for her skin condition, as she was wary of their side effects. She was referred to a psychiatrist for interdisciplinary disease management. She was diagnosed to have a co-occurring generalized anxiety disorder. Psychological counseling was provided, and oral escitalopram 10 mg daily was added to her management plan. She returned after a month with much better control of her skin disease.

Discussion

Prurigo nodularis is a poorly understood, extremely pruritic condition. It can be quite frustrating for the patient and the treating dermatologist because of the lack of adequate treatment response. The medical literature on prurigo nodularis is limited, and some studies on chronic itch have grouped prurigo nodularis with other pruritic dermatological disorders (Whang et al. 2019). Prurigo nodularis has also been linked with lichen simplex chronicus. Some authors consider prurigo nodularis to be a variant of lichen simplex in which the patient scratches the skin rather than rubbing and scratching it (Lotti et al. 2008). Constant picking and scratching leads to excoriations and crusting, later transforming into papules and nodules surrounded by hyperpigmentation, as seen in this patient. The lesions are usually symmetrically distributed, with a predilection for the extensor aspect of extremities, back, and buttocks. Face, palms, and soles are usually spared. As the patients find the interscapular region of the back difficult to scratch, it may be spared; this has been called the butterfly sign, as seen in this patient.

There are no uniform histopathological features, but rather, a constellation of changes in prurigo nodularis. There may be pseudoepitheliomatous hyperplasia; hyperkeratosis; focal parakeratosis; hypergranulosis; vertically arranged collagen fibers in the dermis with increased number of fibroblasts; superficial, perivascular, and interstitial inflammatory infiltrate of histiocytes, lymphocytes, eosinophils, and neutrophils; and increased numbers of capillaries. An increase in dermal nerve fibers with S100 stain may be seen in some lesions.

It has been postulated that overexpression of nerve growth factor in prurigo nodularis lesions leads to heightened perception to itch and touch in patients. Initial studies found neural hyperplasia of dermal nerve fibers in prurigo nodularis lesions. Certain neurochemical changes, such as increased staining for CGRP and substance P, along with a local increase in mast cells have been demonstrated. Those substances could modulate heightened itch perception through release of proinflammatory cytokines such as tumor necrosis factor α and IL-1, -4, -6, -17, -22, and -31 (Molloy et al. 2020; Oetjen et al. 2017). Interestingly, some studies have revealed that the sensory, unmyelinated epidermal nerve fibers (sensory C fibers), which play an important role in the pathogenesis of pruritus, were found to be reduced in prurigo nodularis lesions and perilesional skin. These gains in the understanding of the pathophysiology of prurigo nodularis have led to the development of newer therapeutic modalities to treat this challenging disorder.

Essentially, all conditions that can induce chronic pruritus may lead to the development of prurigo nodularis. It has been associated with underlying chronic disorders such as chronic kidney disease, chronic hepatitis C, HIV infection, chronic obstructive pulmonary disease, congestive heart failure, hypertension, depression, xerosis cutis, and atopic dermatitis (Boozalis et al. 2018; Huang et al. 2020). A judicious plan of management of chronic pruritus in these conditions needs to be formulated, although at times pruritus is persistent and unaffected by therapeutic modalities.

Prurigo nodularis has a profound effect on the patient, considerably impacting multiple domains of quality of life (Janmohamed et al. 2021). Effects on psychological well-being have been documented to be much more intense in prurigo nodularis compared with other chronic cutaneous dermatoses, such as atopic dermatitis and psoriasis (Huang et al. 2020). Furthermore, prurigo nodularis has been associated with mental health illnesses such as depression, OCD, and anxiety (Konuk et al. 2007). From a psychosomatic perspective, emotional stress leads to the sensation of pruritus in predisposed individuals, with the unavoidable urge to scratch the skin, leading to the formation of the distinct skin lesions of prurigo nodularis.

This patient had dry, xerotic skin and co-occurring generalized anxiety disorder that worsened her pruritus. Some studies have found the highest likelihood of prurigo lesions in association with atopic predisposition and atopic dermatitis, and the lesions have been given a distinct name: Besnier prurigo.

Prurigo nodularis is generally a refractory skin disorder, and tackling pruritus is the priority of treating dermatologists to inhibit the itch-scratch-itch cycle. Topical agents such as emollients, potent steroids, calcineurin inhibitors, and the substance P–depleting agent capsaicin have limited success. They have been augmented with oral or intralesional steroids, a combination of oral antihistamines, and neuromodulating agents such as gabapentin and pregabalin, but the response may be inadequate. Phototherapy has been tried with varying success, but in our experience, patient compliance is problematic, as it is difficult to come to the hospital two or three times a week for months, along with the financial burden incurred.

Of possible use in managing prurigo nodularis are immunosuppressive agents such as methotrexate, cyclosporine, mycophenolate mofetil, azathioprine, and thalidomide. They all have considerable side effects and need vigilant monitoring and regular follow-ups. This patient refused immunosuppressive agents for those reasons. Moreover, the response has been found to be short lived once the drug is withdrawn. Newer therapeutic agents include neuropeptide antagonists such as serlopitant and aprepitant, the IL-4/-13 inhibitor dupilumab, and the Janus kinase inhibitor tofacitinib; these are not readily available in developing economies, and affordability is a significant issue (Peng et al. 2022).

Psychological and social factors have been linked with certain cutaneous disorders. Researchers have shown the role of stress and psychoneuroimmunologic factors in dermatological conditions such as prurigo nodularis and lichen simplex chronicus (Lotti et al. 2008). A significant proportion of prurigo nodularis patients have underlying psychiatric disorders, which play a role in the pathogenesis or at least in the perpetuation of prurigo nodularis (Han et al. 2022). Given that prurigo nodularis is a challenging disease to manage, with limited efficacious treatment, physicians need to be vigilant to identify and manage any underlying psychiatric comorbidities. This patient showed significant improvement with psychotherapy combined with pharmacological treatment.

TEACHING POINTS

- Prurigo nodularis is significantly associated with psychiatric comorbidities and decreases quality of life.

- Physicians must rule out systemic causes of prurigo nodularis through careful history, clinical examination, and appropriate laboratory workup.

- Management of prurigo nodularis aims to control not only dermatologic and somatosensory aspects, but also psychological components of the disease.

References

Boozalis E, Tang O, Patel S, et al: Ethnic differences and comorbidities of 909 prurigo nodularis patients. J Am Acad Dermatol 79(4):714.e3–719.e3, 2018 29733939

Han J, Palomino A, Estupinan B, et al: Psychiatric comorbidity in prurigo nodularis and the impact of socioeconomic status. J Clin Aesthet Dermatol 15(6):53–58, 2022 35783571

Huang AH, Canner JK, Khanna R, et al: Real-world prevalence of prurigo nodularis and burden of associated diseases. J Invest Dermatol 140(2):480.e4–483.e4, 2020 31421126

Janmohamed SR, Gwillim EC, Yousaf M, et al: The impact of prurigo nodularis on quality of life: a systematic review and meta-analysis. Arch Dermatol Res 313(8):669–677, 2021 33108524

Konuk N, Koca R, Atik L, et al: Psychopathology, depression and dissociative experiences in patients with lichen simplex chronicus. Gen Hosp Psychiatry 29(3):232–235, 2007 17484940

Lotti T, Buggiani G, Prignano F: Prurigo nodularis and lichen simplex chronicus. Dermatol Ther 21(1):42–46, 2008 18318884

Molloy OE, Kearney N, Byrne N, et al: Successful treatment of recalcitrant nodular prurigo with tofacitinib. Clin Exp Dermatol 45(7):918–920, 2020 32484964

Oetjen LK, Mack MR, Feng J, et al: Sensory neurons co-opt classical immune signaling pathways to mediate chronic itch. Cell 171(1):217–228.e13, 2017 28890086

Peng C, Li C, Zhou Y, et al: Tofacitinib for prurigo nodularis: a case report. Clin Cosmet Investig Dermatol 15:503–506, 2022 35340735

Whang KA, Khanna R, Thomas J, et al: Racial and gender differences in the presentation of pruritus. Medicines (Basel) 6(4):98, 2019 31569651

Case 7-3
Prurigo Nodularis— A Frustrating Malady

Usha N. Khemani, M.D.
Neha Fogla, M.D.

Case Description

A 7-year-old girl presented to our clinic with a complaint of intractable itching associated with lesions over the body on and off for a duration of 3 years. The patient's guardian also reported that the patient was irritable and scratched and picked her skin. The patient's medical history revealed that she had received multiple topical and oral corticosteroids in the past, which provided slight relief in her symptoms but resulted in flare-ups after discontinuation. On examination, multiple discrete erythematous excoriated papules and flesh-colored nodules were present, predominantly over bilateral upper and lower limbs, classically sparing the back (Figure 7–8A and B). Dermoscopy revealed a starburst pattern (Figure 7–9). The nodules also showed hyperpigmentation, scarring, and irregular borders.

Differential Diagnosis

- Prurigo nodularis
- Lichen simplex chronicus
- Hypertrophic lichen planus
- Nodular scabies
- Atopic dermatitis

Diagnosis

A diagnosis of prurigo nodularis was made based on the clinical presentation and classic dermoscopy findings.

Management

The patient was treated with phototherapy, low-dose UVA1, for 23 sessions along with topical corticosteroids, emollients, and oral antihistamines for 6 months, which resulted in significant relief from itching and the resolution of lesions. After assessment with the draw-a-person test and the house-tree-person test, psychotherapy was provided to the patient, after which her behavior showed significant improvement.

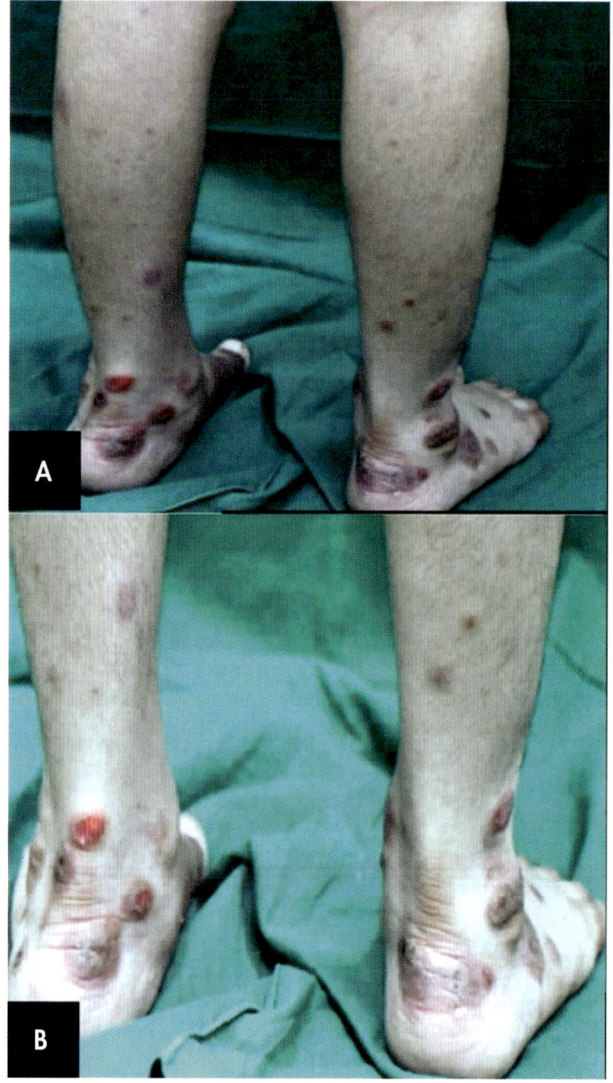

FIGURE 7–8. Excoriated nodules on the legs.
Source. Dr. Usha Khemani.

During follow-up visits, the patient reported a decrease in the intensity and frequency of itching episodes, and the lesions had resolved (Figure 7–10A and B). The hyperpigmented macules persisted, and the patient was advised to continue using emollients and topical corticosteroids. The patient's guardian reported that the child's mood and behavior had significantly improved, and she no longer engaged in scratching and picking of the skin.

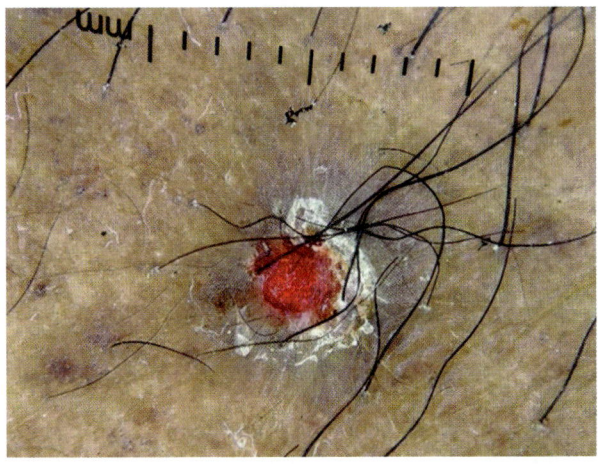

FIGURE 7-9. Dermoscopy suggestive of starburst pattern as seen in prurigo nodularis.

Discussion

UVA1 therapy is an effective treatment option for managing inflammation and itch in patients with prurigo nodularis who do not respond to or cannot tolerate conventional treatments. It can be used in combination with other therapies, such as topical steroids or oral antihistamines, for better outcomes. Because prurigo nodularis can affect a patient's psychological health, leading to anxiety, depression, and social isolation, psychotherapy can be helpful in managing these effects and developing coping strategies (Han et al. 2022). Projective tests such as draw-a-person and house-tree-person are useful in identifying underlying psychological factors that may contribute to prurigo nodularis in children. Combining UVA1 therapy with psychotherapy can provide a comprehensive and effective treatment approach for prurigo nodularis patients, addressing both the physical and psychological aspects of the condition to improve outcomes and enhance overall well-being (Janmohamed et al. 2021).

TEACHING POINTS

- Prurigo nodularis is a challenging condition, particularly in children, and early diagnosis is crucial to prevent chronicity.

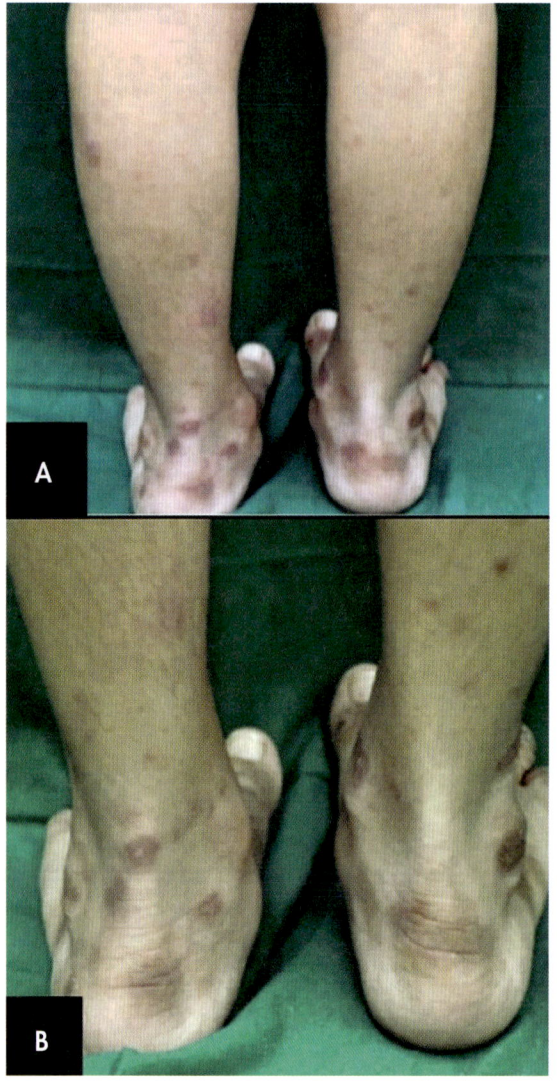

FIGURE 7–10. Lesions healed after UVA1 phototherapy.
Source. Dr. Usha Khemani.

- The starburst pattern observed in dermoscopy aids in distinguishing prurigo nodularis from other nodular skin conditions.
- A multidisciplinary approach, including UVA1 therapy and psychotherapy, can lead to significant symptom relief and improve the quality of life for patients.

References

Han J, Palomino A, Estupinan B, et al: Psychiatric comorbidity in prurigo nodularis and the impact of socioeconomic status. J Clin Aesthet Dermatol 15(6):53–58, 2022 35783571

Janmohamed SR, Gwillim EC, Yousaf M, et al: The impact of prurigo nodularis on quality of life: a systematic review and meta-analysis. Arch Dermatol Res 313(8):669–677, 2021 33108524

Case 7-4
Prurigo Nodularis With Anxiety and Depression

Varsha Gowda, V.M., M.D.
Shrutakirthi D. Shenoi, M.D.
Nidhika V. Sorake, M.D.

Case Description

A 23-year-old woman presented to the dermatology department with complaints of recurrent multiple itchy skin lesions over both arms and legs since childhood. There was history of multiple exacerbations as well as oozing and crusting. A history of atopy was present. The patient had received various topical creams and oral medications with little or no improvement. Dermatological examination revealed multiple hyperpigmented lichenified nodules and plaques of 0.2–1.5 cm^2 over bilateral arms, forearms, and legs, along with excoriations (Figure 7–11A and B).

Differential Diagnosis

- Prurigo nodularis
- Lichen simplex chronicus
- Lichen planus hypertrophicus

Diagnosis

A skin biopsy was performed from lesions of the left arm and leg, and the result showed orthokeratosis with focal parakeratosis, hypergranulosis, and prominent irregular acanthosis with blunt rete ridges in the epidermis. Papillary dermis showed fibrosis with vertically oriented collagen bundles and

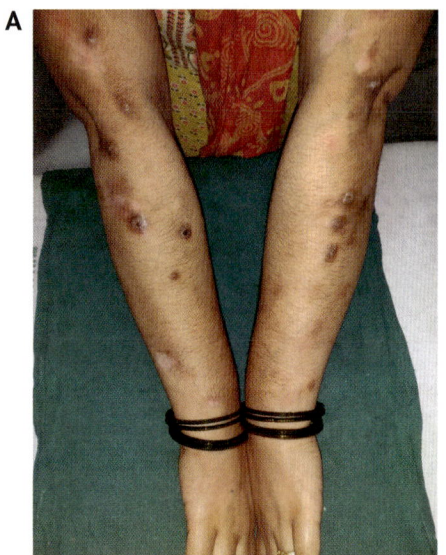

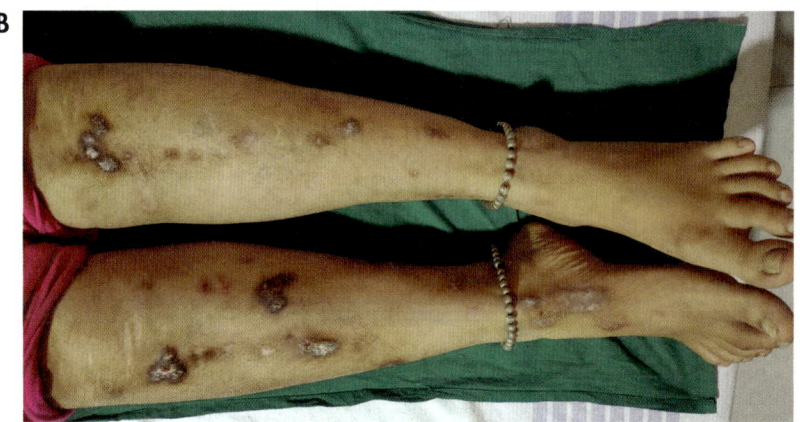

FIGURE 7–11. Hyperpigmented lichenified nodules and plaques over forearms and legs.
Source. Dr. Varsha Gowda.

chronic perivascular inflammatory infiltrate. Complete blood count, urinalysis, random blood sugar, liver function tests, and kidney function tests were within normal limits.

A diagnosis of prurigo nodularis was considered based on clinical and histopathological findings. As the patient complained of low mood and anxiety symptoms, we calculated her Generalized Anxiety Disorder scale and Patient Health Questionnaire scores, which were 16 and 18, respectively, indicative of moderate depression and anxiety. On further psychiatry evaluation, the patient revealed a history of decreased interest in doing daily activities, decreased sleep, on-and-off restlessness, palpitations, headache, increased anger on trivial matters, repeated skin scratching, and removing scabs of skin lesions frequently, for the past few months. There was a history of two episodes of self-harm by consuming multiple tablets of medication. There was no history of hair pulling or skin picking in other areas.

Management

The patient was counseled for lifestyle modifications and prescribed oral fluoxetine 20 mg once daily and oral clonazepam 0.5 mg once daily. Lifestyle measures included attempting to keep her mind busy and cooling the affected areas with chilled flannel on the skin to reduce inflammation and ease the itching. Other measures included keeping the room at a cool temperature and avoiding sleeping with heavy or multiple bedclothes. The patient was instructed to avoid wearing clothes made of synthetic fibers, instead choosing preferably cotton. The patient was also advised to avoid soaps or bath gels that may irritate the skin. The patient was encouraged to apply an emollient at least twice a day and keep her nails short. She was referred to a psychiatrist for habit reversal therapy.

Discussion

Prurigo nodularis is a chronic psychogenic pruritic disorder characterized by intense pruritus, which may be intensified or perpetuated by emotional factors and associated with intrinsic factors, such as local cytokine releases, neuropeptide changes, and inflammatory cell infiltrates (Radmanesh et al. 2011). Patients with prurigo nodularis have a high frequency of psychiatric morbidity, deranged sleep patterns, mood disturbances, anxiety, and depression, which in turn exacerbate the itching (Konuk et al. 2007; Yamamoto et al. 2009). Pruritus itself can significantly impair the quality of life and sleep (Yosipovitch et al. 2000). This patient had difficulty with sleeping and felt depressed.

The exact cause of prurigo nodularis is unknown, but altered function of the immune system and the nerves in the skin is believed to be associated with heightened sensations of itchiness (pruritus) that lead to frequent scratching. Emotional stress and psychological disorders are concurrent factors in some cases. Prurigo nodularis is associated with depression, anxiety, and dissociative disorders that lead to excessive scratching, as in this case (Hughes et al. 2020).

Behavioral modifications and habit reversal therapies play an important role in prurigo nodularis. The first step in habit reversal therapy is to make the patient aware of the habitual element of scratching. It is also important to identify the individual trigger situations and individual scratching profile. Scratching is then replaced by an alternative behavior, such as a competing response (a posture that is anatomically opposite to scratching) or a safe action (clenching fists to a count of 30 and if itch has not subsided, pinching the itchy area instead of scratching) (Grillo et al. 2007). To increase the capacity to deal with itch and decrease frequency of scratching, patients can receive CBT to alter dysfunctional beliefs or behaviors. CBT may be useful in breaking the itch-scratch cycle associated with prurigo nodularis (Bonchak and Lio 2020).

Prurigo nodularis is a benign disorder and has a decent prognosis. The intensity of the itch (which can cause psychological distress), the chronic nature of the ailment, the prolonged duration of therapy, and the potential side effects of the medicine are all barriers to treating prurigo nodularis.

TEACHING POINTS

- Prurigo nodularis is a chronic psychogenic pruritic disorder characterized by intense pruritus, which may be intensified or perpetuated by emotional factors and associated with intrinsic factors, such as local cytokine releases, neuropeptide changes, and inflammatory cell infiltrates.

- SSRIs reduce itch through the attenuation of serotonergic signals, which provide inhibitory inputs to itch pathways in the central nervous system, and hence can be used in prurigo nodularis patients with psychiatric comorbidity.

- Habit awareness and habit reversal therapy, along with cognitive-behavioral therapy, are important aspects of nonpharmacological therapy in treatment of prurigo nodularis.

References

Bonchak JG, Lio PA: Nonpharmacologic interventions for chronic pruritus. Itch 5(1):e31, 2020

Grillo M, Long R, Long D: Habit reversal training for the itch-scratch cycle associated with pruritic skin conditions. Dermatol Nurs 19(3):243–248, 2007 17626502

Hughes J, Woo T, Belzberg M, et al: Association between prurigo nodularis and etiologies of peripheral neuropathy: suggesting a role for neural dysregulation in pathogenesis. Medicines (Basel) 7(1):4, 2020

Konuk N, Koca R, Atik L, et al: Psychopathology, depression and dissociative experiences in patients with lichen simplex chronicus. Gen Hosp Psychiatry 29(3):232–235, 2007 17484940

Radmanesh M, Sharifi M, Shafiei S: Lichen simplex chronicus, neurotic excoriation and nodular prurigo and their correlation with atopy: a case-control study. Iran J Dermatol. 14:25–28, 2011

Yamamoto Y, Yamazaki S, Hayashino Y, et al: Association between frequency of pruritic symptoms and perceived psychological stress: a Japanese population-based study. Arch Dermatol 145(12):1384–1388, 2009 20026846

Yosipovitch G, Goon A, Wee J, et al: The prevalence and clinical characteristics of pruritus among patients with extensive psoriasis. Br J Dermatol 143(5):969–973, 2000 11069504

8

Alopecia Areata

Zeba H. Hafeez, M.D.

Introduction

Alopecia areata is a common autoimmune disorder characterized by non-scarring, and often patchy, hair loss that can affect any hair-bearing area of the body. Alopecia areata has a lifetime risk of ~2%, and the estimated prevalence is 1 in 1,000 people (Strazzulla et al. 2018). Alopecia areata affects all ethnic groups, and both sexes are affected equally. Although alopecia areata may occur at any age, the relative incidence is higher in younger age groups, with the disease most commonly presenting as hair loss in children. Additionally, alopecia areata totalis occurs in 5% of patients with alopecia areata, and 1% of patients may develop alopecia universalis (Otberg and Shapiro 2019).

Etiology and Pathogenesis

Alopecia areata is frequently comorbid with several autoimmune diseases, such as vitiligo, Hashimoto thyroiditis, irritable bowel syndrome, psoriasis/psoriatic arthritis, systemic lupus erythematosus, rheumatoid arthritis, and diabetes mellitus. A major role of gene variants that impact immune responses is implicated in the pathophysiology of the disease (Xing et al. 2014). Serum antibodies to hair follicle tissue are also common. Auto-active cytotoxic CD8 T cells that attack hair follicles, and sometimes nails, and an interferon-γ–driven immune response have been shown to have prominent roles in alopecia areata's pathogenesis (Jabbari et al. 2016; Otberg and Shapiro 2019).

A family history exists in ~20% of alopecia areata cases. A positive family history, childhood onset, ophiasis pattern (band-like hair loss of the fronto-parieto-temporal region), nail changes, and comorbid atopic dermatitis are prognostic of worse outcomes. Identifying a positive family history of alopecia areata and the treatment of comorbid autoimmune diseases may help in managing this condition (MacLean and Tidman 2013; Wang et al. 2018).

Many individuals report experiencing significant emotional stress before the onset of alopecia areata. The perception of stress appears to be a risk factor that could influence the onset and worsening of alopecia areata (Brajac et al. 2003). Antioxidant-oxidant imbalance, which also occurs in many autoimmune diseases, has been shown to be associated with psychological and environmental stress (Acharya and Mathur 2020; Bakry et al. 2014).

Clinical Features

Alopecia areata generally has an acute onset. The disease appears as sharply demarcated, oval or round patches of hair loss, without atrophy (Figure 8–1), with exclamation point hairs (thicker at the apex and progressively thin toward the hair shaft base). Alopecia areata totalis presents with entire scalp hair loss (Figure 8–2), and alopecia universalis involves loss of hair over the entire body. Both alopecia areata totalis and alopecia universalis can occur suddenly or can follow long-standing partial alopecia. Additionally, patches of hair loss can affect the beard. Marie Antoinette syndrome (canities subita) is an acute episode of diffuse alopecia with sudden, "overnight" graying (Navarini et al. 2009). The incidence of nail changes is estimated to be 7%–66% and commonly presents as pitted or sandpaper nails (Chelidze and Lipner 2018).

Diagnosis

In addition to the clinical features detailed above, dermatoscopic evaluation can identify the presence of follicular ostia, exclamation mark hair, cadaver hair (residual hair shafts visible as black dots in the follicular ostia), and yellow dots that confirm the diagnosis (Figure 8–3). Trichoscopic evaluation offers higher magnification to identify these features (Rudnicka et al. 2011). Diffuse alopecia areata can be difficult to diagnose, and in doubtful cases, a scalp biopsy provides confirmation.

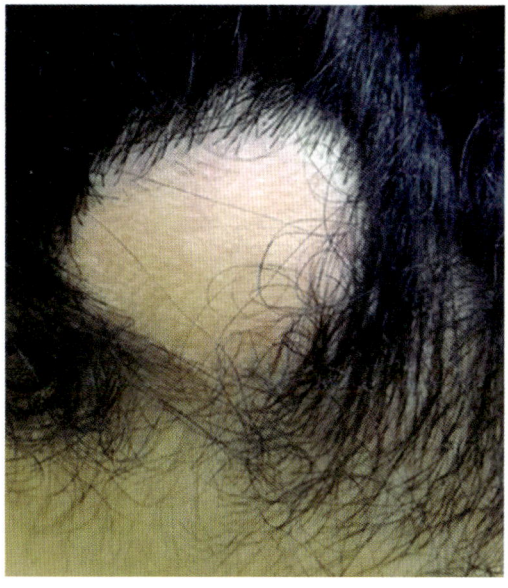

FIGURE 8–1. Sharply demarcated, round patch of hair loss.
Source. Dr. Asmahane Souissi.

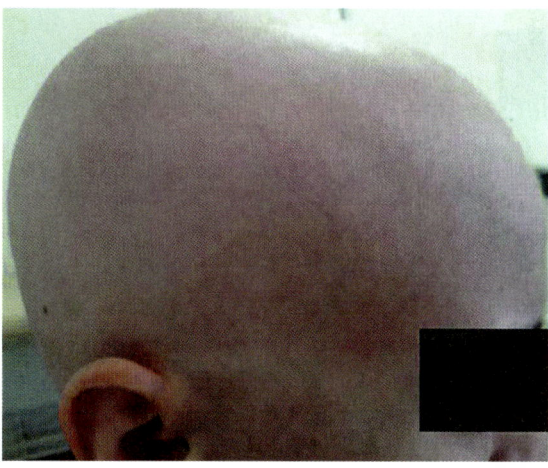

FIGURE 8–2. Alopecia areata totalis.
Source. Dr. Asmahane Souissi.

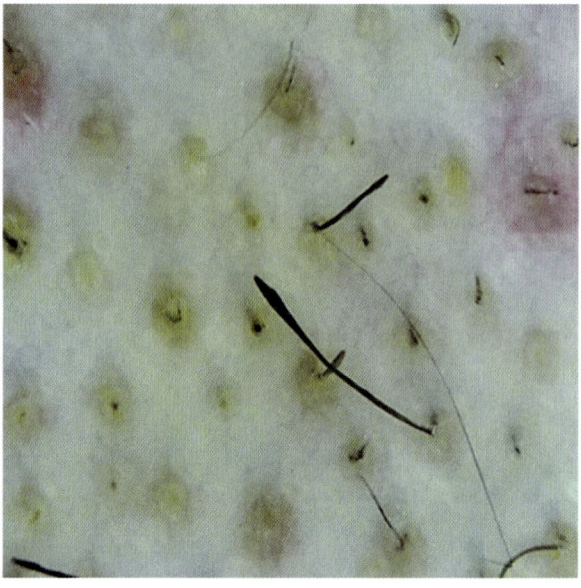

FIGURE 8–3. Trichoscopy of alopecia areata showing exclamation mark hairs, black dots, and yellow dots.
Source. Dr. Asmahane Souissi.

Differential Diagnosis

Table 8–1 shows the differential diagnosis of alopecia areata.

Clinical Course and Prognosis

Alopecia areata has an irregular, relapsing course, with ~25% of affected individuals having a single episode. Hair regrowth can be spontaneous. About 60% of patients have partial regrowth by 1 year. Generally, ~40% of relapses occur within a year, and a significant percentage of patients may relapse after 5 years. Hair that regrows white can change to its natural color over time. Poor prognosis is associated with chronic relapsing course, nail changes, childhood onset, and occiput or hairline involvement.

Psychodermatological Perspective

Alopecia areata can be influenced by psychological factors. Multiple studies conclude that alopecia areata is associated with emotional or physical stress (Matzer et al. 2011; Taheri et al. 2012). Long-standing and extensive alopecia may precipitate serious mental disorders because of the difficulty in

TABLE 8–1. Differential diagnosis of alopecia areata

Temporal triangular alopecia
Tinea capitis
Trichotillomania
Early scarring alopecia
Secondary syphilis
Androgenetic alopecia
Telogen effluvium
Anagen effluvium
Chemotherapy-induced alopecia
Pressure-related alopecia
Aplasia cutis

accepting one's appearance and the social isolation that subsequently occurs. Commonly reported environmental triggers include bereavement, divorce, loss of employment, injury resulting in an impaired quality of life, and social withdrawal. The comorbid mental health conditions most frequently seen with alopecia areata are generalized anxiety disorder, social phobia, body dysmorphic disorder, PTSD, major depressive disorder (MDD), and suicidal ideation (Koo et al. 1994; Kuty-Pachecka 2015).

A population-based retrospective cohort study identified a two-way association between MDD and alopecia areata. Patients with alopecia areata were at risk of developing MDD, and MDD was a significant risk factor for precipitating alopecia areata (Vallerand et al. 2019). About 50% of children and adolescents with alopecia areata were shown to have depression (Ghanizadeh and Ayoobzadehshirazi 2014). Other comorbid conditions identified in children were OCD (35.7%), specific phobia (28.6%), separation anxiety (7.1%), and PTSD (7.1%) (Ghanizadeh 2008; Ghanizadeh and Ayoobzadehshirazi 2014).

In a retrospective case-controlled review of alopecia areata, alopecia areata totalis, and alopecia universalis, a significant association between alopecia universalis and stimulant medication use was found in ADHD patients. Close monitoring was recommended for alopecia universalis patients, as well as discontinuation of stimulants upon signs of worsening disease. No association between stimulant use and other types of hair loss was found (Meaux et al. 2021). Another recent study determined that the risk of alopecia areata in children with ADHD was higher than in those without ADHD. However, there was no statistically significant reduction in the risk of alopecia areata in children who received methylphenidate compared with those who did not (Ho et al. 2021).

Schizophrenia is not commonly seen in patients with alopecia areata, and a negative association with schizophrenia, as well as bipolar disorder, has been reported in the literature (Ghanizadeh and Ayoobzadehshirazi 2014; Tzur Bitan et al. 2022). Additionally, depressive symptoms were more profound in women affected by hair loss compared with men (Ho et al. 2021).

In another study, two patients with alopecia areata manifested self-induced nail trauma or habit tic nail disorder related to psychological stress (Horne et al. 2018). Poor adjustment to alopecia areata was associated with generalized anxiety, depression, dependent personality disorder, and anti-social personality disorder (Kuty-Pachecka 2015; Ruiz-Doblado et al. 2003). Alopecia areata can be comorbid with alexithymia, which presents as diminished emotional awareness, impaired interpersonal relationships, and lack of social cohesiveness (Koo et al. 1994; Kuty-Pachecka 2015; Willemsen et al. 2009). Therefore, it is recommended that alopecia areata patients be evaluated for alexithymia.

Treatment

There is a high rate of spontaneous remission, especially in patients with a brief history and limited scalp involvement. Unfortunately, this occurrence is rare in alopecia areata totalis and alopecia universalis (Otberg and Shapiro 2019). Various treatment modalities are shown in Table 8–2.

A multidisciplinary approach, involving psychiatric evaluation and appropriate dermatologic care, is recommended. Patient education, psychological support, and screening for mental health disorders are important aspects of management. Local alopecia areata support groups and camouflage with wigs increase social confidence, with women reporting more improvement with these interventions than men (Park et al. 2018). Hair pieces, bandanas, false eyelashes, and semipermanent tattoos can also be considered.

Managing negative emotions and insecurities is important, especially at the first onset of hair loss. Appropriate coping mechanisms for regulating emotions could increase the possibility of spontaneous remission of alopecia areata (Matzer et al. 2011). CBT, insight-oriented psychotherapy, individual or group therapy, family therapy, hypnotherapy, psychotherapeutic stress-and-anxiety management techniques, and psychotropic medications have a known therapeutic role in the treatment of alopecia areata (Kuty-Pachecka 2015; Moattari and Jafferany 2022; Vallerand et al. 2019). A case-control study that compared psychotherapy and relaxation training in addition to immunosuppressants versus immunosuppressants alone identified more hair regrowth in patients undergoing psycho-immunotherapy than in those treated with immunosuppressants alone (Toussi et al. 2021).

TABLE 8–2. Treatment of alopecia areata

Topical corticosteroids	Class I and class II topical corticosteroids applied under occlusion or in combination with minoxidil
Intralesional corticosteroids	Preferred therapy for adult patients with <50% scalp involvement
Systemic corticosteroids	Effective but controversial; should not be used routinely, especially as the long-term prognosis is not altered
Platelet-rich plasma injections	Monotherapy or in combination with other therapies
Topical minoxidil 5% solution	Better results when combined with class I and II corticosteroids, or anthralin (minimal efficacy in alopecia areata totalis and alopecia universalis)
Prostaglandin analogs	Monotherapy or as adjunct mainly in alopecia areata of eyelashes/eyebrows
Anthralin	An irritant; may have a nonspecific (anti-Langerhans cell) immunomodulating effect
Topical immunotherapy	The purpose of treatment is to cause contact dermatitis
Photo(chemo)therapy	Ultraviolet B light, oral and topical administration of psoralen followed by ultraviolet A irradiation; risk of various skin cancers, including melanoma
Cyclosporine	4–6 mg/kg/day benefits some patients
Janus kinase inhibitors	Oral baricitinib, tofacitinib, oral ruxolitinib can induce full hair growth in widespread alopecia areata
Nonmedical treatment	Extensive hair loss of scalp can be camouflaged with wigs, hair pieces, or bandanas; semipermanent tattooing for loss of eyebrows

Source. Adapted from Otberg and Shapiro 2019.

Depressed patients, when treated with antidepressants, have a lower risk of having alopecia areata compared with those not taking an antidepressant. Doxepin, imipramine, and paroxetine have been useful in small clinical trials (Cipriani et al. 2001; García-Hernández et al. 1999; Perini et al. 1994). Generally, selective serotonin reuptake inhibitors (SSRIs) are considered to be effective. However, antidepressants, especially SSRIs, may cause hair loss in some patients (Krasowska et al. 2007; Moattari and Jafferany 2022). In a small group of depressed patients, the combination of triamcinolone injections and citalopram significantly improved patches of alopecia areata compared with those who received only steroid injections (Abedini et al. 2014).

References

Abedini H, Farshi S, Mirabzadeh A, et al: Antidepressant effects of citalopram on treatment of alopecia areata in patients with major depressive disorder. J Dermatolog Treat 25(2):153–155, 2014 23339335

Acharya P, Mathur MC: Oxidative stress in alopecia areata: a systematic review and meta-analysis. Int J Dermatol 59(4):434–440, 2020 31875951

Bakry OA, Elshazly RM, Shoeib MA, et al: Oxidative stress in alopecia areata: a case-control study. Am J Clin Dermatol 15(1):57–64, 2014 23839259

Brajac I, Tkalcic M, Dragojević DM, et al: Roles of stress, stress perception and trait-anxiety in the onset and course of alopecia areata. J Dermatol 30(12):871–878, 2003 14739513

Chelidze K, Lipner SR: Nail changes in alopecia areata: an update and review. Int J Dermatol 57(7):776–783, 2018 29318582

Cipriani R, Perini GI, Rampinelli S: Paroxetine in alopecia areata. Int J Dermatol 40(9):600–601, 2001 11737460

García-Hernández MJ, Ruiz-Doblado S, Rodriguez-Pichardo A, et al: Alopecia areata, stress and psychiatric disorders: a review. J Dermatol 26(10):625–632, 1999 10554427

Ghanizadeh A: Comorbidity of psychiatric disorders in children and adolescents with alopecia areata in a child and adolescent psychiatry clinical sample. Int J Dermatol 47(11):1118–1120, 2008 18986440

Ghanizadeh A, Ayoobzadehshirazi A: A review of psychiatric disorders comorbidities in patients with alopecia areata. Int J Trichology 6(1):2–4, 2014 25114444

Ho HY, Wong CK, Wu SY, et al: Increased alopecia areata risk in children with attention-deficit/hyperactivity disorder and the impact of methylphenidate use: a nationwide population-based cohort study. Int J Environ Res Public Health 18(3):1286, 2021 33535410

Horne MI, Rieder EA, Vincenzi C, et al: Alopecia areata and habit tic deformities. Skin Appendage Disord 4(4):323–325, 2018 30410907

Jabbari A, Cerise JE, Chen JC, et al: Molecular signatures define alopecia areata subtypes and transcriptional biomarkers. EBioMedicine 7:240–247, 2016 27322477

Koo JY, Shellow WV, Hallman CP, et al: Alopecia areata and increased prevalence of psychiatric disorders. Int J Dermatol 33(12):849–850, 1994 7883407

Krasowska D, Szymanek M, Schwartz RA, et al: Cutaneous effects of the most commonly used antidepressant medication, the selective serotonin reuptake inhibitors. J Am Acad Dermatol 56(5):848–853, 2007 17147971

Kuty-Pachecka M: Psychological and psychopathological factors in alopecia areata. Psychiatr Pol 49(5):955–964, 2015 26688846

MacLean KJ, Tidman MJ: Alopecia areata: more than skin deep. Practitioner 257(1764):29–32, 2013 24383154

Matzer F, Egger JW, Kopera D: Psychosocial stress and coping in alopecia areata: a questionnaire survey and qualitative study among 45 patients. Acta Derm Venereol 91(3):318–327, 2011 21290087

Meaux TA, McMahon PM, Jones GN, et al: Association of alopecia areata with attention-deficit/hyperactivity disorder stimulant medication: a case-control study. Ochsner J 21(2):139–142, 2021 34239372

Moattari CR, Jafferany M: Psychological aspects of hair disorders: consideration for dermatologists, cosmetologists, aesthetic, and plastic surgeons. Skin Appendage Disord 8(3):186–194, 2022 35707291

Navarini AA, Nobbe S, Trüeb RM: Marie Antoinette syndrome. Arch Dermatol 145(6):656, 2009 19528420

Otberg N, Shapiro J: Alopecia areata, in Fitzpatrick's Dermatology, 9th Edition. Edited by Kang S, Amagai M, Bruckner AL, et al. New York, McGraw Hill, 2019, pp 1517–1522

Park J, Kim DW, Park SK, et al: Role of hair prostheses (wigs) in patients with severe alopecia areata. Ann Dermatol 30(4):505–507, 2018 30065604

Perini G, Zara M, Cipriani R, et al: Imipramine in alopecia areata: a double-blind, placebo-controlled study. Psychother Psychosom 61(3–4):195–198, 1994 8066157

Rudnicka L, Olszewska M, Rakowska A, et al: Trichoscopy update 2011. J Dermatol Case Rep 5(4):82–88, 2011 22408709

Ruiz-Doblado S, Carrizosa A, García-Hernández MJ: Alopecia areata: psychiatric comorbidity and adjustment to illness. Int J Dermatol 42(6):434–437, 2003 12786868

Strazzulla LC, Wang EHC, Avila L, et al: Alopecia areata: disease characteristics, clinical evaluation, and new perspectives on pathogenesis. J Am Acad Dermatol 78(1):1–12, 2018 29241771

Taheri R, Behnam B, Tousi JA, et al: Triggering role of stressful life events in patients with alopecia areata. Acta Dermatovenerol Croat 20(4):246–250, 2012 23317485

Toussi A, Barton VR, Le ST, et al: Psychosocial and psychiatric comorbidities and health-related quality of life in alopecia areata: a systematic review. J Am Acad Dermatol 85(1):162–175, 2021 32561373

Tzur Bitan D, Berzin D, Kridin K, et al: The association between alopecia areata and anxiety, depression, schizophrenia, and bipolar disorder: a population-based study. Arch Dermatol Res 314(5):463–468, 2022 34089375

Vallerand IA, Lewinson RT, Parsons LM, et al: Assessment of a bi-directional association between major depressive disorder and alopecia areata. JAMA Dermatol 155(4):475–479, 2019 30649133

Wang S, Ratnaparkhi R, Piliang M, et al: Role of family history in patchy alopecia areata. Dermatol Online J 24(10):13030/qt0n19r7ps, 2018 30677822

Willemsen R, Haentjens P, Roseeuw D, et al: Alexithymia in patients with alopecia areata: educational background much more important than traumatic events. J Eur Acad Dermatol Venereol 23(10):1141–1146, 2009 19368614

Xing L, Dai Z, Jabbari A, et al: Alopecia areata is driven by cytotoxic T lymphocytes and is reversed by JAK inhibition. Nat Med 20(9):1043–1049, 2014 25129481

Case 8-1
Alopecia Areata Associated With Trichotillomania

Asmahane Souissi, M.D.
Wejden Fakhfekh, M.D.
Mourad Mokni, M.D.

Case Description

A 17-year-old girl with no relevant medical history presented with a 6-month history of hair loss diagnosed as alopecia areata and treated with intralesional corticosteroids for 1 month, with no improvement. She reported that she initially developed a small bald patch on the right parietal region of the scalp that progressively increased in size. Clinical examination showed an irregular large patch of nonscarring alopecia on the right parietal, temporal, and occipital regions of the scalp (Figure 8–4). The underlying skin was of normal appearance with no scaling and no inflammation. There was no involvement of other hair-bearing areas. Nails were normal, and the rest of the physical examination was unremarkable. The patient was accompanied by her brother. She was anxious and apprehensive regarding the lack of improvement despite treatment and asked for further investigations. She has been avoiding public places and covering her head all the time, even at home. Her continued anxiety and social avoidance limited her activity, and she stopped visiting or seeing her friends.

Differential Diagnosis

- Alopecia areata
- Trichotillomania
- Traction alopecia
- Tinea capitis

Diagnosis

After performing trichoscopy at the central area of the patchy alopecia, we noted black dots, broken hairs, exclamation mark hairs, tapered hairs, and yellow dots, consistent with the diagnosis of alopecia areata (Figure 8–5). A

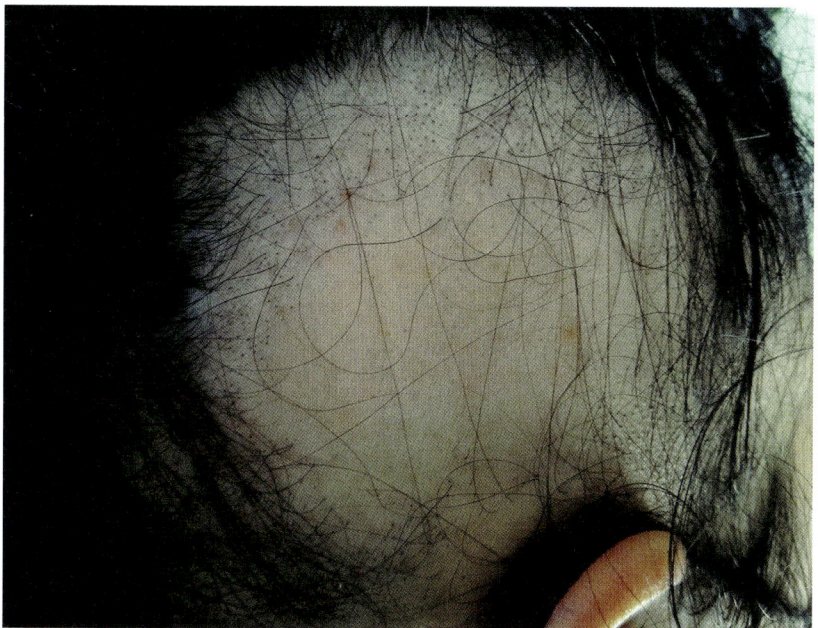

FIGURE 8–4. Irregular large patch of nonscarring alopecia on the right parietal, temporal, and occipital regions of the scalp.
Source. Dr. Asmahane Souissi.

dermoscopic examination of the marginal part of the alopecia patch demonstrated a chaotic trichoscopic pattern with multiple broken hairs of varying lengths, and hemorrhagic suffusions highly suggestive of the diagnosis of trichotillomania (Figure 8–6). The patient denied hair pulling but admitted that she feels constantly anxious. The brother affirmed that he did not notice that his sister was manipulating her hair. According to clinical and trichoscopic findings, we concluded that the patient had alopecia areata in the central area of hair loss, and she was pulling hairs surrounding the alopecia areata patch. The diagnosis of alopecia areata combined with trichotillomania was made.

Management

The patient was reassured and referred to a psychiatrist for psychological counseling and therapy.

Discussion

Co-occurrence of alopecia areata and trichotillomania is uncommon. Few cases have been reported in the literature (Bhalla et al. 2003; Brzezinski et al. 2016; Cua et al. 2021; Ise et al. 2014; Trüeb and Cavegn 1996). Tricho-

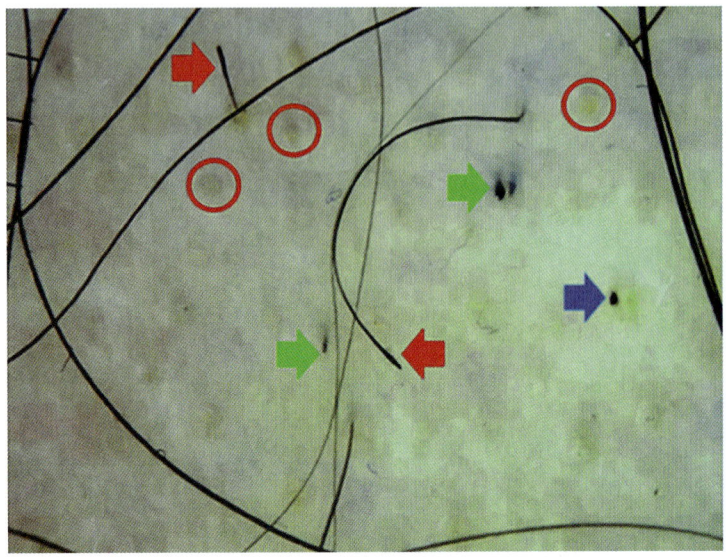

FIGURE 8–5. Dermoscopy of the central area of hair loss: black dots (blue arrows), broken hair (green arrows), exclamation mark hairs (red arrows), and yellow dots (red circles), consistent with the diagnosis of alopecia areata.
Source. Dr. Asmahane Souissi.

tillomania is an obsessive-compulsive related disorder characterized by repetitive hair pulling from the scalp and other hair-bearing areas. Hair pulling causes significant distress and functional impairment. Patients tend to pull hair in response to negative emotions such as anxiety, sadness, and anger (Grant and Chamberlain 2016). The relationship between alopecia areata and trichotillomania is unclear. It has been suggested that trichotillomania may result from scratching alopecia areata patches (Trüeb and Cavegn 1996).

In this case, the patches of trichotillomania were localized at the periphery of alopecia areata hair loss. Alopecia areata was probably the triggering factor for trichotillomania in this patient. Pulling hair may serve as a coping mechanism to release tension and feelings of anxiety. On trichoscopy, the presence of broken hairs in a chaotic arrangement at the periphery of the patchy alopecia was the key for diagnosing trichotillomania. Trichoscopy is very helpful in distinguishing alopecia areata and trichotillomania. In alopecia areata, trichoscopic findings include yellow dots, black dots, exclamation mark hairs, and vellus hairs, whereas in trichotillomania, trichoscopy reveals broken hairs of varying lengths and shapes (Kaczorowska et al. 2021;

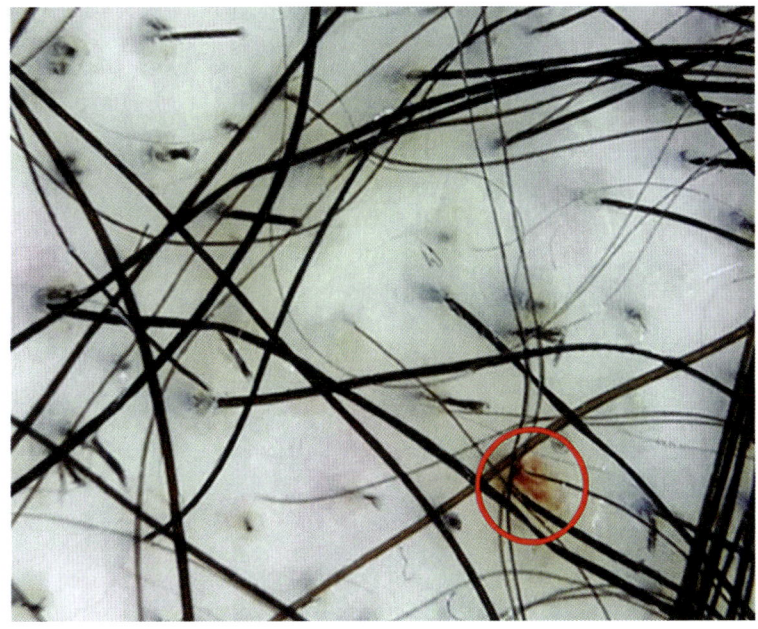

FIGURE 8–6. Dermoscopy of the marginal area of the patchy alopecia: broken hairs of varying lengths and hemorrhagic suffusion (red circle), consistent with the diagnosis of trichotillomania.
Source. Dr. Asmahane Souissi.

Waśkiel et al. 2018). In addition, the presence of follicular microhemorrhages is very suggestive of traumatic plucking (Ise et al. 2014). Trichoscopy was a useful tool for detecting hidden trichotillomania to accelerate psychological management and prevent mental sequelae.

TEACHING POINTS

- Physicians should be aware of the potential association of alopecia areata and trichotillomania.
- This case highlights the importance of trichoscopic findings to make an accurate diagnosis of both alopecia areata and trichotillomania and to provide appropriate psychological management.

References

Bhalla M, Sarkar R, Arun P, et al: Trichotillomania. Indian Pediatr 40(1):52–56, 2003 12554920

Brzezinski P, Cywinska E, Chiriac A: Report of a rare case of alopecia areata coexisting with trichotillomania. Int J Trichology 8(1):32–34, 2016 27127375

Cua VCS, Lizarondo FPJ, Silva CY: Trichotillomania masked by diffuse alopecia areata: a case report. Acta Med Philipp 55(5): 2021

Grant JE, Chamberlain SR: Trichotillomania. Am J Psychiatry 173(9):868–874, 2016 27581696

Ise M, Amagai M, Ohyama M: Follicular microhemorrhage: a unique dermoscopic sign for the detection of coexisting trichotillomania in alopecia areata. J Dermatol 41(6):518–520, 2014 24815359

Kaczorowska A, Rudnicka L, Stefanato CM, et al: Diagnostic accuracy of trichoscopy in trichotillomania: a systematic review. Acta Derm Venereol 101(10):adv00565, 2021 34184065

Trüeb RM, Cavegn B: Trichotillomania in connection with alopecia areata. Cutis 58(1):67–70, 1996 8823553

Waśkiel A, Rakowska A, Sikora M, et al: Trichoscopy of alopecia areata: an update. J Dermatol 45(6):692–700, 2018 29569271

Case 8–2
Alopecia Areata and Psychological Comorbidity

Prajwal Pudasaini, M.D.
Sushil Paudel, M.D.
Sadiksha Adhikari, M.D.
Prashanta Pudasaini, M.D.

Case Description

A 25-year-old man presented with multiple patches of hair loss over the scalp for 3 years. He had a history of recurrent small patches of hair loss over the parieto-occipital region. Hair loss started with an initial small patch over the occipital region that regrew spontaneously within a month. Two months later, similar well-circumscribed patches developed over the occipitoparietal scalp.

On examination, multiple diffuse discrete patches of hair loss were present over the occipitoparietal scalp (Figure 8–7), with easily pluckable hair and exclamation hair seen in the margin of the patch. The largest patch, measuring 0.5 cm and roughly oval in shape, was present over the occipitoparietal scalp 2 cm above the occipital protuberance. Trichoscopy showed short vellus hairs, black dots, broken hairs, and exclamation mark hairs in the periphery. Occasional tapered hairs were also seen (Figures 8–8 through 8–10).

The patient was stressed and depressed about his hair loss, which had been relapsing and remitting for years. He had lost interest in activities that he used to enjoy in the past. He had difficulty falling asleep. He denied any suicidal ideation. The patient had frequent mood swings and anger since the hair loss began, which had affected his college performance. Hair loss had also affected his daily activities and work productivity. He felt stressed most of the time, and the hair loss further exacerbated his physical and mental stress. He was unable to express this feeling of stress to anyone. This prolonged stress and accentuated hair loss affected his quality of life. The patient was given general precautions to avoid repeated rubbing of hair along with counseling about the disease, its natural course, and its prognosis. The patient was counseled and reassured about the possibility of spontaneous remission and the recalcitrant nature if lesions persist for longer durations.

Given the diffuse nature of the disease and the associated psychological comorbidity, the patient was started on 40 mg prednisolone, with the dose tapered over a period of 6 weeks, along with topical clobetasole propionate cream and minoxidil solution for 2 months. Significant hair growth was seen with treatment, except for a few on-and-off discrete patches that were treated with intralesional triamcinolone acetonide 5 mg/mL. Psychosocial counseling was done with proper referral to a psychiatrist. The patient was started on fluoxetine 20 mg at night for 2 months, and significant improvement in his depressive symptoms were seen with therapy. The patient became symptom free and experienced significant improvement in his psychological comorbidity of not being able to express his emotions (alexithymia) and mood changes 2 months into treatment, highlighting the need for concomitant psychotherapy in the treatment of alopecia areata, as in this case.

Differential Diagnosis

- Trichotillomania
- Alopecia areata
- Tinea capitis
- Secondary syphilis

Diagnosis

Alopecia areata was diagnosed with clinical history, examination, and trichoscopy. Cutaneous diagnosis included concurrent diagnosis of psychological comorbidities of depression, social withdrawal, and alexithymia. Biopsy was deferred in our case, which can be performed to confirm and rule out other causes such as scarring alopecia.

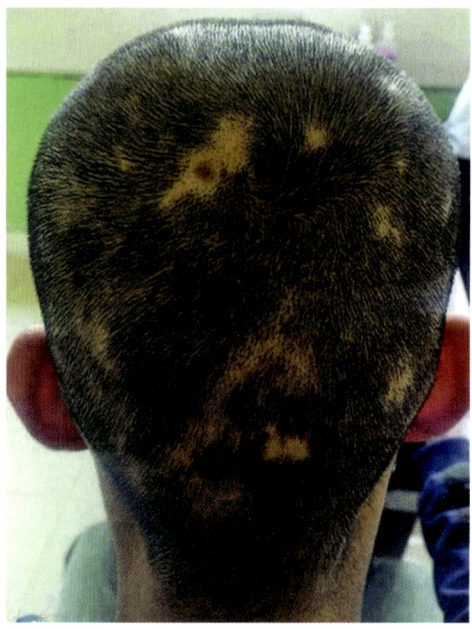

FIGURE 8–7. Alopecia areata: multiple discrete diffuse patches of hair loss over occipitoparietal scalp region.
Source. Dr. Prajwal Pudasaini.

Management

Management of the case was conducted with a multidisciplinary approach. General measures of treatment included proper counseling about the disease and its course and reassurance about spontaneous resolution in a large proportion of cases. Psychosocial counseling, patient support groups, and educational training programs were incorporated after in-house consultation with psychiatry. The patient received intralesional triamcinolone acetonide injection 5 mg/mL for a recalcitrant patch along with oral prednisolone.

Systemic treatment included a tapering course of oral prednisolone starting with 40 mg for 6 weeks. An SSRI (fluoxetine 20 mg for 2 months) was also prescribed after psychiatric review for the associated depressive symptoms and psychological counterpart.

Discussion

Alopecia areata is an autoimmune disorder that manifests with well-circumscribed patchy hair loss over scalp, beard, and other hair-bearing sites of the body. In a large proportion of patients, these lesions tend to remit spontaneously, whereas they may persist with further new patches in a few individuals in due course (Dy and Whiting 2011). In this case, the per-

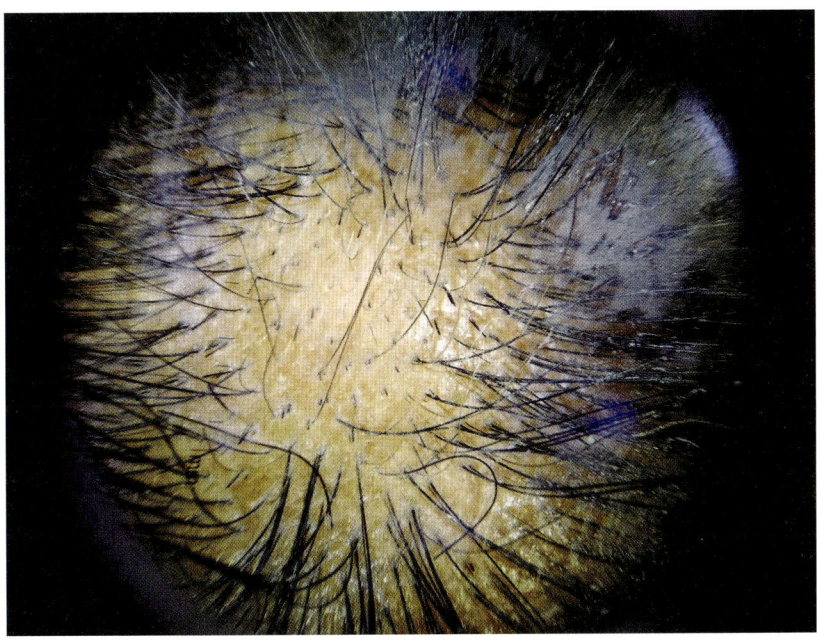

FIGURE 8–8. Trichoscopy of alopecia areata with findings of broken hair and exclamation mark hair in the periphery of the patch.
Source. Dr. Prajwal Pudasaini.

sistent and recalcitrant nature of the disease was further complicated by the associated emotional and psychological changes. Psychological changes can be induced or exacerbated in alopecia areata, as in many other instances of hair loss disorders (Marahatta et al. 2020). Prolonged duration of disease in this patient and the associated stress induced the vicious cycle of hair loss and psychological accentuation manifesting with mood changes, low self-esteem, and anger. Avoidance of social encounters and gatherings by the patient also suggested psychological comorbidities. Further, this tumult of psychological manifestation was expressed in the form of depressive symptoms. These psychological comorbidities were largely attributed to the neuro/immuno/cutaneous axis and associated cytological interplay. The amount of data on anxiety and depression associated with alopecia areata adds significant focus on the importance of psychotherapy, psychological medications, and CBT in alopecia areata patients with comorbidities.

The associated depressive symptoms in our patient warranted a thorough examination including assessment for suicidal ideation. Depression is one of the most common causes of suicide in the world (Darwin et al. 2018). The patient was also started on the SSRI fluoxetine (20 mg per day) for 2

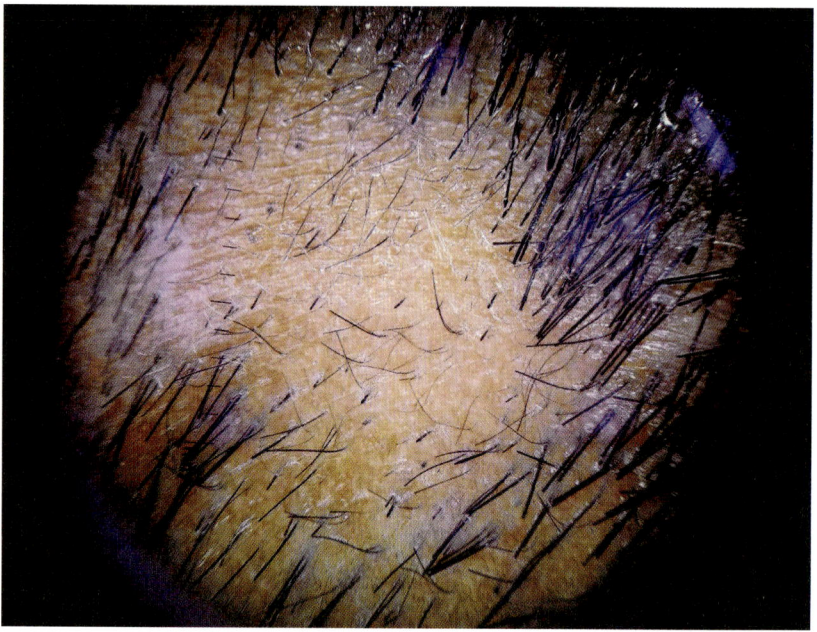

FIGURE 8–9. Trichoscopy with vellus hair in the center and exclamation mark hair in the periphery, 1 month after treatment.
Source. Dr. Prajwal Pudasaini.

months, along with psychological counseling, after which he showed improvement in the depressive symptoms and associated stress. Psychotherapy was incorporated alongside treatment of the primary cause—alopecia areata—with a tapering dose of oral prednisolone 40 mg per day over 6 weeks, along with intralesional triamcinolone injection 5 mg/mL over the recalcitrant patch. Although the administration of oral prednisolone is a second-line treatment, the associated psychological comorbidity and the prolonged nature of the disease warranted its use. A vigilant clinical acumen, use of dermoscopy, and assessment of concomitant psychological disorders form a multimodal treatment approach involving medical and psychotherapy.

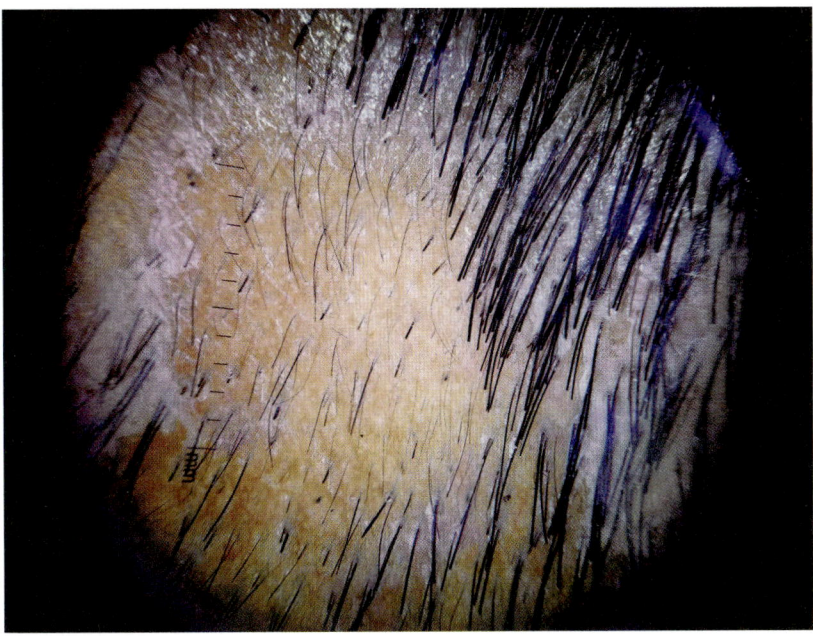

FIGURE 8–10. Trichoscopy 2 months posttreatment, with findings of significant vellus hair growth.
Source. Dr. Prajwal Pudasaini.

TEACHING POINTS

- In a significant proportion of patients, alopecia areata is associated with psychological comorbidities such as anxiety and depression.

- Among many comorbidities, depression is the most serious because of its direct correlation to suicidal ideation and suicide.

- Early assessment of concomitant psychiatric comorbidities such as anxiety and depression can prevent hazardous complications.

- Education for patients and practicing clinicians is valuable, given the subtle findings associated with these two interrelated clinical entities.

- A holistic approach to treatment of alopecia areata should address both the physical disease and the psychological counterpart with appropriate psychosomatic counseling and psychotropic medications.

References

Darwin E, Hirt PA, Fertig R, et al: Alopecia areata: review of epidemiology, clinical features, pathogenesis, and new treatment options. Int J Trichology 10(2):51–60, 2018 29769777

Dy LC, Whiting DA: Histopathology of alopecia areata, acute and chronic: why is it important to the clinician? Dermatol Ther 24(3):369–374, 2011 21689247

Marahatta S, Agrawal S, Adhikari BR: Psychological impact of alopecia areata. Dermatol Res Pract 24:8879343, 2020 33424962

Case 8-3
Holistic Management of Alopecia Areata—A Case-Based Approach

Maria Angeliki Gkini, M.D., M.Sc., Ph.D.

Case Description

A 38-year-old woman presented to the dermatology outpatient clinic with alopecia areata, formerly diagnosed and treated by another dermatologist. She was first diagnosed with alopecia areata in 2019, with no response to treatment since then. She had tried topical and systemic treatments, including topical and intralesional corticosteroids, systemic oral prednisolone pulses, and a 3-month course of topical calcineurin inhibitors. At her appointment, she had been using only clobetasol propionate lotion once a day.

Her medical history included idiopathic juvenile arthritis and atopic dermatitis in childhood. She did not report other autoimmune conditions, such as vitiligo or Hashimoto disease. She did not smoke and had no history of alcohol or recreational drug misuse. The patient is a pharmacist and is married with two children. She had been going through a very stressful period as she returned to work after maternity leave, and was finding it hard to balance work and family life.

On examination, the patient had severe alopecia areata. The hair pull test was positive. Severity of Alopecia Tool (SALT) score was >50, with alopecia patches also on the body (Figure 8–11A and B). She had ophiasis-pattern scalp hair loss, a negative prognostic factor for alopecia areata. Dermatology

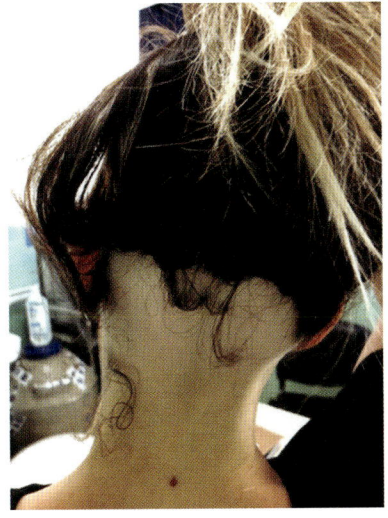
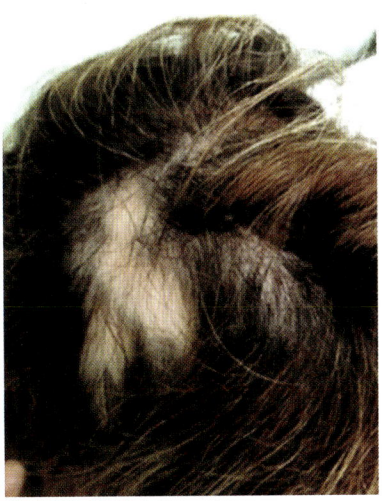

FIGURE 8-11. Severe alopecia areata in a 38-year-old woman before treatment.
Source. Dr. Maria Angeliki Gkini.

Quality of Life Index (DLQI) score was 30, indicative of a significant impairment in her quality of life; PHQ-9 (Patient Health Questionnaire/9 items) and GAD-7 (generalized anxiety disorder/7 items) scores were 20 for both, indicative of significant anxiety and depression. During the consultation, the patient was tearful and avoided eye contact. She seemed very distressed and reported active suicidal ideation without a plan.

Differential Diagnosis

- Alopecia areata
- Androgenic alopecia
- Scarring alopecia
- Secondary syphilis
- Tinea capitis
- Trichotillomania

Diagnosis

In this case, the diagnosis was clear. The history and pattern of hair loss and trichoscopy confirmed the diagnosis. On trichoscopy, the patient showed typical features of alopecia areata, including yellow and black dots, exclamation mark hairs, and some short vellus hair. Results of all other lab work, including syphilis serology, were negative. The patient was diagnosed with alopecia areata with comorbid anxiety and depression.

Management

The patient was prescribed escitalopram 20 mg daily along with CBT for psychiatric comorbidities. In terms of treatment options for her alopecia areata, topical immunotherapy (diphenylcyclopropenone [DPCP]) was impractical because of the need for frequent hospital visits and the presence of multiple body lesions. Cyclosporine could have a beneficial effect, but it is a short-term treatment. Off-label treatment with other agents, such as methotrexate or azathioprine, could be tried with variable results. Therefore, the patient was an ideal candidate for baricitinib, the first FDA-approved treatment for severe alopecia areata.

Blood and imaging tests, as per Janus kinase (JAK) inhibitor pretreatment guidelines, were unremarkable. The patient was informed in detail of the safety profile of the medication, including potential serious adverse events, and she provided written informed consent. An application for funding for baricitinib (Olumiant) was approved, and the patient was started on oral baricitinib 4 mg once a day.

At the 1-month follow-up, the SALT score was reduced significantly to almost 25, with many newly grown white hairs. Her DLQI score dropped to 5. PHQ-9 and GAD-7 scores were both 4, and the patient was feeling much better (Figure 8–12). Her blood tests remained normal.

At the 6-month follow-up, the patient was still in complete remission, without any lesions of alopecia areata. SALT, DLQI, PHQ-9, and GAD-7 scores were 0 (Figure 8–13A and B). Escitalopram was stopped, and the patient was still doing well 2 months later. Monitoring blood tests remained unremarkable.

Discussion

This case describes a patient with severe alopecia areata and psychological comorbidities, successfully treated with a combined psychodermatology approach, including oral baricitinib 4 mg daily, escitalopram 20 mg daily, and CBT. Interestingly, this patient responded very quickly and successfully to the baricitinib treatment, whereas two phase 3 trials with baricitinib for alopecia areata showed a slower onset of action and response to medication. This response could potentially be related to the multidisciplinary approach and management of stress, or simply to the unpredictable course of the disease, as well as other potential factors.

Alopecia areata is a chronic autoimmune condition that causes nonscarring hair loss, affecting 0.2% of the population worldwide (Toussi et al. 2021). Newer data support its systemic nature. Psychiatric and psychosocial comorbidities are common (Gkini and Jolliffe 2021). Hair loss has a signif-

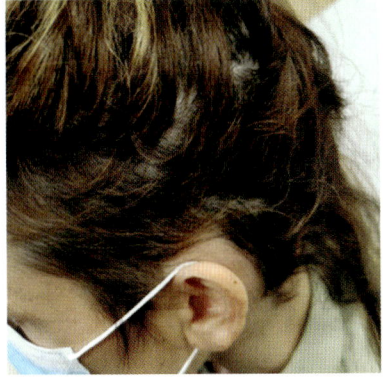
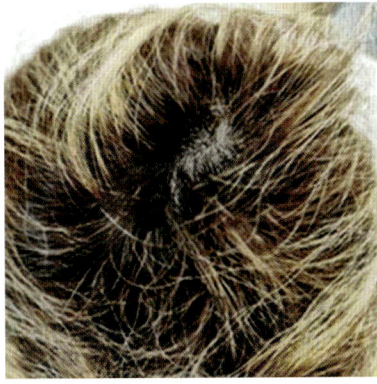

FIGURE 8–12. Full hair regrowth after 3 months of combined treatment with baricitinib, escitalopram, and CBT. Many newly grown hairs present on the occipital scalp are still white.
Source. Dr. Maria Angeliki Gkini.

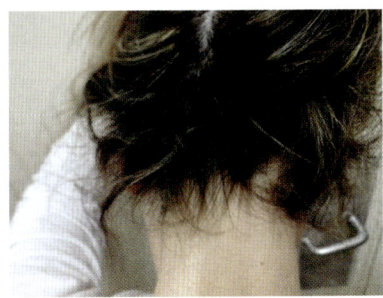
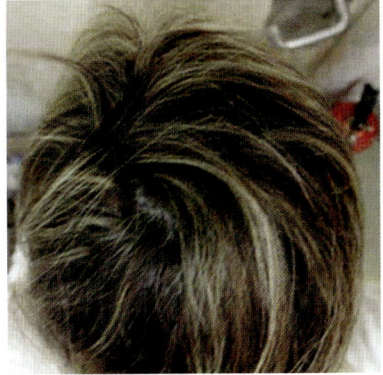

FIGURE 8–13. Patient successfully treated for 6 months. A few hairs on the occipital area of the scalp remain white.
Source. Dr. Maria Angeliki Gkini.

icant impact on the lives of patients, who may present with low self-esteem, poor self-image, depression, alexithymia, or even suicidal ideation. Screening for psychiatric and psychosocial comorbidities and a holistic approach plan are crucial for management of the hair disorder itself and its comorbidities (Jafferany and Patel 2020). Finally, the recent availability of new treatment options (JAK inhibitors) in hair diseases will hopefully change the landscape of this disorder (King et al. 2022).

Further studies are needed to assess the efficacy of a combined psychodermatology approach in patients with alopecia areata treated with advanced treatments.

TEACHING POINTS

- Alopecia areata has strong associations with psychiatric comorbidities that need specific treatments, such as antidepressants.
- Multiple scoring systems exist to determine the effect a dermatological disorder has on a patient's life (e.g., DLQI, SALT, PHQ-9, GAD-7).
- The availability of novel treatment options, such as Janus kinase inhibitors, will hopefully change the landscape of psychotrichology.

References

Gkini MA, Jolliffe V: Hair disorders and impact on quality of life, in Psychodermatology in Clinical Practice. Edited by Bewley A, Lepping P, Taylor RE. Cham, Switzerland, Springer, 2021, pp 283–300

Jafferany M, Patel A: Trichopsychodermatology: the psychiatric and psychosocial aspects of hair disorders. Dermatol Ther 33(1):e13168, 2020 31714654

King B, Ohyama M, Kwon O, et al: Two phase 3 trials of baricitinib for alopecia areata. N Engl J Med 386(18):1687–1699, 2022 35334197

Toussi A, Barton VR, Le ST, et al: Psychosocial and psychiatric comorbidities and health-related quality of life in alopecia areata: a systematic review. J Am Acad Dermatol 85(1):162–175, 2021 32561373

Case 8-4
Alopecia Areata in an Infant Triggered by Admission to Intensive Care Unit

Asmahane Souissi, M.D.
Wejden Fakhfekh, M.D.
Zohra Fitouri, M.D.

Case Description

An 8-month infant was referred from the pediatric department for alopecia of the vertex and occipital regions. It appeared after 2-week hospitalization in an ICU for acute respiratory distress syndrome. Clinical examination showed an 8-cm-diameter patch of nonscarring alopecia on the vertex and occipital regions. The underlying skin was of normal appearance with no scaling and no inflammation (Figure 8–14). The hair pull test was negative. There was no involvement of other hair-bearing areas. Physical and dermatological examination was otherwise unremarkable.

Differential Diagnosis

- Pressure alopecia
- Alopecia areata

Diagnosis

Trichoscopy examination of the patchy alopecia demonstrated broken hairs and exclamation mark hairs consistent with the diagnosis of alopecia areata (Figure 8–15). A family history of autoimmune diseases and atopy revealed that the father had a patch of nonscarring alopecia of the temporal region of the scalp consistent with alopecia areata (Figure 8–16). The diagnosis of alopecia areata was made.

Management

The patient was treated with topical corticosteroids for 3 months. The evolution was favorable, with total hair regrowth.

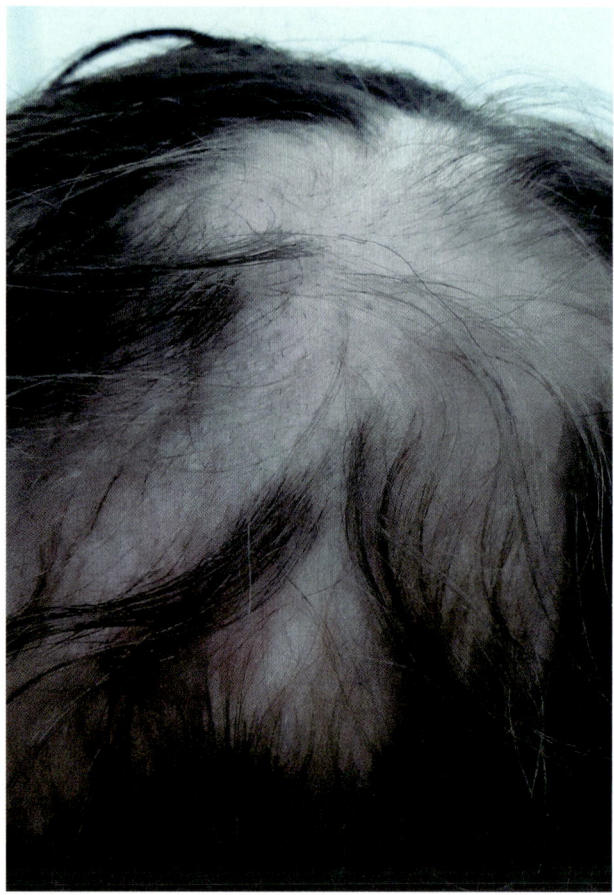

FIGURE 8–14. A patch of nonscarring alopecia on the vertex and occipital regions.
Source. Dr. Asmahane Souissi.

Discussion

Alopecia areata is an acquired autoimmune disease with multifactorial etiology. Multiple studies provide evidence supporting an autoimmune response to hair follicles, in addition to environmental factors (Zhou et al. 2021). Psychological stress has been recognized as a pathogenic trigger in alopecia areata. Stressful life events may have an impact at the onset or before exacerbation of alopecia areata (Ahn et al. 2023; Manolache and Benea 2007). In this case, hospitalization in intensive care was a stressful situation involved in triggering alopecia areata.

Alopecia Areata 235

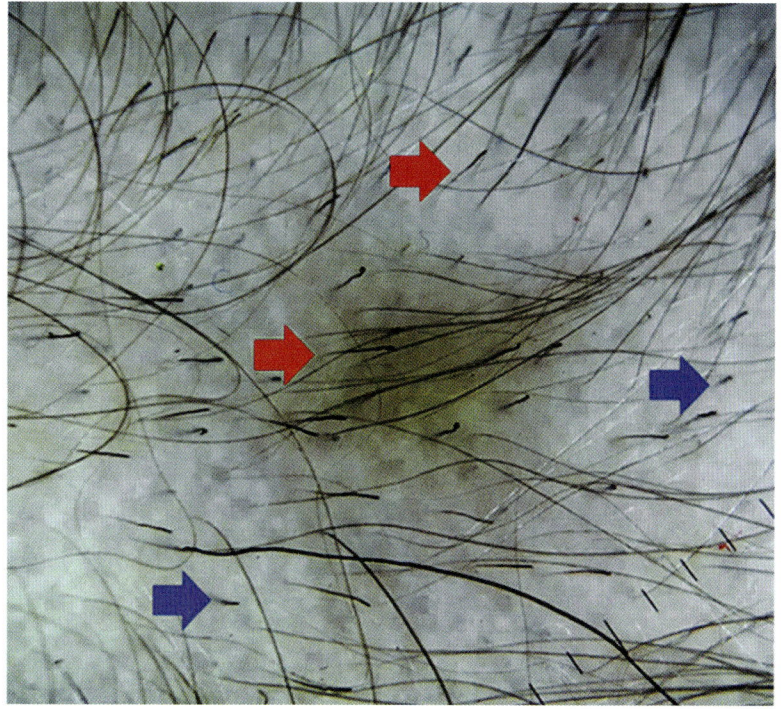

FIGURE 8–15. Broken hairs (blue arrows) and exclamation mark hairs (red arrows).
Source. Dr. Asmahane Souissi.

The diagnosis of alopecia areata in this patient was challenging, because the involvement of occipital area associated with supine immobilization was highly suggestive of pressure alopecia (Ramot et al. 2014). Trichoscopy was useful to make the proper diagnosis. Some trichoscopic findings may be seen in both conditions, such as black and yellow dots and short vellus hair. However, the presence of multiple exclamation mark hairs was consistent with alopecia areata (Waśkiel et al. 2018).

The age of onset is another peculiarity of this case—alopecia areata is uncommon before the age of 2 years. An early age of onset may reflect genetic factors, because a positive family history of alopecia areata or other autoimmune disease is more common in infantile alopecia areata (Crowder et al. 2002). The occurrence of alopecia areata after an ICU stay in an infant less than 2 years of age with a father's history of alopecia areata illustrates the combination of genetic factors and environmental influence.

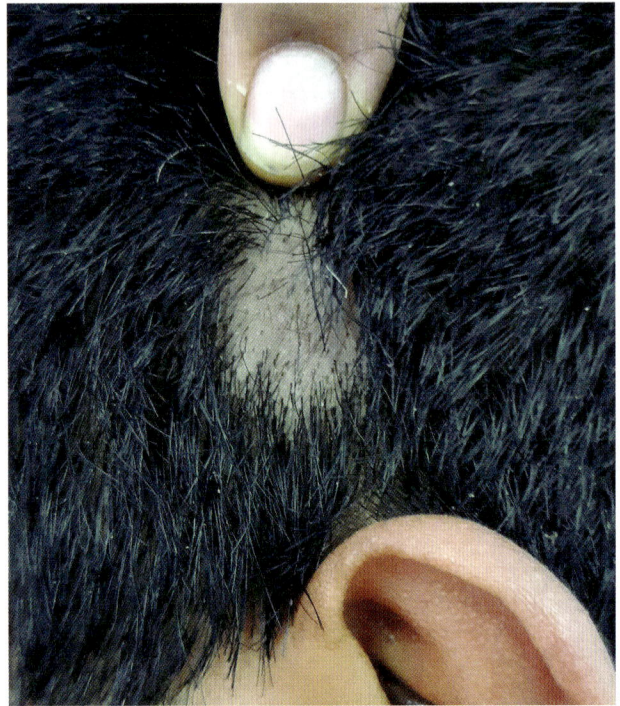

FIGURE 8–16. A patch of alopecia areata of the temporal region of the father's scalp.
Source. Dr. Asmahane Souissi.

TEACHING POINTS

- This case highlights the role of stressful situations in triggering alopecia areata.
- On a predisposed genetic background, environmental factors may be determining in the onset of alopecia areata.
- Alopecia areata can occur at a young age, as early as 8 months.

References

Ahn D, Kim H, Lee B, et al: Psychological stress-induced pathogenesis of alopecia areata: autoimmune and apoptotic pathways. Int J Mol Sci 24(14):11711, 2023 37511468

Crowder JA, Frieden IJ, Price VH: Alopecia areata in infants and newborns. Pediatr Dermatol 19(2):155–158, 2002 11994183

Manolache L, Benea V: Stress in patients with alopecia areata and vitiligo. J Eur Acad Dermatol Venereol 21(7):921–928, 2007 17659001

Ramot Y, Renert-Yuval Y, Maly A, et al: Patches of hair loss on the occipital scalp. J Dtsch Dermatol Ges 12(10):918–920, 2014 24903057

Waśkiel A, Rakowska A, Sikora M, et al: Trichoscopy of alopecia areata: an update. J Dermatol 45(6):692–700, 2018 29569271

Zhou C, Li X, Wang C, et al: Alopecia areata: an update on etiopathogenesis, diagnosis, and management. Clin Rev Allergy Immunol 61(3):403–423, 2021 34403083

Case 8–5
Anxiety and Depression Associated With Alopecia Areata

Dipali Rathod, M.D.
Ruchi Hemdani, M.D.

Case Description

A 23-year-old woman presented with a history of gradual loss of hair for the last 2–3 years. It started off with a few small patches of hair loss on the frontal region of the scalp, which gradually progressed to involve the entire scalp. The patient was greatly affected by her current situation and appeared anxious and depressed while narrating her history. There was no other history in terms of any stressful event or acute illness preceding the hair loss. There was no hair loss from any other part of the body. There was no recent or past history of any other illness, and none of the family members had similar complaints.

On further inquiry, the patient acknowledged that the alopecia affected her identity to an extent that she stopped socializing. Her appearance had taken a toll on her emotionally and mentally, leading to personal and social problems. Her dating prospects were damaged because of the state of her hair, and this led to her increasing psychological distress. She had already visited various doctors for her hair treatment, but in vain. She had lost hope of ever growing back her hair.

On examination, there were well-circumscribed, oval-shaped, smooth patches and areas of hair loss covering almost the entire scalp, with the frontotemporal region, vertex, and occipital area being affected the most (Figure 8–17A–D). These patches coalesced to form larger patches. The posterior scalp was relatively less involved, with fewer lesions, and some patches had white hair. There was no underlying scaling, atrophy, or pigmentation. The patient was otherwise healthy, with no skin or nail changes. On trichoscopic examination, there were black dots, yellow dots, broken hair, vellus hairs, a few pigtail hairs, and coudability hairs. There was no scaling or atrophy or pigmentation on magnified view, ruling out scarring alopecia.

Differential Diagnosis

- Alopecia areata
- Trichotillomania
- Tinea capitis

Diagnosis

With the history of progressive patchy hair loss and clinical examination showing nonscarring alopecia along with trichoscopy findings, the diagnosis of alopecia areata was made. Trichoscopy helped to confirm alopecia areata, showing black dots, yellow dots, broken hair, vellus hairs, pigtail hairs, and coudability hair.

Management

Once the diagnosis was confirmed, the patient was reassured and counseled regarding her hair loss. She was made aware of the course of disease and expected results, along with the various therapeutic options. Laboratory investigations, such as complete blood cell count, ferritin, thyroid function tests, and other serum chemistry, were all within normal limits. The patient was started on DPCP application along with simultaneous positive reassurance at every visit to tackle anxiety. After the DPCP patch test, she developed mild erythema and a few papules on the test area. She was then treated with gradually increasing concentrations of DPCP.

The patient was diligent in applying DPCP and reported mild improvement with some hair growth within 3 weeks of application, which kept improving steadily, along with her anxiety/depression. She followed up regularly for a duration of 9 months; by that time, she had good results, with the hair covering almost all the patches of her scalp (Figure 8–18A and B). During her follow-up, we could appreciate that the hair also grew in length, and she was less anxious and, more importantly, not affected by her looks anymore.

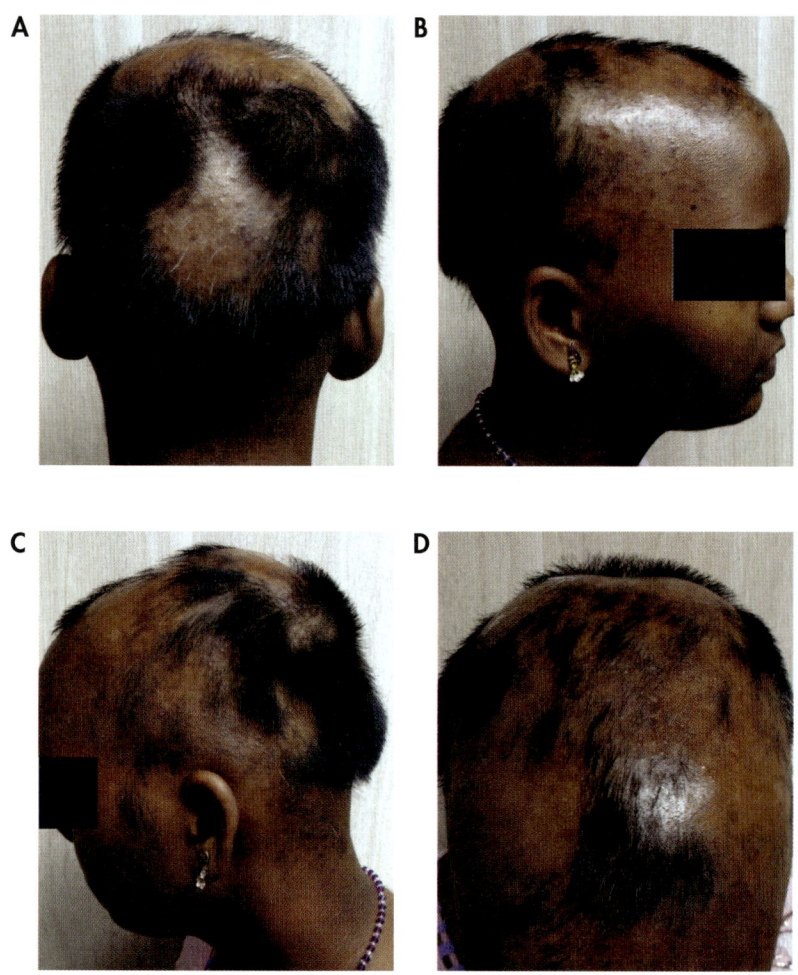

FIGURE 8–17. Well-circumscribed, oval-shaped, smooth patches of hair loss affecting the frontotemporal region, vertex, and occipital area, almost depicting an ophiasis pattern.
Source. Dr. Dipali Rathod.

Discussion

Alopecia areata is a chronic inflammatory disorder of autoimmune origin. The prevalence is estimated to be 1.7% (Hunt and McHale 2005). It has been reported that almost 40% of women with alopecia have some interpersonal issues, and ~63% have career difficulties (Chiang et al. 2015). The extent of alopecia has been related to the degree of psychological distress. Patients are generally reluctant to take medications because of stigma and

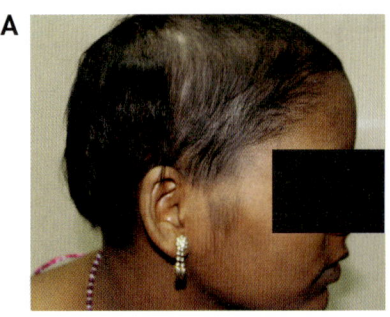 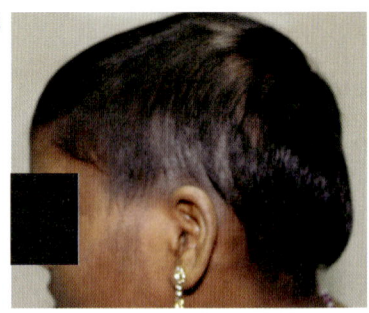

FIGURE 8-18. Almost full coverage of the scalp with black, dense, shiny hair.
Source. Dr. Dipali Rathod.

concerns about dependence or side effects. In this case, simple reassurance with positive feedback on seeing the growth of hair took care of the patient's anxiety associated with hair loss. Stress is a big risk factor and perpetuator in this condition, as losing hair creates additional stress, which further aggravates the disease. Therefore, the vicious cycle needs to be broken.

There are limited treatment options for alopecia areata, including topical and oral therapies with steroids. JAK-STAT inhibitors are the latest treatments. DPCP has been found to be an effective topical immunotherapeutic modality in patients who have failed to respond to other therapies or have extensive disease. A good outcome is seen in patients with less severe disease at baseline. Limitations with using DPCP include its preparation, availability, unclear duration of application, and side effects (itching, rash, local lymphadenopathy), which need to be explained to the patient in detail. Psychoeducation and counseling are very important in the treatment of this condition by decreasing stress and easing the patient mentally, favoring a good therapeutic response, as observed in this case.

TEACHING POINTS

- Psychological repercussions of alopecia areata can be devastating.
- The most common differential diagnosis includes trichotillomania and tinea capitis.

- The treatment of alopecia areata comprises psychotherapy and topical or systemic medications.

References

Chiang KS, Mesinkovska NA, Piliang MP, et al: Clinical efficacy of diphenylcyclopropenone in alopecia areata: retrospective data analysis of 50 patients. J Investig Dermatol Symp Proc 17(2):50–55, 2015 26551948

Hunt N, McHale S: The psychological impact of alopecia. BMJ 331(7522):951–953, 2005 16239692

Body-Focused Repetitive Behavioral Disorders

Usha N. Khemani, M.D.
Neha Fogla, M.D.

Introduction

Body-focused repetitive behavior disorders (BFRBDs) are a group of obsessive-compulsive spectrum disorders that involve recurrent, repetitive behaviors concentrated on the body, along with repeated efforts to minimize or halt these behaviors (Yasir and Kanwal 2023). These behaviors include nail biting, skin picking, and hair pulling and are found in the obsessive-compulsive and related disorders (OCRD) category of DSM-5-TR (American Psychiatric Association 2022; Greenberg 2019). They were once considered benign "nervous habits," but it is now recognized that BFRBDs can lead to negative outcomes, including medical and aesthetic problems, as well as socioemotional difficulties (La Buissonnière-Ariza et al. 2021; McGuire et al. 2012). Furthermore, BFRBDs may be either a primary or secondary component of skin and hair disorders and can occur in all age ranges (McGuire et al. 2012). The diagnosis of a BFRBD must involve a dermatologist, a psychiatrist, and a primary care provider.

Epidemiology

The epidemiology of BFRBDs varies depending on the specific behavior being studied. The data vary greatly due to many patients not seeking clinical help, as these behaviors are often perceived as harmless, and there is a lack of awareness about them. However, in general, these conditions tend to have an onset in early adolescence and affect females more than males. One study found that the overall prevalence of BFRBDs is 22%, with females being affected more than males (13.9% and 8.1%, respectively) (Siddiqui et al. 2012). Furthermore, hair pulling and nail biting have been found to cause greater distress in females, whereas teeth grinding was more prevalent in males (Houghton et al. 2018). The majority of individuals seeking treatment for their symptoms are females ((Bohne et al. 2005; Lochner et al. 2017).

The prevalence of skin picking, otherwise known as excoriation disorder, in young people is 10%–40%, with 8.3% experiencing significant distress and interference associated with it (McGuire et al. 2012). In one study, prevalence estimates of excoriation disorders were found to be 1.4%–5.4% (Hayes et al. 2009). Excoriation disorders may occur at any age, but generally have their onset in adolescence, typically coinciding with the onset of puberty. Similarly, nail biting is prevalent in 5%–45% of youth, with 7.3% experiencing significant distress and interference associated with it. The prevalence of hair-pulling behaviors in adults is as much as 15.3% and in 10.5% of young people (McGuire et al. 2012).

In a study on clinical correlates and prevalence of BFRBDs, skin picking was found to be the most reported BFRBD. The study found that 38% of patients reported some level of skin picking, and 16% reported elevated levels of skin picking, followed by nail biting, with 34% reporting some level, and 17% reporting elevated levels. Hair pulling was less common, with 8% of the sample reporting some level and 4% reporting elevated levels (La Buissonnière-Ariza et al. 2021).

One study revealed significant differences between child and parental reports of BFRBDs. Although 15% of the children reported distress and impairment associated with BFRBDs, only 4.5% of parents directly observed the behaviors in their children (La Buissonnière-Ariza et al. 2021). The results suggest that there may be significant differences between parent and child reports of child BFRBDs. Children may be more aware of their behaviors and emotions in certain contexts, such as school, and may underreport them to their parents. Conversely, parents may observe some behaviors that are not necessarily evident to their child or may interpret behaviors differently. These differences highlight the importance of considering multiple perspectives when assessing BFRBDs and other psychiatric symptoms in youth.

Overall, while the epidemiology of BFRBs varies depending on the specific behavior being studied, these conditions tend to have onset in early adolescence and affect females more than males. Further research is needed to better understand the underlying causes and risk factors associated with these behaviors.

Association With Other Psychiatric Conditions

The emotional regulation theory, which is one of the most common theories of BFRBD etiology, suggests that BFRBDs are related to modulating our emotional experience. According to this theory, it is expected that individuals with greater levels of affective dysregulation such as anxiety or depression would be more likely to engage in repetitive behaviors and vice versa. Studies have indicated that different repetitive behaviors such as nail biting and skin picking are associated with higher levels of anxiety and depression. This suggests that BFRBDs may be linked with other psychiatric conditions and can be considered a potential marker for emotional distress or mental health problems (Teng et al. 2004).

The association between BFRBDs and other psychiatric conditions is complex and multifaceted. OCD and body dysmorphic disorder are more common in individuals with eating disorders compared with the general population, as are mood and anxiety disorders. Some studies have found an increased risk of mortality associated with these disorders (Kondziolka and Hudak 2008; O'Sullivan et al. 1999). Children with BFRBDs, specifically trichotillomania, report high rates of psychiatric comorbidity with anxiety disorders, ADHD, and oppositional defiant disorder. They often endorse a history of other body-focused behaviors, such as thumb sucking, nail biting, lip biting, and cheek chewing (McGuire et al. 2012).

In children and adolescents with anxiety disorders or OCD, there is a high prevalence of BFRBDs, which are present to some level in 55% and are associated with significant distress and impairment in 27%. Young people with higher BFRBD severity were found to present with higher behavioral avoidance and anxiety sensitivity, as well as higher child-reported separation anxiety, generalized anxiety, and panic symptom severity (La Buissonnière-Ariza et al. 2021).

Individuals who have first-degree relatives with BFRBDs are more likely to suffer from BFRBDs themselves and may have more severe outcomes from these disorders (Redden et al. 2016), indicated by an increased amount of time spent performing these behaviors. Furthermore, individuals who have first-degree relatives with BFRBDs are also more likely to have other comorbid psychiatric conditions such as ADHD and family members with substance use disorders (Skurya et al. 2020).

Overall, the relationship between BFRBDs and other psychiatric conditions is complex and requires further research to fully understand. However, it is clear that individuals with BFRBDs are at a higher risk of developing other mental health disorders and require a comprehensive treatment approach.

Classification

The World Health Organization ICD-11 Working Group on the Classification of Obsessive-Compulsive and Related Disorders suggested that BFRBDs be classified under the OCRD cluster, which includes trichotillomania and skin-picking disorder. DSM-5-TR (American Psychiatric Association 2022) categorized trichotillomania and excoriation (skin-picking) disorder under the OCRD grouping and BFRBD under other specified forms of OCRD (Stein and Woods 2014). BFRBD symptom criteria are similar to those of trichotillomania (see Box 5–1 in Chapter 5) and excoriation (skin-picking) disorder (see Box 9–1).

Box 9–1. Diagnostic Criteria for Excoriation (Skin-Picking) Disorder

A. Recurrent skin picking resulting in skin lesions.
B. Repeated attempts to decrease or stop skin picking.
C. The skin picking causes clinically significant distress or impairment in social, occupational, or other important areas of functioning.
D. The skin picking is not attributable to the physiological effects of a substance (e.g., cocaine) or another medical condition (e.g., scabies).
E. The skin picking is not better explained by symptoms of another mental disorder (e.g., delusions or tactile hallucinations in a psychotic disorder, attempts to improve a perceived defect or flaw in appearance in body dysmorphic disorder, stereotypies in stereotypic movement disorder, or intention to harm oneself in nonsuicidal self-injury).

Source. Reprinted from American Psychiatric Association: *Diagnostic and Statistical Manual of Mental Disorders*, 5th Edition, Text Revision. Washington, DC, American Psychiatric Association, 2022, p. 367. Copyright © 2022 American Psychiatric Association. Used with permission.

Clinical Features

BFRBDs are a group of disorders that involve self-injurious behaviors directed toward the body. These behaviors can be seen clinically as repeated and persistent behaviors resulting in skin lesions, hair loss, or other physical damage to the body; common examples include nail biting, skin picking, hair pulling, and lip biting. To diagnose a BFRBD, clinicians must be able to recognize the characteristic behaviors associated with the disorder. Patients may demonstrate attempts to decrease or stop the repetitive behavior, and negative effects may result from the behaviors, such as social or occupational impairment or distress.

Recognizing the clinical features of BFRBDs is important for accurate diagnosis and effective treatment. Early intervention can prevent long-term physical and emotional damage caused by these disorders (Skurya et al. 2020). Clinical judgment is crucial in making the diagnosis; however, there is no defined frequency or duration for the disorder. Some patients may be aware of their behaviors, and others may engage subconsciously. Co-occurring behaviors, such as trichotillomania and skin-picking disorder, are also common and may complicate the diagnosis.

Skin-picking disorder (excoriation disorder) is a mental disorder that often begins during adolescence and causes significant emotional distress and impairment in daily functioning. Despite attempts to stop, the individual continues to pick at their skin, leading to skin lesions and scarring. Common comorbidities include anxiety disorders and depression. Feelings of shame and lack of control are common (Eskeland et al. 2021)

Trichotillomania is a chronic condition that involves recurrent hair pulling leading to noticeable hair loss, significant distress, and impairment. The disorder is characterized by an inability to resist the impulse to pull hair, followed by a sense of relief or gratification in some cases. Hair is usually pulled from the scalp, eyebrows, or eyelashes (Hossain et al. 2022). The triggers for hair pulling can be physical, emotional, or cognitive, including factors such as the appearance and sensation of the hair, anxiety, boredom, or tension. It is important to note that the diagnosis of trichotillomania should not be made if the hair pulling is in response to a delusion or a hallucination or if there is preexisting inflammation of the skin (Grant and Stein 2014).

Nail biting (onychophagia) is a common BFRB characterized by the compulsive and repetitive biting of the nails. While it is often considered a harmless habit, clinical nail biting can lead to bleeding, scarring, and infection in the fingers (Figure 9–1). The severity of onychophagia can range from mild to severe and can cause serious social and emotional problems, such as low self-esteem and anxiety. It is believed to affect as many as 20%–

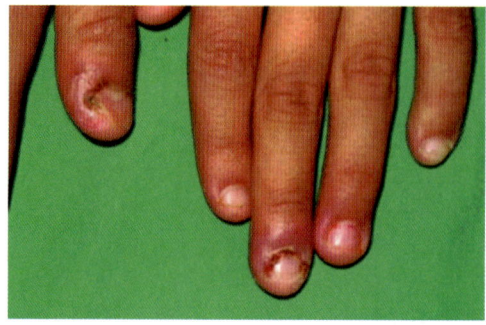

FIGURE 9–1. Nail and cuticle biting.
Source. Dr. Hamida Turki.

30% of the general population, with a higher prevalence, up to 45%, in children (Halteh et al. 2017). However, the true prevalence may be higher due to underreporting out of shame and embarrassment. Onychophagia typically begins in childhood but can also occur in adulthood, and men and women are affected equally. The behavior can be conscious or subconscious—the individual may not even be aware of it. Nail biting is often associated with stress and anxiety, and the habit may be used as a coping mechanism (Skurya et al. 2020).

Cheek biting is a repetitive and self-injurious behavior in which an individual bites their buccal mucosa (inner cheeks), resulting in injury and ulcers. This disorder is associated with other psychiatric disorders and is more prevalent in adults (10.1%) than in children (1%–7%) (Sarkhel et al. 2011). Similar disorders include lip chewing and tongue chewing (Skurya et al. 2020).

Teeth grinding (bruxism), characterized by grinding or clenching of teeth, is another BFRB that can cause distress. Bruxism can occur while an individual is awake (diurnal bruxism) or during sleep (nocturnal bruxism). The prevalence of bruxism is not well known, but studies have reported rates ranging from 8% to 31.4% (Manfredini et al. 2013). Oral examination may lead to a diagnosis of bruxism, and treatment may involve a multidisciplinary approach that includes both medical and mental health professionals (Skurya et al. 2020).

Nose picking (rhinotillexomania) is a behavior that, when performed excessively, may turn into a pathological condition. Research has shown that as many as 91% of individuals surveyed engage in nose picking. Among adolescents, up to 17% consider themselves to have a problem with nose picking, and 14% exhibit other repetitive behaviors, such as hair pulling and nail biting (Jefferson and Thompson 1995). The pathological form of this disorder may lead to frequent nosebleeds, ulcers, and even deformities in the nasal canal (Skurya et al. 2020).

BFRBDs and OCD are similar but have enough differences to be considered separate disorders. BFRBDs do not respond to the same medications as OCD, and whereas OCD involves obsessions that increase anxiety and compulsions that reduce it, BFRBs serve a self-regulating function and often provide pleasure. Both BFRBDs and OCD are treated with CBT; OCD can be treated with exposure and response prevention techniques, in addition to CBT.

Measurement of Severity

Assessing a BFRBD clinically remains the primary method to determine its severity, as no definitive measurement approach exists (La Buissonnière-Ariza et al. 2021). Some scoring systems have been proposed:

- Clinical Global Impression-Severity (CGI-S): a one-item clinician rating of severity (La Buissonnière-Ariza et al. 2021).
- Behavior Assessment System for Children, 2nd Edition, Behavioral and Emotional Screening System (BASC-2 BESS): a 30-item self-report questionnaire completed by the child or parent (La Buissonnière-Ariza et al. 2021).
- Repetitive Body-Focused Behavior Scale (RBBS): a 33-item questionnaire assessing the presence, severity, and associated consequences of skin picking, nail biting, and hair pulling behaviors (La Buissonnière-Ariza et al. 2021).
- Massachusetts General Hospital Hairpulling Scale (MGH-HPS): a 7-item clinician-rated scale that assesses hair-pulling severity and impairment (Keuthen et al. 1995).
- Skin Picking Scale (SPS): a 16-item self-report questionnaire that assesses the severity and functional impairment of skin-picking behavior; it rates the frequency, intensity, and interference of skin picking as well as the degree of distress associated with the behavior (Keuthen et al. 2001).

Complications

BFRBs can have both physical and psychological complications. Frequent engagement in these behaviors may be distressing and physically damaging, but only a minority of individuals with pathological BFRBs experience actual functional impairment from their symptoms. Those affected by BFRBs do often experience chronic, mild-to-moderate distress and physical consequences, which may lead to shame, embarrassment, anxiety, and depression (Weingarden and Renshaw 2015).

In addition to the psychological consequences, BFRBs can cause physical harm, such as infections, raw areas, scarring, and even serious physical disfigurement (Lochner et al. 2017; Odlaug and Grant 2008). Trichotillomania can result in hair loss and other complications; trichophagia, in which the patient eats their hair, can lead to the formation of a trichobezoar, a mass of hair that becomes trapped in the gastrointestinal tract (Skurya et al. 2020).

BFRBs can also lead to psychosocial difficulties, including social embarrassment, avoidance of situations or activities where skin lesions can be detected, and loss of productivity in work, as patients might spend a lot of time in repetitive picking or camouflaging (Flessner and Woods 2006). Individuals with trichotillomania may experience low self-esteem and social anxiety due to loss of hair.

It is possible that individuals with pathological BFRBs typically function normally but experience mild to moderate distress and physical consequences. This may explain why many affected individuals do not seek medical treatment or receive advice from health care professionals to address their symptoms, except in cases of teeth grinding that can be easily identified during routine check-ups by dental professionals (Tsiggos et al. 2008). Medical professionals may not be aware of their patients' pathological BFRBs unless they have severe physical complications such as extreme hair loss, infected lesions, missing nails, or scabs on lips (Houghton et al. 2018; Tucker et al. 2011; Weingarden and Renshaw 2015).

Overall, medical professionals may be unaware that their patient has a pathological BFRB. Even when they are aware, medical professionals may not be well trained in how to assess and treat these disorders. This underscores the need for increased awareness and education regarding BFRBs, among both medical professionals and the public.

Treatment

BFRBDs are challenging conditions to treat and often require a combination of psychotherapeutic and pharmacological interventions. Several treatment options have been proposed, including behavioral therapies, medications, and alternative treatments (Farhat et al. 2020; Lochner et al. 2017).

Psychotherapy

Behavioral therapy with habit reversal training (BT-HRT) has the largest treatment benefit and should be considered first-line treatment for trichotillomania (Gupta and Gargi 2012). Other individual psychotherapeutic approaches, particularly acceptance and commitment therapy (ACT) and approach avoidance therapy (AAT), have also been tried, with limited success. Group behavioral therapy, cognitive bias dysfunction, response inhibition training, and decoupling are other psychotherapeutic treatments that may be helpful.

Psychopharmacology

N-acetylcysteine (NAC), an amino acid derivative and glutamate modulator, is typically administered at 1,200 mg twice a day and has shown some evidence in treating hair-pulling symptoms. In some reported cases, olanzapine (20 mg/day) has been found to be effective in treating hair pulling. Selective serotonin reuptake inhibitors (SSRIs) such as citalopram (20 mg/day), fluoxetine (55 mg/day), escitalopram (30 mg/day), or fluvoxamine (300 mg/day) have shown some evidence in treating BFRBDs, notably with skin-picking symptoms.

Other treatments have been attempted, including inositol, an isomer of glucose, which may be useful in treating excoriation disorders. Naltrexone, milk thistle, and antipsychotics have also been reported to have variable success. Alternative treatments such as yoga, aerobic exercise, acupuncture, and hypnosis have been proposed as monotherapy or adjuncts to psychotherapy or pharmacotherapy for treating excoriation disorders.

It is important to note that referral to specialists should be considered in severe or treatment-resistant cases (Hossain et al. 2022). Although some pharmacological and behavioral treatment options are available, more research and clinical trials are needed to improve the care for patients with these disorders.

Conclusion

BFRBDs are often misunderstood and overlooked as benign nervous habits, yet they can significantly impact an individual's physical, emotional, and social well-being. Dermatologists and primary care providers play a crucial role in diagnosing and treating BFRBDs, especially when these behaviors are associated with skin or hair disorders. It is essential to raise awareness among the public and health care professionals about BFRBDs, their negative consequences, and the importance of early intervention to improve the quality of life of individuals with BFRBDs. Seeking help from qualified mental health professionals or medical providers is crucial for individuals with BFRBDs to receive a proper diagnosis and appropriate treatment plan. Educating medical professionals about BFRBDs, proper assessment, and treatment referral is important to manage pathological BFRBs. HRT is the mainstay of treatment in disorders such as trichotillomania or skin-picking disorder.

References

American Psychiatric Association: Diagnostic and Statistical Manual of Mental Disorders, 5th Edition, Text Revision. Washington, DC, American Psychiatric Association, 2022

Bohne A, Keuthen N, Wilhelm S: Pathologic hairpulling, skin picking, and nail biting. Ann Clin Psychiatry 17(4):227–232, 2005 16402755

Eskeland SO, Moen E, Meland KJ, et al: Skin picking disorder. Tidsskr Den Nor Laegeforen 141(18), 2021 34911273

Farhat LC, Olfson E, Nasir M, et al: Pharmacological and behavioral treatment for trichotillomania: an updated systematic review with meta-analysis. Depress Anxiety 37(8):715–727, 2020 32390221

Flessner CA, Woods DW: Phenomenological characteristics, social problems, and the economic impact associated with chronic skin picking. Behav Modif 30(6):944–963, 2006 17050772

Grant JE, Stein DJ: Body-focused repetitive behavior disorders in ICD-11. Br J Psychiatry 36(Suppl 1):59–64, 2014 25388613

Greenberg E: 51.1 Pulling and picking: body-focused repetitive behavior disorders. J Am Acad Child Adolesc Psychiatry 58(10):S72, 2019

Gupta S, Gargi PD: Habit reversal training for trichotillomania. Int J Trichology 4(1):39–41, 2012 22628990

Halteh P, Scher RK, Lipner SR: Onychophagia: a nail-biting conundrum for physicians. J Dermatolog Treat 28(2):166–172, 2017 27387832

Hayes SL, Storch EA, Berlanga L: Skin picking behaviors: an examination of the prevalence and severity in a community sample. J Anxiety Disord 23(3):314–319, 2009 19223150

Hossain R, Leung-Yee J, Sinyor M: Body-focused repetitive disorders. CMAJ 194(40):E1381, 2022 36252988

Houghton DC, Alexander JR, Bauer CC, et al: Body-focused repetitive behaviors: more prevalent than once thought? Psychiatry Res 270:389–393, 2018 30300869

Jefferson JW, Thompson TD: Rhinotillexomania: psychiatric disorder or habit? J Clin Psychiatry 56(2):56–59, 1995 7852253

Keuthen NJ, O'Sullivan RL, Ricciardi JN, et al: The Massachusetts General Hospital (MGH) Hairpulling Scale: 1. Development and factor analyses. Psychother Psychosom 64(3–4):141–145, 1995 8657844

Keuthen NJ, Wilhelm S, Deckersbach T, et al: The Skin Picking Scale: scale construction and psychometric analyses. J Psychosom Res 50(6):337–341, 2001 11438115

Kondziolka D, Hudak R: Management of obsessive-compulsive disorder-related skin picking with gamma knife radiosurgical anterior capsulotomies: a case report. J Clin Psychiatry 69(8):1337–1340, 2008 18816157

La Buissonnière-Ariza V, Alvaro J, Cavitt M, et al: Body-focused repetitive behaviors in youth with mental health conditions: a preliminary study on their prevalence and clinical correlates. Int J Ment Health 50(1):33–52, 2021

Lochner C, Roos A, Stein DJ: Excoriation (skin-picking) disorder: a systematic review of treatment options. Neuropsychiatr Dis Treat 13:1867–1872, 2017 28761349

Manfredini D, Winocur E, Guarda-Nardini L, et al: Epidemiology of bruxism in adults: a systematic review of the literature. J Orofac Pain 27(2):99–110, 2013 23630682

McGuire JF, Kugler BB, Park JM, et al: Evidence-based assessment of compulsive skin picking, chronic tic disorders and trichotillomania in children. Child Psychiatry Hum Dev 43(6):855–883, 2012 22488574

Odlaug BL, Grant JE: Clinical characteristics and medical complications of pathologic skin picking. Gen Hosp Psychiatry 30(1):61–66, 2008 18164942

O'Sullivan RL, Phillips KA, Keuthen NJ, et al: Near-fatal skin picking from delusional body dysmorphic disorder responsive to fluvoxamine. Psychosomatics 40(1):79–81, 1999 9989126

Redden SA, Leppink EW, Grant JE: Body focused repetitive behavior disorders: significance of family history. Compr Psychiatry 66:187–192, 2016 26995252

Sarkhel S, Praharaj SK, Akhtar S: Cheek-biting disorder: another stereotypic movement disorder? J Anxiety Disord 25(8):1085–1086, 2011 21889295

Siddiqui EU, Naeem SS, Naqvi H, et al: Prevalence of body-focused repetitive behaviors in three large medical colleges of Karachi: a cross-sectional study. BMC Res Notes 5(1):614, 2012 23116460

Skurya J, Jafferany M, Everett GJ: Habit reversal therapy in the management of body focused repetitive behavior disorders. Dermatol Ther 33(6):e13811, 2020 32542916

Stein DJ, Woods DW: Stereotyped movement disorder in ICD-11. Br J Psychiatry 36(Suppl 1):65–68, 2014 25388614

Teng EJ, Woods DW, Marcks BA, et al: Body-focused repetitive behaviors: the proximal and distal effects of affective variables on behavioral expression. Journal of Psychopathology and Behavior Assessment 26(1):55–64, 2004

Tsiggos N, Tortopidis D, Hatzikyriakos A, et al: Association between self-reported bruxism activity and occurrence of dental attrition, abfraction, and occlusal pits on natural teeth. J Prosthet Dent 100(1):41–46, 2008 18589073

Tucker BTP, Woods DW, Flessner CA, et al: The Skin Picking Impact Project: phenomenology, interference, and treatment utilization of pathological skin picking in a population-based sample. J Anxiety Disord 25(1):88–95, 2011 20810239

Weingarden H, Renshaw KD: Shame in the obsessive compulsive related disorders: a conceptual review. J Affect Disord 171:74–84, 2015 25299438

Yasir W, Kanwal S: The role of age and gender in developing body-focused repetitive behavior disorders among adolescents. Journal of Social Sciences Review 3(1):562–571, 2023

Case 9–1
Onychotillomania

Matilde Iorizzo, M.D., Ph.D.
Marcel C. Pasch, M.D., Ph.D.

Case Description

A 58-year-old man sought a dermatological consultation because of long-standing nail dystrophy of the right thumbnail (Figure 9–2). He was otherwise healthy, did not smoke, and was not taking any medications. He was a left-handed mechanic, but he did not recall any specific trauma responsible for the dystrophy. Skin, scalp, and mucosae examinations were normal. No symptoms were referred by the patient except for stinging and pain due to nail bed and hyponychium fissures. These symptoms were the main reason for the consultation and are very common in manual workers who perform wet work or come into contact with irritants or solvents, but the discomfort experienced by the subjects may render many subtle tasks difficult and even impossible.

Differential Diagnosis

- Malignancy
- Mycotic infection
- Nail trauma
- Onychotillomania

Diagnosis

Because this was a monodactylic nail dystrophy in an adult patient without any explanation, it was necessary to rule out malignancy. An easily treatable mycotic infection should also be ruled out in a case like this, but it was impossible to collect material. For these reasons, a biopsy was the most appropriate examination to start with. A lateral longitudinal biopsy was performed with additional staining for fungal organisms. PAS stain was negative, and the pathologist ruled out an underlying malignancy. Epithelial

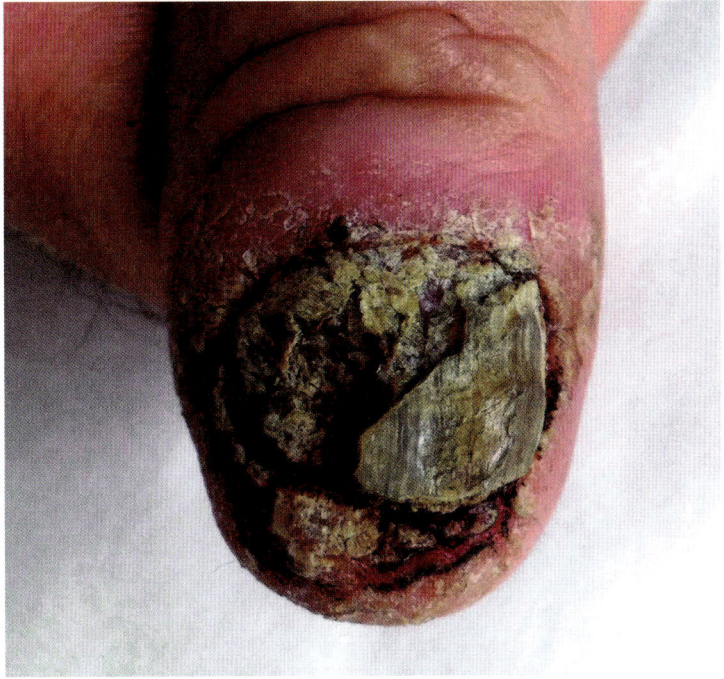

FIGURE 9–2. Patient presenting with total nail plate dystrophy, painful nail bed fissures, and chronic paronychia.
Source. Dr. Matilde Iorizzo.

hyperplasia, hyperkeratosis, hypergranulosis, hemorrhages within the stratum corneum, and minimal inflammation were compatible with onychotillomania. After facing the diagnosis, the patient refused to accept the causative relationship between his behavior and the onychodystrophy. Onychotillomania can be defined as a compulsive and self-induced trauma of the nail unit leading to nonspecific nail dystrophy. Most patients have psychiatric comorbidities, such as depression, anxiety disorders, or OCD, and often deny their habits. The patient's wife acknowledged that her husband had an anxious personality but never visited a therapist.

Management

Even though the diagnosis was denied and rejected by the patient, treatment was welcomed. There are two main approaches to onychotillomania treatment: nonpharmacologic and pharmacologic. The nonpharmacological methods include behavioral modification, stimulus control, and HRT. Occlusive dressing 24 hours a day for at least 3 months is another possibility. Local antiseptics and antimicrobial ointments may help to settle secondary infections when necessary. Mild topical steroids may help to reduce inflammation when present. The motivation and compliance of the patient is al-

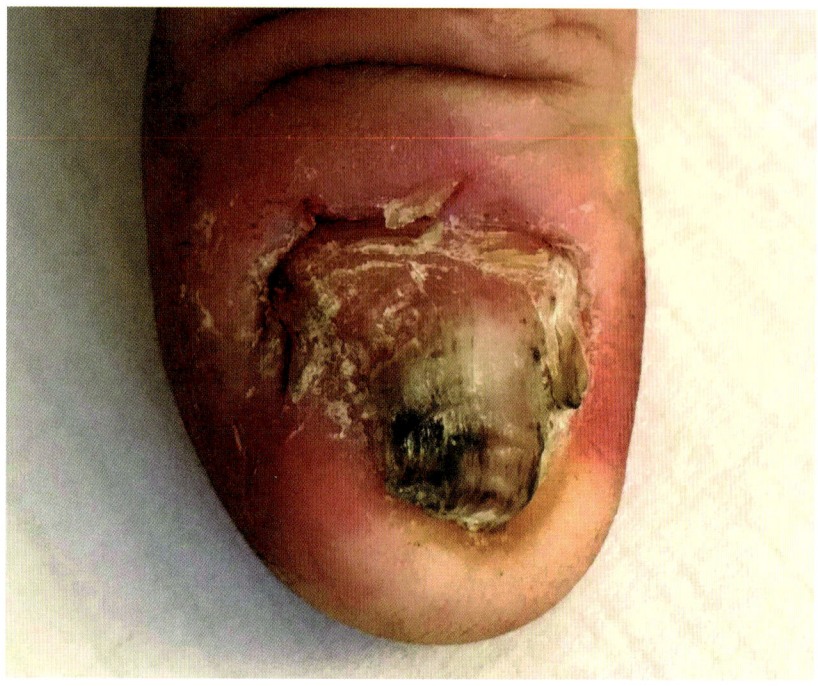

FIGURE 9–3. The same patient as in Figure 9–2 after 3 months of treatment: daily occlusive dressing and a short course of methylprednisolone aceponate cream (overnight for 1 month).
Source. Dr. Matilde Iorizzo.

ways necessary for a successful outcome (Figure 9–3). The literature also describes the use of cyanoacrylate glues or gel nails, but they should be advised with reluctance owing to the potential risk of developing allergic contact dermatitis from acrylates. In severe forms, the pharmacological method is probably the best option: oral NAC 1,200–2,400 mg/day has been described as beneficial in BFRBDs and has a good safety profile. In this case, the patient chose occlusive dressing, and there was obvious but incomplete improvement.

Discussion

Onychotillomania and onychophagia are psychodermatological disorders related to the nails. Both are chronic nail conditions categorized as BFRBDs and share the same complications, including damage to the nails, paronychia, and secondary bacterial and viral infections.

Onychophagia, or habitual nail biting, is a very common problem in children and young adults and usually involves all fingers. Onychotillomania is much rarer. It can be defined as self-induced damage of the nail unit, either by recurrent picking or pulling at elements of the nails, leading to nonspecific nail dystrophy or nail extraction (Halteh et al. 2017). Patients usually experience tension before and relief after nail manipulation. Other related disorders include onychotemnomania (cutting nails extremely short), onychodaknomania (nail biting to enjoy the pain), and onychoteiromania (very thin nails caused by excessive rubbing) (Singal and Daulatabad 2017). Most patients diagnosed with onychotillomania have psychiatric comorbidities, specifically depression, anxiety disorders, or OCD (Halteh et al. 2017). Referral to a psychiatrist may be indicated. In some cases, the habit is denied out of dissociation or shame, but in others it is confirmed and justified by countless reasons.

In the majority of cases, the diagnosis of onychotillomania is made clinically. Signs vary according to the different self-induced, compulsive or impulsive, direct trauma that can be inflicted by utensils (such as scissors, nail files, knives), teeth, or other nails. Indirect damage by causing matrix dysfunction is another possibility and may be due to repeatedly pushing back the cuticle of a digit using another finger. Onychotillomania can mimic many nail diseases depending on the creativity of the patient to inflict the trauma (Lee and Lipner 2022; Maddy and Tosti 2018; Reese et al. 2013). For this reason, onychotillomania is not characterized by specific and diagnostic signs and has no specific differential diagnosis. Histology is also not very specific, but at a minimum inflammation and findings consistent with trauma, such as entrapped red blood cells and unambiguous epidermal hyperplasia, must be present for reasonably reliable confirmation (Chen et al. 2022). Dermoscopy may be extremely helpful in supporting the clinical suspicion: total or partial absence of the nail plate, wavy lines, obliquely oriented nail bed hemorrhages, crusts, scales, and grayish nail bed pigmentation are the most common dermoscopic features described (Chen et al. 2022; Maddy and Tosti 2018). Wavy lines are longitudinal white, reddish purple, brown, or black pigmented lines that appear to be on different planes, with a wavy appearance due to uneven or absent nail plate growth after recurring trauma.

Even though the clinical picture in onychotillomania is not probative of the diagnosis, there are clinical pictures that are strongly suggestive. In onychotillomania, erosions of the nail folds are often present, sometimes accompanied by tranverse ridges, thinning, macrolunula, and generalized dystrophy. In more conscious forms of self-damage, sharp instruments are used to produce dermatitis artefacta of the nail unit (Figure 9–4). At the mild end of the spectrum is a habit tic, the nervous habit of pushing back the cuticle. This is usually done unconsciously and results in a groove in the center of the nail plate, with associated transverse ridges and depressions

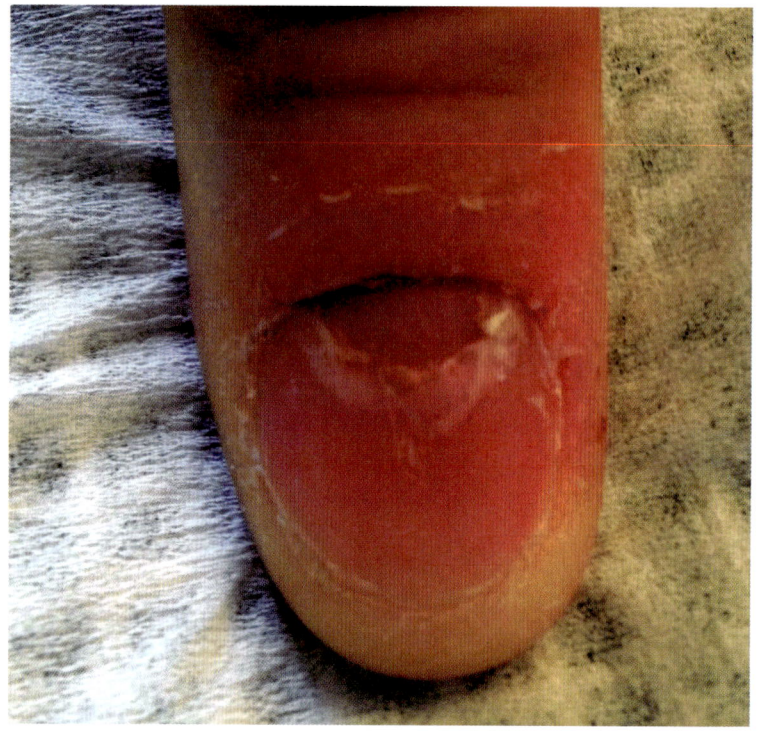

FIGURE 9–4. Dermatitis artefacta due to proximal trimming of the plate.
Source. Dr. Matilde Iorizzo.

(washboard nails) (Figures 9–5 and 9–6), sometimes accompanied by longitudinal melanonychia. Patients often deny this and do not understand how it is possible to develop nail plate dystrophy through manipulation of the cuticle with the nail-forming matrix underneath. The manual removal of single (Figures 9–7 and 9–8) or multiple (Figures 9–9, 9–10, and 9–11) nail plates is often justified by patients as mandatory due to abnormal appearance or signs—too thin, too thick, dystrophic, and painful.

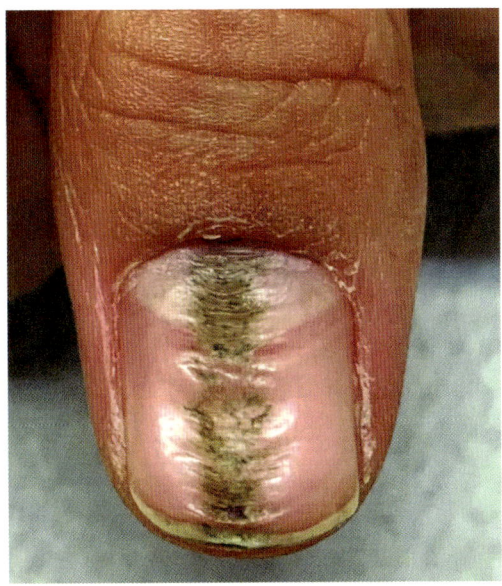

FIGURE 9–5. Longitudinal furrow with transverse grooves due to the habit tic of pushing back the cuticle.
Source. Dr. Matilde Iorizzo.

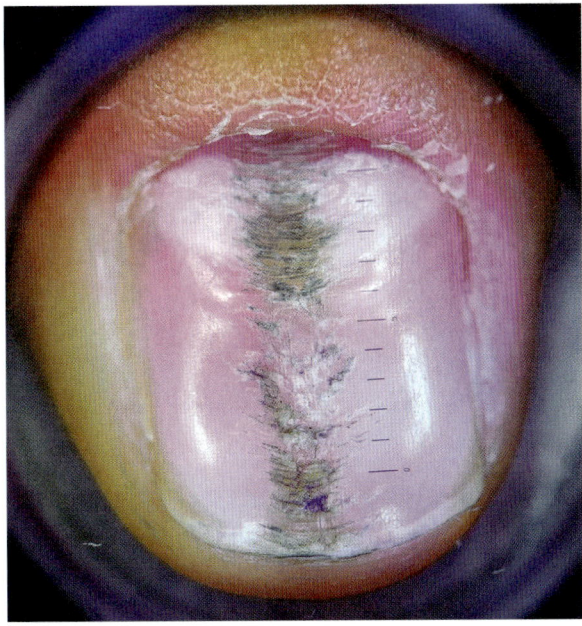

FIGURE 9–6. Dermoscopy view (×20) of the dystrophy in Figure 9–5.
Source. Dr. Matilde Iorizzo.

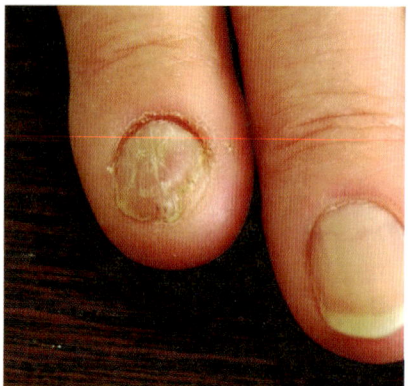

FIGURE 9–7. Self-induced nail plate peeling.
Source. Dr. Matilde Iorizzo.

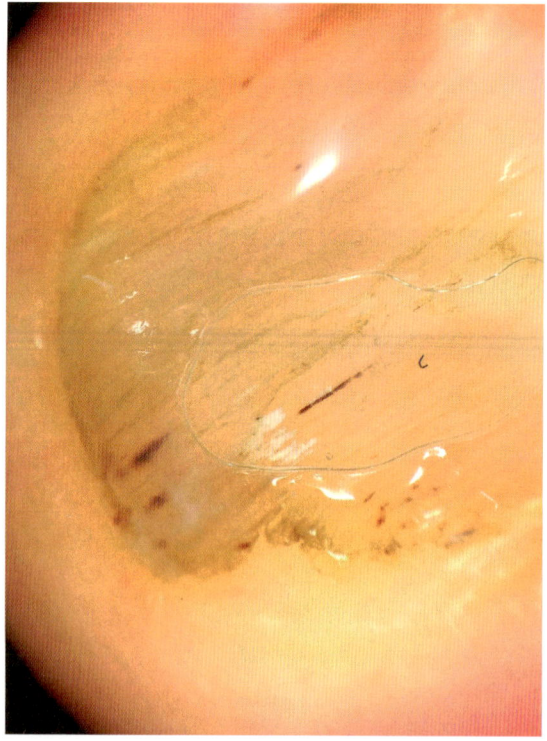

FIGURE 9–8. Dermoscopy (×20) picture of the same patient as in Figure 9–7 showing wavy lines and hemorrhages.
Source. Dr. Matilde Iorizzo.

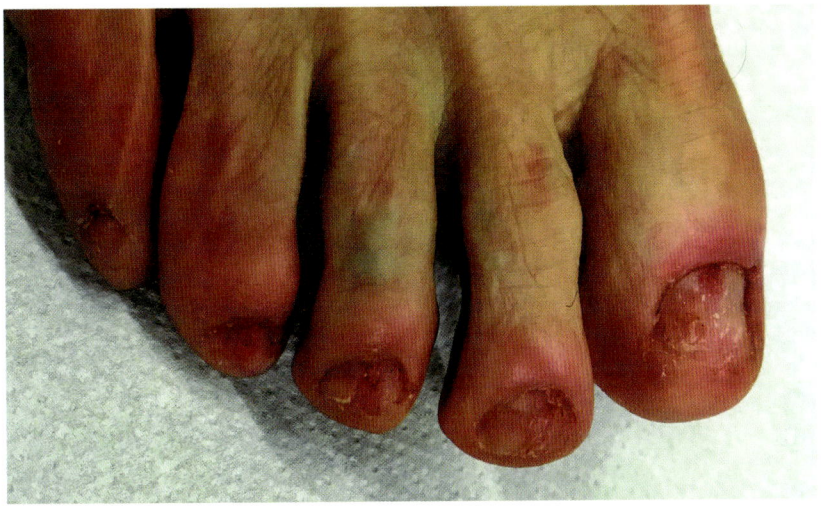

FIGURE 9–9. Manual removal of nail plates. All toenails have been removed.
Source. Dr. Matilde Iorizzo.

Pharmacological or nonpharmacological (CBT) treatments for onychotillomania are possible and will often need to be combined for a good treatment outcome. Unfortunately, treatment is often unsuccessful because subjects refuse to accept the causative relationship between their behavior and the onychodystrophy. When the patient acknowledges an element of self-damage, they may comply with the use of an occlusive and protective dressing over the tip of the digit 24 hours a day for 2–3 months. In the first month, it may be motivating for the patient to combine the dressing with a moderate-potency topical steroid to suppress any inflammation, because many patients are often more likely to accept that they need to contribute themselves if a somatic treatment is prescribed in parallel. In severe forms of onychophagia and onychotillomania, behavioral therapy (Silber and Haynes 1992); oral NAC (Lee and Lipner 2022; Nguyen et al. 2022; Nwankwo and Jafferany 2019); the antidepressants clomipramine, sertraline, or amitriptyline; and the antipsychotics pimozide or thioridazine (Halteh et al. 2017; Pacan et al. 2014a; Singal and Daulatabad 2017) may be beneficial and indicated in select cases.

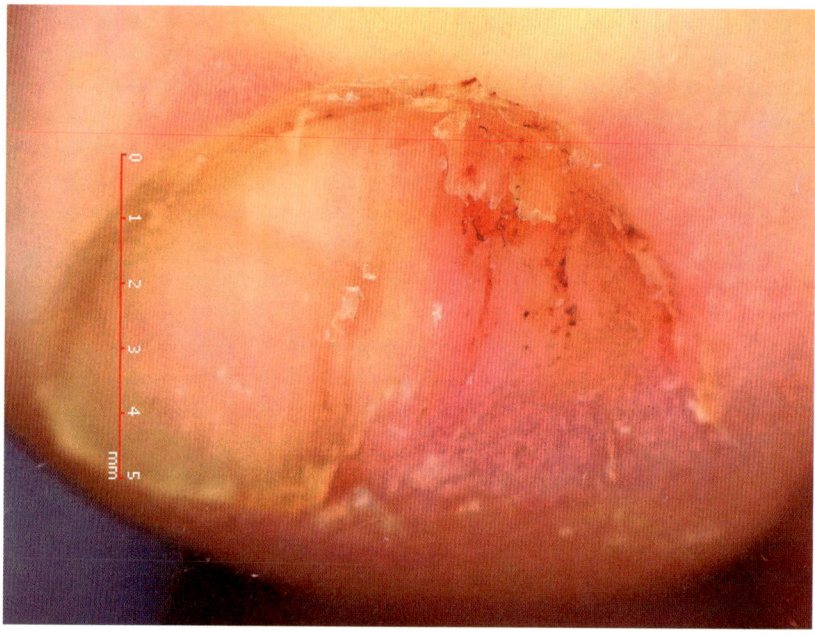

FIGURE 9–10. Dermoscopy (×20) picture of the same patient as in Figure 9–9 showing wavy lines and fresh hemorrhages. A nail plate partially torn is also visible.
Source. Dr. Mustafa Esen.

TEACHING POINTS

- Onychotillomania is a self-induced disorder that should not be underevaluated because it can be associated with underlying psychological dysfunction.

- Nail dystrophies are usually asymmetric.

- Onychotillomania is a mimic—it can be misdiagnosed as onychomycosis or as an inflammatory disease.

- Histopathological findings are nonspecific and often require clinical correlation.

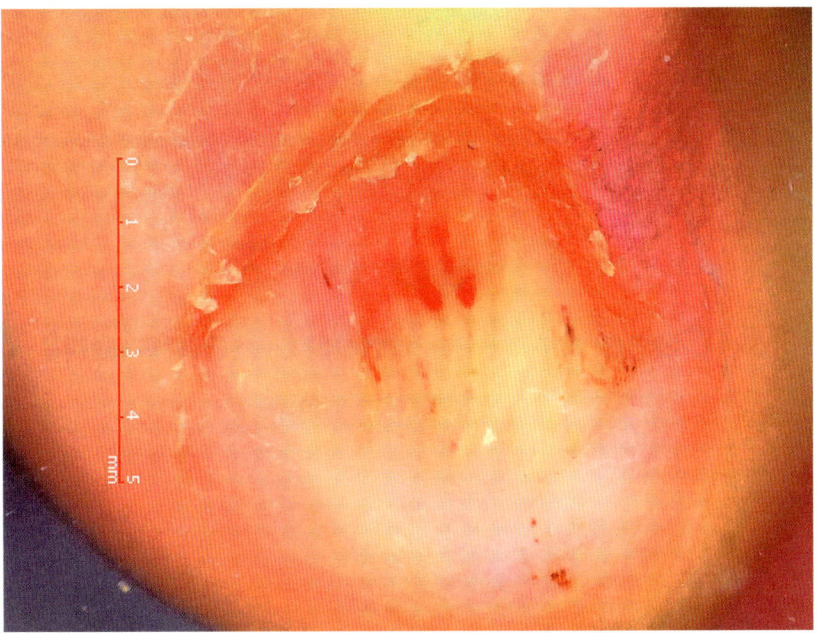

FIGURE 9–11. Dermoscopy (×20) picture of the same patient as in Figure 9–9 showing wavy lines and fresh hemorrhages.
Source. Dr. Mustafa Esen.

References

Chen Y, Pradhan S, Lyu L, et al: Clinical and dermoscopic characteristics of onychophagia and onychotillomania: a retrospective study of 63 cases. Clin Exp Dermatol 47(5):961–963, 2022 34905226

Halteh P, Scher RK, Lipner SR: Onychotillomania: diagnosis and management. Am J Clin Dermatol 18(6):763–770, 2017 28488241

Lee DK, Lipner SR: The potential of N-acetylcysteine for treatment of trichotillomania, excoriation disorder, onychophagia, and onychotillomania: an updated literature review. Int J Environ Res Public Health 19(11):6370, 2022 35681955

Maddy AJ, Tosti A: Dermoscopic features of onychotillomania: a study of 36 cases. J Am Acad Dermatol 79(4):702–705, 2018 29660424

Nguyen B, Hawash AA, Tosti A: Oral N-acetylcysteine in the treatment of onychotillomania. Dermatol Ther 35(8):e15605, 2022 35620921

Nwankwo CO, Jafferany M: N-Acetylcysteine in psychodermatological disorders. Dermatol Ther 32(5):e13073, 2019 31444827

Pacan P, Grzesiak M, Reich A, et al: Onychophagia and onychotillomania: prevalence, clinical picture, and comorbidities. Acta Derm Venereol 94(1):67–71, 2014 23756561

Reese JM, Hudacek KD, Rubin AI: Onychotillomania: clinicopathologic correlations. J Cutan Pathol 40(4):419–423, 2013 23398617

Silber KP, Haynes CE: Treating nailbiting: a comparative analysis of mild aversion and competing response therapies. Behav Res Ther 30(1):15–22, 1992 1540108

Singal A, Daulatabad D: Nail tic disorders: manifestations, pathogenesis, and management. Indian J Dermatol Venereol Leprol 83(1):19–26, 2017 27320768

Case 9-2
A Case of Treatment-Resistant Onychophagia

Mustafa Esen, M.D.
Ayşe Serap Karadag, M.D.

Case Description

A 34-year-old man was admitted to the dermatology clinic with complaints of bilateral fractures and deformities in all fingernails. On examination, subungual hyperkeratosis, periungual peeling, inflammation, and cuticle damage were detected, along with separation of the distal nail plaque in all bilateral fingernails (Figure 9–12). Dermatoscopic examination revealed separations of the distal nail plate, subungual splinter hemorrhage, subungual hyperkeratosis, and periungual crusting and peeling (Figure 9–13). The patient had a history of taking multiple antidepressants, including paroxetine, fluoxetine, aripiprazole, and fluvoxamine, together with alternative treatments of gum chewing, use of bitter nail polish, and receiving manicures.

Differential Diagnosis

- Nail dystrophy
- Onychotillomania
- Onychophagia
- Onychomycosis

Diagnosis

The patient said that the habit of nail biting had been going on since childhood and was exacerbated by emotional stress. He had a history of anxiety disorder and depression. His older sister and brother had OCD, and his mother had depression. His routine lab work results were within normal

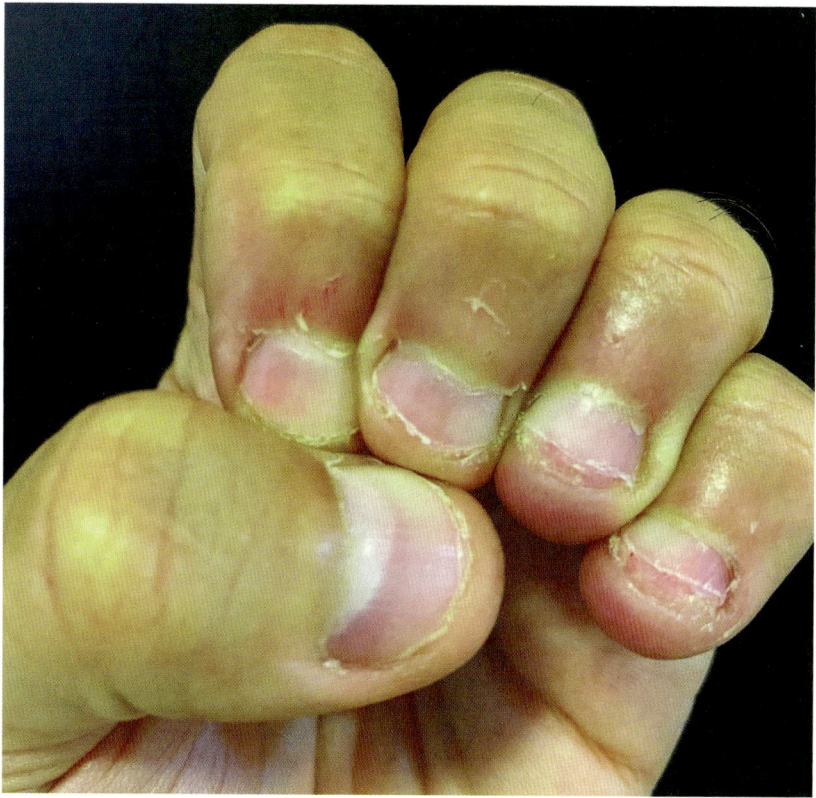

FIGURE 9–12. Subungual hyperkeratosis, periungual peeling and inflammation, along with cuticle damage in all bilateral fingernails.
Source. Dr. Mustafa Esen.

limits. The onychophagia diagnosis was made with the current clinical and dermatoscopic findings.

Management

A psychiatric consultation was requested, with the diagnosis of onychophagia. He was given CBT and fluoxetine 40 mg daily to address his anxiety and nail-biting symptoms. At a 6-month follow-up, the patient's symptoms had decreased considerably.

Discussion

Onychophagia is a psychodermatological disease characterized by recurrent widespread nail breaking and biting (Sachan and Chaturvedi 2012). It starts at an early age, and its frequency decreases with adolescence and after

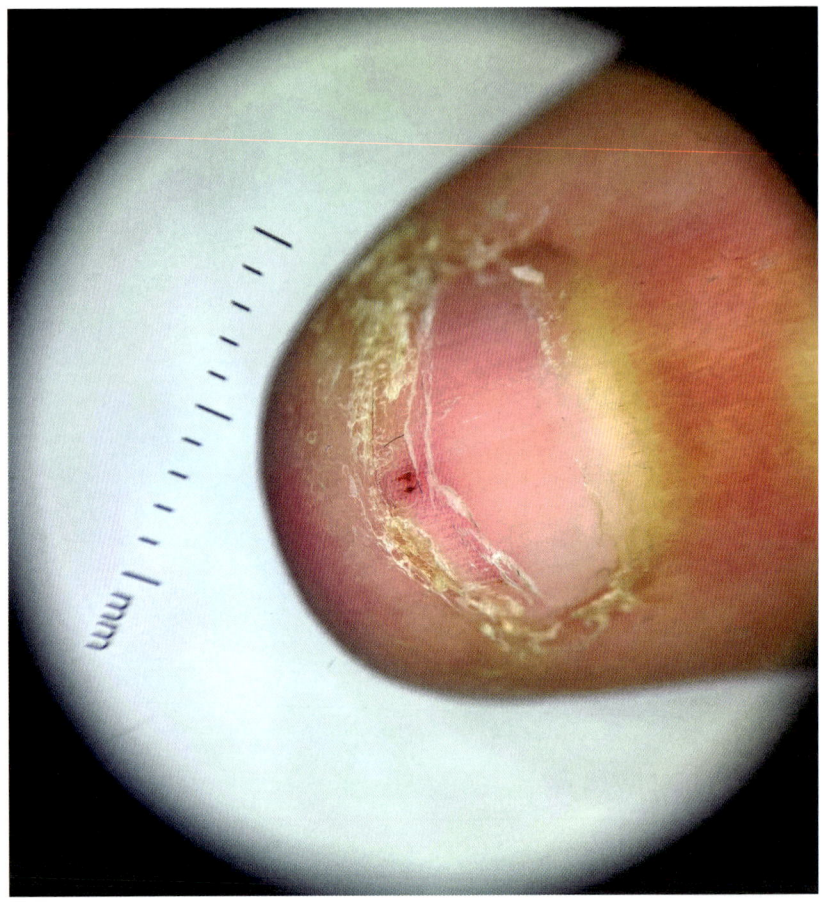

FIGURE 9–13. Separation of the distal nail plaque, subungual splinter hemorrhage, subungual hyperkeratosis, and periungual crusting and peeling.
Source. Dr. Mustafa Esen.

the age of 18 (Malone and Massler 1952). In the United States, the frequency in children ages 3–6 was reported to be 23% (Foster 1998). Although there is no difference in frequency between males and females during childhood, it is more common in males at later ages (Pacan et al. 2014a).

Psychiatric comorbidities are common in onychophagia. In one study with children and adolescents, it was found that psychiatric comorbidity was associated with two-thirds of children with onychophagia (Ghanizadeh 2008). The etiology of onychophagia is not well known (Ghanizadeh 2011). It is suggested to be associated with psychosexual development and obsessions related to the oral phase (Pearson 1948). It was also reported that onychophagia emerges as a habit that helps alleviate feelings of anxiety and loneliness, especially in children who are deprived of a sense of security, love, and close relationships (Pelc and Jaworek 2003).

This patient was initially treated with the diagnoses of depression and anxiety disorder. In clinical and dermatoscopic terms, lamellar onychoschisis, saw-tooth nail, subungual hyperkeratosis, crusting, peeling, separation of distal nail plate, longitudinal fissure, pitting, punctate leukonychia, longitudinal melanonychia, macrolunula, subungual splinter hemorrhage, cuticula, and matrix injury can be seen in onychophagia. Separation of the distal nail plate, subungual hyperkeratosis, periungual peeling and inflammation, and cuticle damage were observed in this patient. Psoriasis, eczema, lichen planus, Darier's nail involvement, and congenital nail abnormalities must be considered in the differential diagnosis of onychophagia (Chen et al. 2022). The diagnosis is often made based on clinical presentation, history of the patient, information from the patient's relatives, and dermoscopic examination. This patient was diagnosed with onychophagia given the present clinical appearance (Figure 9–12), recurrent nail-biting history since childhood, and dermoscopic findings (Figure 9–13).

The treatment approaches of onychophagia are not clear. Previous studies have reported that psychopharmacotherapy is effective in 60%–70% of cases (Pacan et al. 2014a). HRT, a subtype of CBT, is effectively used in impulse-control disorders such as trichotillomania and pathological skin picking. SSRIs, antipsychotics, tricyclic antidepressants, and NAC have been tried with variable success. Reducing environmental triggers, the use of gloves or bandages, chewing gum, bitter polish, and consistent manicures are alternative adjuvant treatments (Kaya et al. 2012; Magid et al. 2017; Pacan et al. 2014b; Velazquez et al. 2000). The treatment of onychophagia must be multidisciplinary, with pharmacology and CBT as well as the involvement of a dermatologist, psychiatrist, pediatrician, and dentist. In patients who have higher rates of anxiety, depression, OCD, and many other pathologies, the deterioration in quality of life and social interaction must not be ignored.

TEACHING POINTS

- Onychophagia is commonly seen in children and young adults.
- Dermoscopic findings could be helpful in the diagnosis.

- Habit reversal therapy is the most useful evidence-based treatment.
- Anxiety is the most common psychiatric comorbidity associated with onychophagia.

References

Chen Y, Pradhan S, Lyu L, et al: Clinical and dermoscopic characteristics of onychophagia and onychotillomania: a retrospective study of 63 cases. Clin Exp Dermatol 47(5):961–963, 2022 34905226

Foster LG: Nervous habits and stereotyped behaviors in preschool children. J Am Acad Child Adolesc Psychiatry 37(7):711–717, 1998 9666626

Ghanizadeh A: Association of nail biting and psychiatric disorders in children and their parents in a psychiatrically referred sample of children. Child Adolesc Psychiatry Ment Health 2(1):13, 2008 18513452

Ghanizadeh A: Nail biting: etiology, consequences and management. Iran J Med Sci 36(2):73–79, 2011 23358880

Kaya MC, Mahmut B, Yasin B: Add on aripiprazole for the treatment of onychophagia: a case report. Psychiatry and Clinical Psychopharmacology 22(1 Suppl):S160, 2012

Magid M, Mennella C, Kuhn H, et al: Onychophagia and onychotillomania can be effectively managed. J Am Acad Dermatol 77(5):e143–e144, 2017 29029927

Malone AJ, Massler M: Index of nailbiting in children. J Abnorm Psychol 47(2):193–202, 1952 14937953

Pacan P, Grzesiak M, Reich A, et al: Onychophagia and onychotillomania: prevalence, clinical picture and comorbidities. Acta Derm Venereol 94(1):67–71, 2014a 23756561

Pacan P, Reich A, Grzesiak M, et al: Onychophagia is associated with impairment of quality of life. Acta Derm Venereol 94(6):703–706, 2014b 24535041

Pearson GHJ: The psychology of finger-sucking, tongue-sucking, and other oral habits. Am J Orthod 34(7):589–598, 1948 18873353

Pelc AW, Jaworek AK: [Interdisciplinary approach to onychophagia] [in Polish]. Przegl Lek 60(11):737–739, 2003 15058046

Sachan A, Chaturvedi TP: Onychophagia (nail biting), anxiety, and malocclusion. Indian J Dent Res 23(5):680–682, 2012 23422619

Velazquez L, Ward-Chene L, Loosigian SR: Fluoxetine in the treatment of self-mutilating behavior. J Am Acad Child Adolesc Psychiatry 39(7):812–814, 2000 10892222

Case 9–3
Pseudo-Knuckle Pads: A Bridge to Psychodermatology

Mezni Line, M.D.
Khallaayoune Mehdi, M.D.
Farah El Hadadi, M.D.
Meziane Mariame, M.D.
Senouci Karima, M.D.

Case Description

A healthy 15-year-old girl presented to the dermatology outpatient clinic for painless, indurated skin lesions over the metacarpal and proximal interphalangeal joints on several digits of the right hand. The patient and her parents denied any comorbid psychiatric disorders, history of trauma on her fingers, or unusual hobbies or sports. During the consultation, a pattern of repeated behaviors of crossing hands, rubbing, biting, and chewing her hands on a daily basis to relieve anxiety was noted. She reported that the behavior started 3 years ago because of academic pressure. At first, the habit was associated with her reaction to a stressful condition (such as an exam period), but gradually it became more habitual and unconscious. She tried various behavioral modifications, such as covering her hands, without any benefit.

On physical examination, we observed asymmetric, slightly hyperpigmented, well-circumscribed, smooth, dome-shaped fibrous plaques over joints on the dorsal surfaces of the hands (Figures 9–14 and 9–15).

Differential Diagnosis

- Subcutaneous granuloma annulare
- Gottron papules
- Gouty tophi
- Pachydermodactyly
- Rheumatoid nodules
- Synovitis
- Erythema elevatum diutinum
- Foreign body granulomas
- Tumor
- Warts

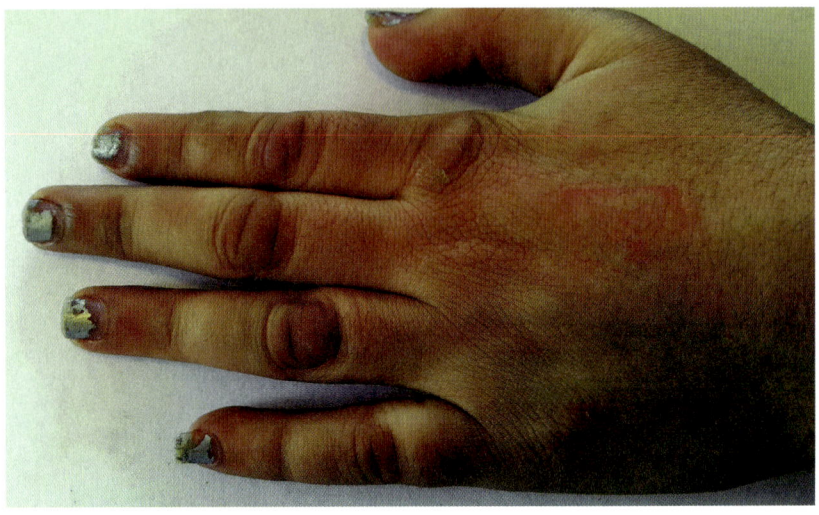

FIGURE 9–14. Pseudo-knuckle pads over proximal interphalangeal and metacarpal joints.
Source. Dr. Mezni Line.

- Osteoarthritis with Heberden nodules

Diagnosis

A skin biopsy showed epidermal and dermal changes. Mild acanthosis, hyperkeratosis, and papillomatosis along with hyperplasia of collagen were noted. The patient was referred to a psychiatrist, who made the diagnosis of BFRBD.

Management

The patient was treated with topical keratolytic ointment (high-dose salicylic acid and urea), and psychotherapy was recommended. The patient showed significant improvement at a 6-month follow-up.

Discussion

Knuckle pads, first described by Garrod in 1893, are also known as athlete's nodules, subcutaneous fibroma, keratosis supracapitularis, discrete keratoderma, heloderma, tylositas articuli, and Garrod pads. They are described as discrete fibromatosis, observed as well-defined, mobile, dome-shaped nodules, or plaque-like lesions, frequently localized on the proximal interphalangeal joints over the dorsal surface of fingers more than toes. They may also affect the metacarpophalangeal or distal interphalangeal joints.

Body-Focused Repetitive Behavioral Disorders

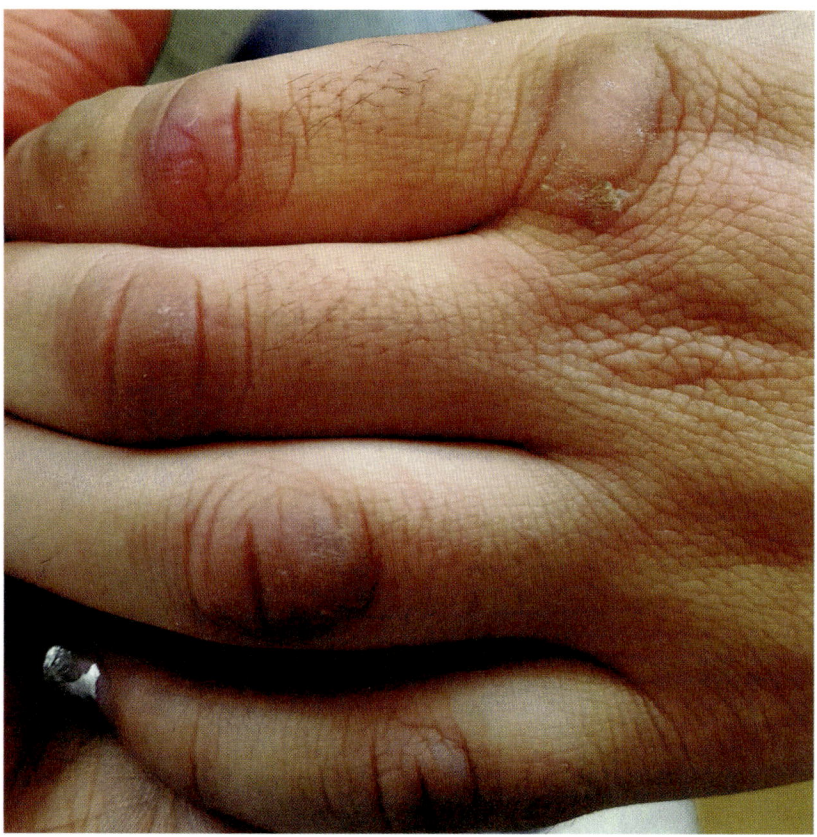

FIGURE 9–15. Asymmetric, slightly hyperpigmented and scaly, well-circumscribed nodules over joints on the dorsal surface of the hand.
Source. Dr. Mezni Line.

The skin can be indurated, flesh colored, or hyperpigmented. The lesions are asymptomatic and not associated with rheumatologic symptoms. Knuckle pads may appear at any age, are permanent, and grow over time (Tamborrini et al. 2012). Inherited (primary) knuckle pads should be differentiated from secondary (acquired) knuckle pads.

Most of the inherited cases are idiopathic; however, some may be associated with fibromatosis disorders (e.g., palmar Dupuytren contracture, plantar ledderhose disease) and Peyronie disease (Tamborrini et al. 2012). Some studies have reported a familial occurrence (Tamborrini et al. 2012). Primary knuckle pads may be a hallmark of different genetic syndromes along with a myriad of clinical symptoms, such as Bart-Pumphrey syndrome, epidermolysis palmoplantar keratoderma, acrokeratoelastoidosis of Costa, and camptodactyly (Tamborrini et al. 2012). It has also been described along with finger pebbles in the context of metabolic syndrome and type 2 diabetes (Saylam Kurtipek et al. 2015).

Secondary knuckle pads, called pseudo-knuckle pads, should be recognized separately as clinical, and management approaches are different. They appear at a younger age, and lesions are hyperkeratotic secondary to chronic friction or repeated trauma, as well as psychiatric disturbances (e.g., chewing or sucking fingers, bulimia nervosa) or along with occupational or athletic activities such as boxing or surfing.

The diagnosis is made based on clinical features; however, further investigations may be considered to rule out differential diagnosis. Ultrasound shows a subcutaneous hypoechoic nodule without vascularization on color Doppler, and pathology of the knuckle pads reveals hyperkeratosis, acanthosis, and proliferation of myofibroblasts, with a decrease of elastic filaments in the deep dermis (Tamborrini et al. 2012).

Recognizing and understanding the psychosocial and occupational context of lesions is critical for the diagnosis and provides the optimal management of its underlying cause. In this case, the patient had been repeatedly rubbing, biting, and chewing the hands because of severe anxiety. BFRBDs are a group of problematic and destructive behaviors directed toward the body (e.g., trichotillomania, onychophagia, cuticle biting, lip biting, nail biting, and cheek biting), most often beginning in late childhood or adolescence (Siddiqui et al. 2012). They are recurrent, undesired, and often designed to remove part of the body (Siddiqui et al. 2012).

Individuals with BFRBDs report the inability to control their behavior and a range of physical and psychological sequelae along with maladaptive emotion regulation mechanisms. Therapy for pseudo-knuckle pads is challenging and should be approached gently, because aggressive procedures may induce keloid formation. First-line treatment is based on education to avoid repetitive trauma and irritation by wearing protective gloves and modifying professional or vocational activities. Topical emollients, keratolytics, and intralesional corticosteroids or fluorouracil injections may be used, with variable success. Psychotherapeutic treatment includes a combination of psychotropic medications and CBT. CBT often involves HRT and exposure response prevention (Koo and Lebwohl 2001).

TEACHING POINTS

- The primary form of knuckle pads is unrelated to trauma, although the secondary type, pseudo-knuckle pads, may be considered a form of callosity that appears after repeated friction.

- They are commonly described in children with obsessive behaviors as "chewing pads," and in adults as an occupational disorder.

- Clinical and occupational history is important in reaching the diagnosis.

- In addition to dermatological treatment, cognitive-behavioral therapy, particularly habit reversal therapy, is useful in treatment.

References

Koo J, Lebwohl A: Psycho dermatology: the mind and skin connection. Am Fam Physician 64(11):1873–1878, 2001 11764865

Saylam Kurtipek G, Kutlu O, Duran C, et al: Frequency of metabolic syndrome in patients with knuckle pads. J Dermatol 42(12):1165–1168, 2015 26119428

Siddiqui EU, Naeem SS, Naqvi H, et al: Prevalence of body-focused repetitive behaviors in three large medical colleges of Karachi: a cross-sectional study. BMC Res Notes 5:614, 2012 23116460

Tamborrini G, Gengenbacher M, Bianchi S: Knuckle pads: a rare finding. J Ultrason 12(51):493–498, 2012 26672439

Case 9-4
Chronic Wound Secondary to Skin Picking Mistaken for Fungal Infection

Meera Aladawi, M.D., M.Sc.
Dimitre Dimitrov, M.D., Ph.D.
Tarek Shahrour, M.D.

Case Description

A 20-year-old man in a wheelchair was referred to the wound clinic with a diagnosis of fungal infection with secondary irritation and wound formation, resulting from concomitant severe itching. The patient was vague regarding the skin problem, and he stated that he couldn't remember how long ago the problem appeared. On physical examination, well-defined erosive and ulcerated lesions with various degrees of maceration and a yellow-green scanty secretion were present. The lesions demonstrated crusting, desquamation, and scars at different stages of healing. The changes were situated on the scrotum and left inguinal groin (Figures 9–16 and 9–17).

Differential Diagnosis

- Fungal infection
- Syphilitic chancre
- Dermatitis artefacta
- Skin-picking disorder

Diagnosis

The lesions displayed were not found to be characteristic of a fungal infection. In fact, the entire appearance was suggestive of skin manipulation and self-inflicted skin changes on thighs, arms, and genital areas. Swabs for bacterial and fungal infections were negative. A detailed history was taken, including targeted questions regarding self-manipulation. The questions were carefully chosen to obtain the information sensitively and without being confrontational. The main goal of the interview was to establish rapport with the patient. The patient was initially reluctant, but after receiving an explanation that what he is experiencing is a recognized problem experi-

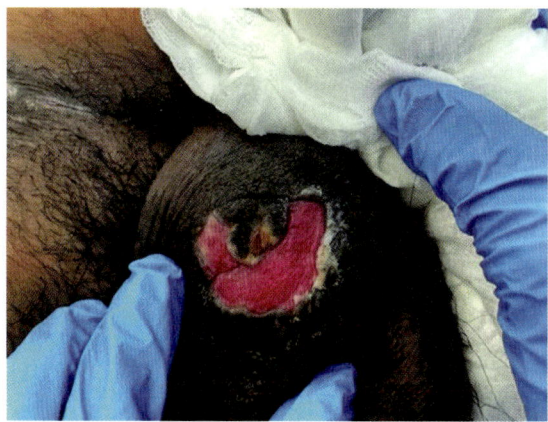

FIGURE 9–16. Lesion on the scrotum at the first visit.
Source. Dr. Meera Aladawi.

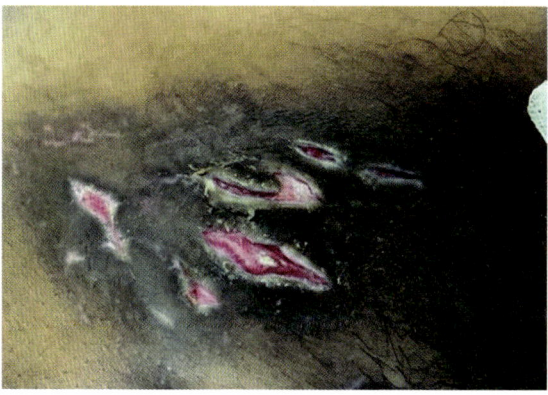

FIGURE 9–17. Lesion on the left inguinal area at the first visit.
Source. Dr. Meera Aladawi.

enced by many people, he relaxed and agreed to discuss the issue further. He admitted to self-manipulating his skin and stated that the lesions mostly resulted from sitting incorrectly. He believed being in bed made them worse than being in a wheelchair. He also reported problems with sleeping.

During the detailed discussion of psychosocial aspects of his life, the patient disclosed that he lost his family during a car accident when he was 3 years old. Since that time, he has been living with other relatives and is unhappy with his living situation. During later visits, he disclosed more details about some interfamilial problems. He has been in a wheelchair since the accident, with restricted activity, difficulties in visiting friends and relatives, and a permanent need for assistance in his activities of daily living. He disclosed that most of his social contacts are virtual.

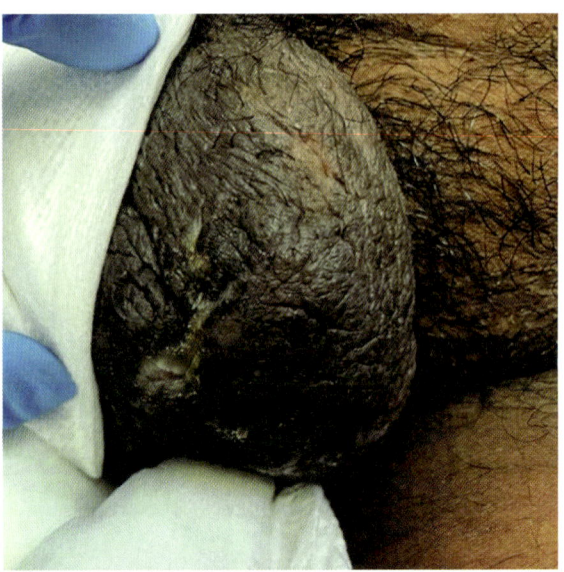

FIGURE 9–18. Lesion on the scrotum after 12 weeks of SSRI treatment.
Source. Dr. Meera Aladawi.

As part of his complete assessment, the patient completed the following questionnaires: Dermatology Life Quality Index, Generalized Anxiety Disorder-7 items (GAD-7), and Patient Health Questionnaire-9 items (PHQ-9). The results showed mild to moderate depression and anxiety. The patient described that his wish to pick the skin is usually preceded by a lightheaded feeling and heavy breathing. The patient reported that the skin picking happens many times a day, sometimes >100 times. He also feels the need to pick his skin when he is sexually aroused.

Management

The patient received topical povidone-iodine spray, nano-silver spray, silver hydrofiber dressing, and povidone iodine nonadherent dressing, without any major benefit. Subsequently, the patient was offered HRT, which he declined. Based on his history of depression and anxiety, confirmed by PHQ-9 and GAD-7, he was started on escitalopram 10 mg daily. The patient's mood and other depressive symptoms greatly improved, and his skin lesions improved dramatically (Figures 9–18 and 9–19).

Discussion

Chronic wounds are defined as wounds that fail to proceed through the normal phases of wound healing in an orderly and timely manner (Frykberg

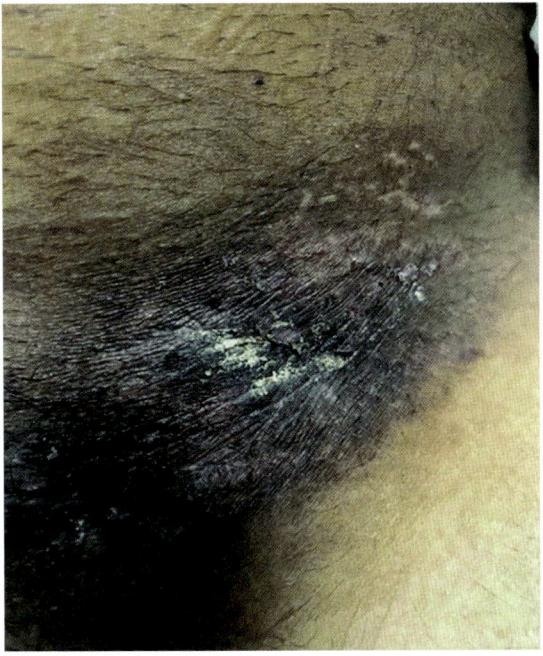

FIGURE 9–19. Lesion on the left inguinal area after 12 weeks of SSRI treatment.
Source. Dr. Meera Aladawi.

and Banks 2015). A wound that does not improve to 50% of its size within 4 weeks is often considered chronic. The most common types of chronic wounds include ulcers, infectious wounds, ischemic wounds, surgical wounds, and wounds from radiation poisoning (Werdin et al. 2008). Clarifying a wound's etiology, as well as underlying and associated conditions, is of paramount importance regarding its proper management. Skin-picking disorder or excoriative disorder is a condition that leads to repetitive picking of the skin, causing soft tissue damage (Hawatmeh and Al-Khateeb 2017). Individuals pick their skin—consciously or unconsciously—to the extent that they produce bleeding, scarring, disfigurement, persistent sores, and ulcers and may need surgery and skin grafting to avoid progression to life-threatening conditions (Ravipati et al. 2021). An association with distress, anxiety, and depression due to picking and lower quality of life have been reported in the medical literature (Torales et al. 2021).

Proper management of skin-picking disorder requires a multidisciplinary team to address the patient's various needs and deliver complex and holistic treatment. In addition to direct skin treatment, a number of both psychopharmacological and psychotherapeutic approaches have been used.

Topical wound treatment usually includes a variety of antiseptics, antibiotics, and epithelializing agents. SSRIs, lamotrigine, glutamatergic agents such as NAC and riluzole, and opioid antagonists such as naltrexone have been tried in skin-picking disorders (Torales et al. 2020). A pilot study examined the use of topiramate (Lochner et al. 2017). A number of articles have pointed out the benefits of SSRIs in treating skin picking, with varying levels of success (Lochner et al. 2017; Jafferany and Osuagwu 2017; Jafferany and Patel 2019; Torales et al. 2020).

This patient demonstrated depression and thus was started on escitalopram. The establishment of good rapport with the patient and a multidisciplinary approach in treatment are important in such cases.

TEACHING POINTS

- Avoiding confrontation is a key factor during the process of caring for skin-picking patients.
- A multidisciplinary team approach is crucial in management.
- Screening tools and questionnaires might be helpful in identifying concomitant underlying mental health conditions.

References

Frykberg RG, Banks J: Challenges in the treatment of chronic wounds. Adv Wound Care (New Rochelle) 4(9):560–582, 2015 26339534

Hawatmeh A, Al-Khateeb A: An unusual complication of dermatillomania. Quant Imaging Med Surg 7(1):166–168, 2017 28275574

Jafferany M, Osuagwu FC: Use of topiramate in skin-picking disorder: a pilot study. Prim Care Companion CNS Disord 19(1): 2017 28129492

Jafferany M, Patel A: Skin-picking disorder: a guide to diagnosis and management. CNS Drugs 33(4):337–346, 2019 30877621

Lochner C, Roos A, Stein DJ: Excoriation (skin-picking) disorder: a systematic review of treatment options. Neuropsychiatr Dis Treat 13:1867–1872, 2017 28761349

Ravipati P, Conti B, Chiesa E, et al: Dermatillomania: strategies for developing protective biomaterials/cloth. Pharmaceutics 13(3):341, 2021 33808008

Torales J, Díaz NR, Barrios I, et al: Psychodermatology of skin picking (excoriation disorder): a comprehensive review. Dermatol Ther 33(4):e13661, 2020 32447793

Torales J, Díaz NR, Barrios I, et al: Hair-pulling disorder (trichotillomania): etiopathogenesis, diagnosis and treatment in a nutshell. Dermatol Ther 34(1):e13466, 2021 33015928

Werdin F, Tenenhaus M, Rennekampff HO: Chronic wound care. Lancet 372(9653):1860–1862, 2008 19041788

Case 9–5
Obsessive-Compulsive Disorder With Repeated Hand Washing and Onset of Fingernail Onychomycosis

Prajwal Pudasaini, M.D.
Sushil Paudel, M.D.
Sadiksha Adhikari, M.D.

Case Description

A 27-year-old woman presented to the clinic with complaints of yellow discoloration and loss of distal fingernails of her little fingers bilaterally for the past 5 months. The patient had a repeated history of hand washing >20 times a day for >6 years. She had repeated thoughts to wash off dirt and germs from her hands, which she knows is abnormal, but she said she had no control over it. She had a sense of urgency and impulse to wash her hands as she thought that her hands were frequently contaminated. She also had a history of chronic repeated nail biting, particularly of both little fingers. She used to bite her nails during times of stress. The patient reported relief and satisfaction after washing her hands. Additionally, she had a history of yellowish discoloration of the nail and separation of the nail plate from the nail bed.

On examination, onychodystrophy with yellow discoloration, distal onycholysis, and nail loss were seen over bilateral nail plates of the little fingers (Figures 9–20, 9–21, and 9–22). The patient had a habit of biting her nails (without eating them). The patient had a history of OCD and took fluoxetine 20 mg for the past 6 years.

Differential Diagnosis

- Traumatic onychodystrophy
- Onychotillomania
- Onychomycosis

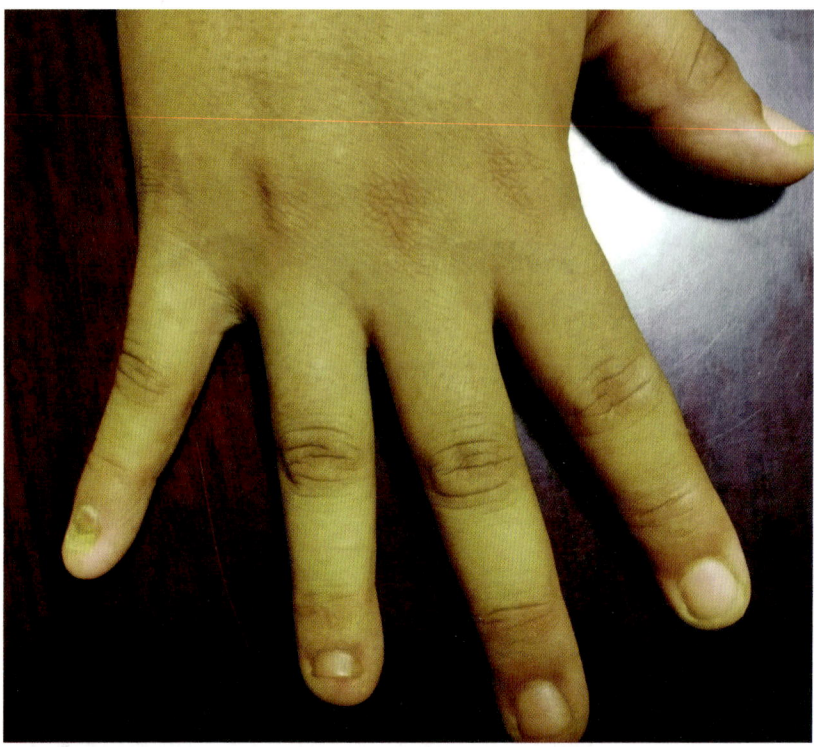

FIGURE 9–20. Onychodystrophy with distal loss of nail plate and yellowish discoloration of nail plate of right little finger.
Source. Dr. Prajwal Pudasaini.

Diagnosis

Onychoscopy showed longitudinal ridges, longitudinal striae, and jagged edge of proximal nail fold (Figure 9–23). Mycological examination showed sparse septate hyphae typical of dermatophyte infection. The diagnosis of onychomycosis was made due to consistent moisture and wet hands.

Management

To address the psychological component of the patient's problems, she was enrolled in HRT three times per week. The patient continued with fluoxetine 20 mg daily and added itraconazole weekly pulse for 2 months and amorolfine nail lacquer two times per week. There was an improvement in nail texture and nail morphology after treatment. Significant improvement was noted during the 2-month follow-up and beyond, and she remained symptom free. The patient experienced significant improvement in symptoms, such as a decrease in repeated thoughts and impulses to wash her hands.

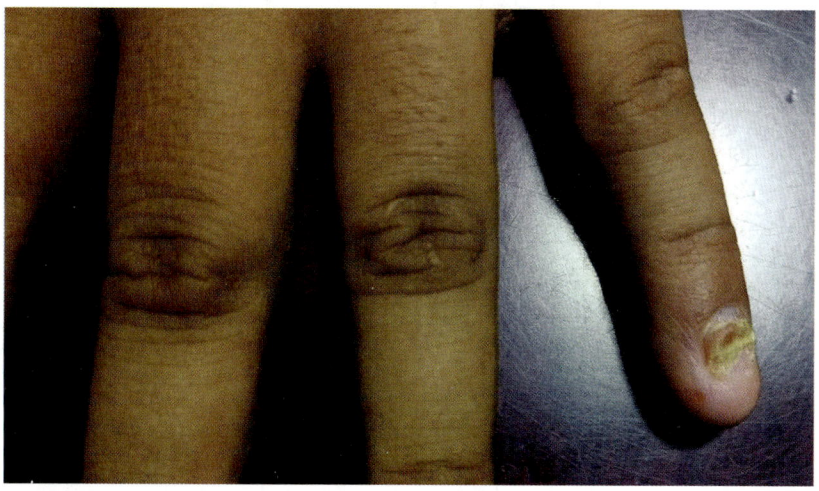

FIGURE 9–21. Onychodystrophy of left little finger.
Source. Dr. Prajwal Pudasaini.

Discussion

Onychomycosis associated with OCD can be diagnosed with a careful clinical history and examination. Underlying psychiatric comorbidities such as family discord, BFRBDs, anxiety, depression, and OCD should be identified and managed accordingly (Singal and Daulatabad 2017). BFRBs associated with onychotillomania and subsequent nail pathology make diagnosis easier (Cohen 2022). Onychomycosis due to OCD can mimic a variety of other conditions, and biopsy is rarely needed to differentiate onychomycosis from other nail pathologies. Dermoscopy is useful to corroborate findings of onychomycosis with its clinical presentation, as in this patient. Characteristic features of onychomycosis in dermoscopy may include longitudinal ridges along the nail bed, longitudinal striae, leukonychia, yellow-brown pigmentation over lateral and distal nail plate edges, subungual hyperkeratosis, and jagged proximal nail fold (Yorulmaz and Yalcin 2018).

Management of onychomycosis associated with OCD should involve a multidisciplinary approach (Singal and Daulatabad 2017). Treatment should include assessment of underlying psychological comorbidity (depression, anxiety, BFRBDs, OCD, and family discord) (Cohen 2022). Psychotherapy, particularly HRT, is an integral part of the therapeutic regimen (Lee and Lipner 2022). SSRIs such as fluoxetine, dapoxetine, and sertraline form an important part of treatment in those with comorbid OCD (Singal and Daulatabad 2017). Treatment with SSRIs may take several months to

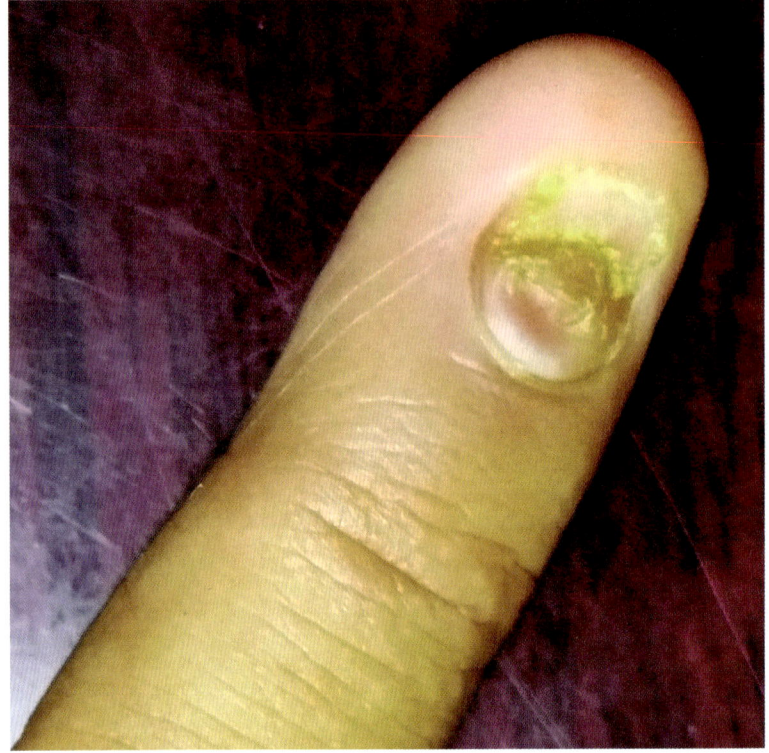

FIGURE 9–22. Onychodystrophy with distal loss of nail plate and yellowish discoloration of nail plate of left little finger.
Source. Dr. Prajwal Pudasaini.

effect therapeutic change. Recurrence, often a challenge, may need reinitiation of therapy.

TEACHING POINTS

- Onychomycosis associated with repeated hand washing due to OCD presents with yellowish-white discoloration of the nail plate, distal onycholysis, and subungual hyperkeratosis.
- Underlying OCD and habit disorders exacerbate this condition, which may lead to nail pathologies.

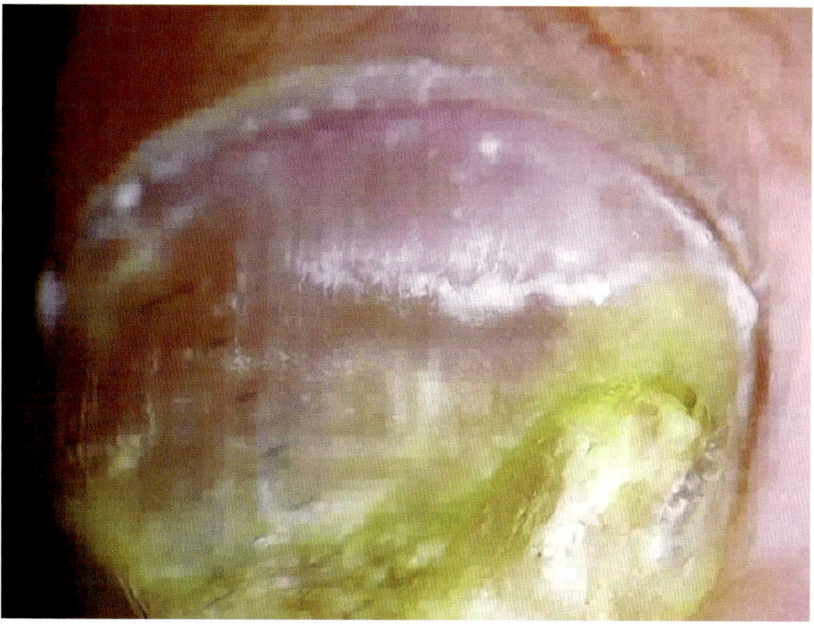

FIGURE 9–23. Longitudinal ridges along nail bed, longitudinal striae, leukonychia, yellowish brown pigmentation over lateral and distal nail plate edges, and subungual hyperkeratosis.
Source. Dr. Prajwal Pudasaini.

- Assessment of underlying psychological conditions and incorporation of psychotherapy help prevent this chronic condition.
- Assessment of psychological causes, comorbidities, and complications forms an important part of the therapeutic regimen, along with psychotherapy.

References

Cohen PR: Nail-associated body-focused repetitive behaviors: habit-tic nail deformity, onychophagia, and onychotillomania. Cureus 14(3):e22818, 2022 35382180

Lee DK, Lipner SR: Update on diagnosis and management of onychophagia and onychotillomania. Int J Environ Res Public Health 19(6):3392, 2022 35329078

Singal A, Daulatabad D: Nail tic disorders: manifestations, pathogenesis, and management. Indian J Dermatol Venereol Leprol 83(1):19–26, 2017 27320768

Yorulmaz A, Yalcin B: Dermoscopy as a first step in the diagnosis of onychomycosis. Postepy Dermatol Alergol 35(3):251–258, 2018 30008642

Case 9-6
Concomitant Onychophagia and Dermatotillomania Successfully Treated With Habit Reversal as Monotherapy

Sara Al Janahi, M.D., M.Sc.
Dimitre Dimitrov, M.D., Ph.D.
Shaden Abdelhadi, M.D.

Case Description

A 17-year-old girl was referred to the dermatology clinic for management of chronic dyshidrotic eczema. She had received various topical steroids, topical antibiotics, and emollients for 2 years, without any benefit. The patient denied excessive exposure to irritants. Her medical history was unremarkable.

On examination, there were multiple erosions and ulcers, of different depths and stages of healing, over the periungual skin, with areas of postinflammatory hyperpigmentation. She also had onychodystrophy, mostly of the thumbnails. There was a shortening of the nail plates. The patient was embarrassed about the appearance of her fingers and provided us with a photo that she felt best represented her condition (Figure 9-24).

A variety of screening tools were used to evaluate psychological percussion of her lesions. The tools used were Skin-Picking Scale, Dermatology Life Quality Index, Screen for Anxiety-Related Disorders (SCARED) for the child, Center for Epidemiological Studies Depression Scale for Children, and 6-item Stigmatization scale. All scales demonstrated significant anxiety and depression. The instruments for the mother included Family Dermatology Life Quality Index and SCARED for the parent, also indicating stress and anxiety in the mother. This was having a moderate effect on the quality of life of the patient and stress in the family. Therefore, a referral to a mental health specialist was recommended, but the patient declined.

Of note, the slight discrepancy between the patient's and her mother's scores on the SCARED questionnaire was significant. Seemingly, the mother was not aware of her child's underlying anxiety, despite their close relationship.

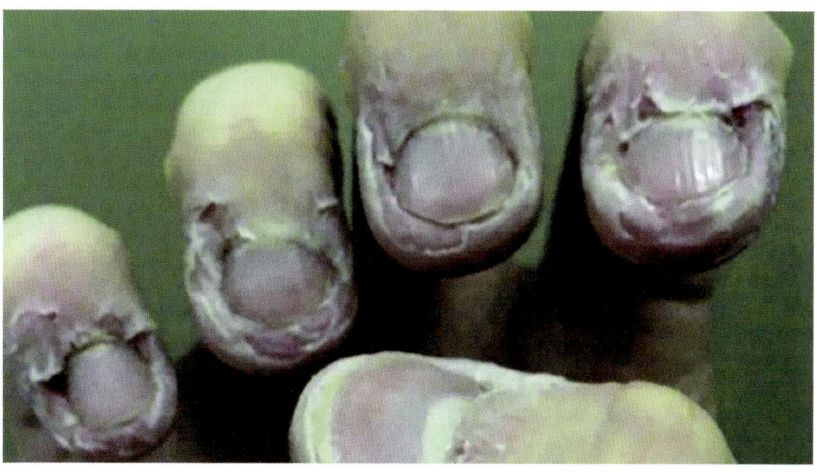

FIGURE 9–24. Image provided by the patient of hands before HRT.
Source. Dr. Sara Al Janahi.

Differential Diagnosis

- Self-induced dermatosis
- Contact dermatitis
- Dyshidrotic eczema
- Onychomycosis

Diagnosis

On further inquiry, the patient admitted that she often bit her nails and pulled the skin around the nails until she bled. She associated this with changes in her life over the past 2 years. It was clear that her symptoms were due to onychophagia and dermatotillomania.

Management

Habit reversal training (HRT) was initiated, along with topical antibiotics and moisturizers, which the patient declined to apply. A few weeks later, a significant reduction in skin picking and nail biting was clinically evident. She consented to us taking a photograph (Figure 9–25).

Discussion

Skin picking and onychophagia may coexist. Both diagnoses are BFRBDs and classified as obsessive-compulsive spectrum disorders. Although psy-

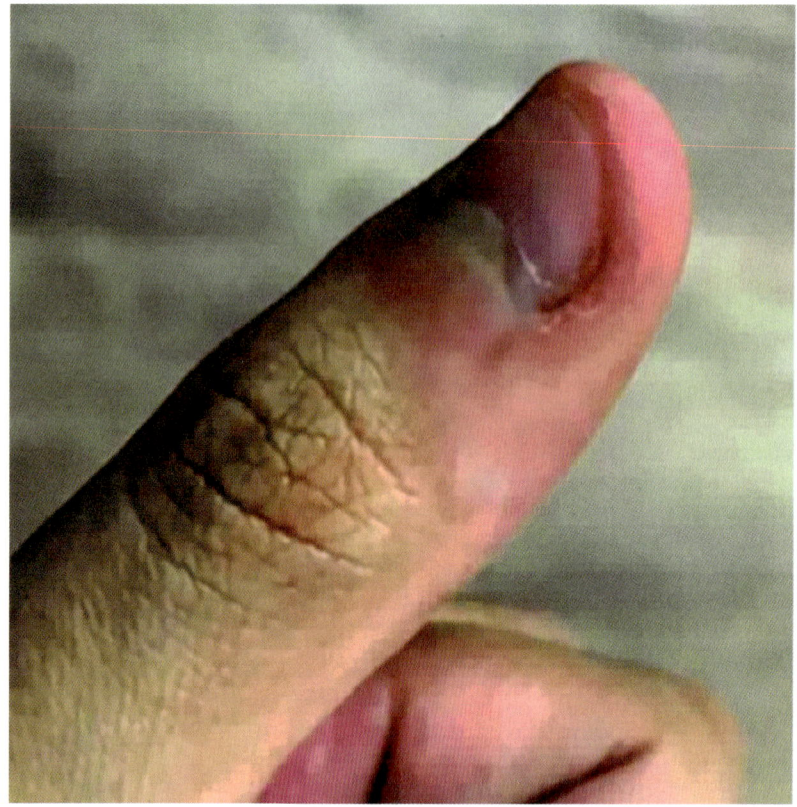

FIGURE 9–25. The patient's thumb 3 months after HRT.
Source. Dr. Sara Al Jahani.

chotropic medications such as SSRIs have been tried, HRT is the mainstay of treatment. HRT is an effective behavior-modification technique, proven to be beneficial in managing a variety of conditions, usually combined with conventional medical therapies (Skurya et al. 2020). In selected cases, it is successful as a monotherapy. This case illustrates the success of HRT in chronic, refractory, self-inflicted conditions even as monotherapy. Multiple factors are required when selecting a candidate for HRT, such as the patient's own motivation and a supportive home environment. We believe that our patient's level of motivation contributed to the successful results she achieved.

TEACHING POINTS

- Health care providers should consider self-inflicted dermatoses and actively inquire about self-destructive behaviors.
- Habit reversal training (HRT) is a valuable option in combination with other traditional therapies.
- In selected patients, HRT may be effective as a monotherapy.
- Patients with self-inflicted skin changes should be evaluated for underlying mental health conditions.
- Family members should not be the only source of information when assessing patients with self-inflicted dermatoses.

References

Skurya J, Jafferany M, Everett GJ: Habit reversal therapy in the management of body focused repetitive behavior disorders. Dermatol Ther 33(6):e13811, 2020 32542916

Case 9-7
Long-Term Pathological Skin Picking Leading to Severe Skin Damage

Mateusz K. Mateuszczyk, M.D.
Joanna Maj, M.D.
Jacek C. Szepietowski, M.D.

Case Description

A 66-year-old woman with a history of depression presented to the dermatology department for skin picking that started ~30 years earlier. On examination, she had numerous, extensive, deep ulcers, excoriations, and scars on her face, neck, arms, and legs (Figures 9–26, 9–27, and 9–28). The patient

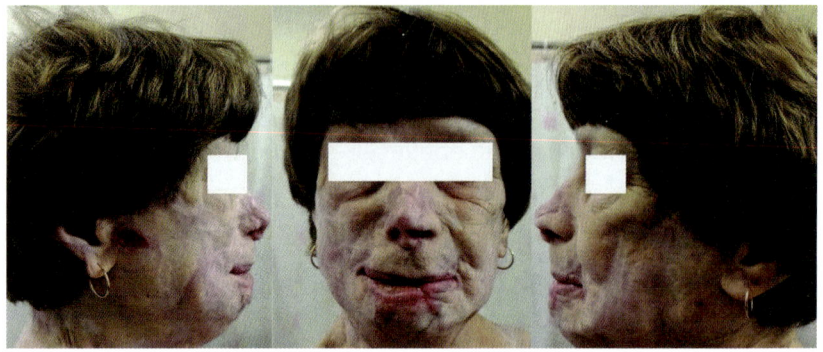

FIGURE 9–26. Ulcers and scars, deforming the face.
Source. Dr. Mateusz Mateuszczyk.

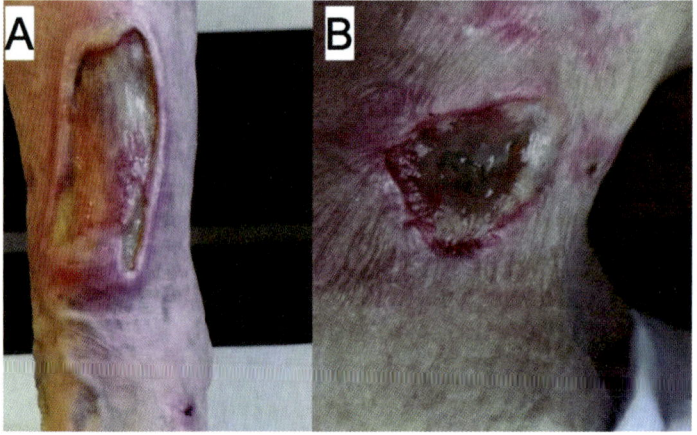

FIGURE 9–27. Deep nonhealing ulcers on the left shin (A) and neck (B).
Source. Dr. Mateusz Mateuszczyk.

reported severe itching. The patient admitted inducing lesions through scratching, which temporarily relieved the itch, and attempts to refrain from scratching were associated with an increase in internal tension and frustration. According to the patient, itching initially occurred on normal skin, and subsequent scratching led to the development of patches, nodules, ulcers, and scars. At the time of admission, she was taking oral quetiapine 25 mg/day, escitalopram 10 mg/day, and bisoprolol 5 mg/day.

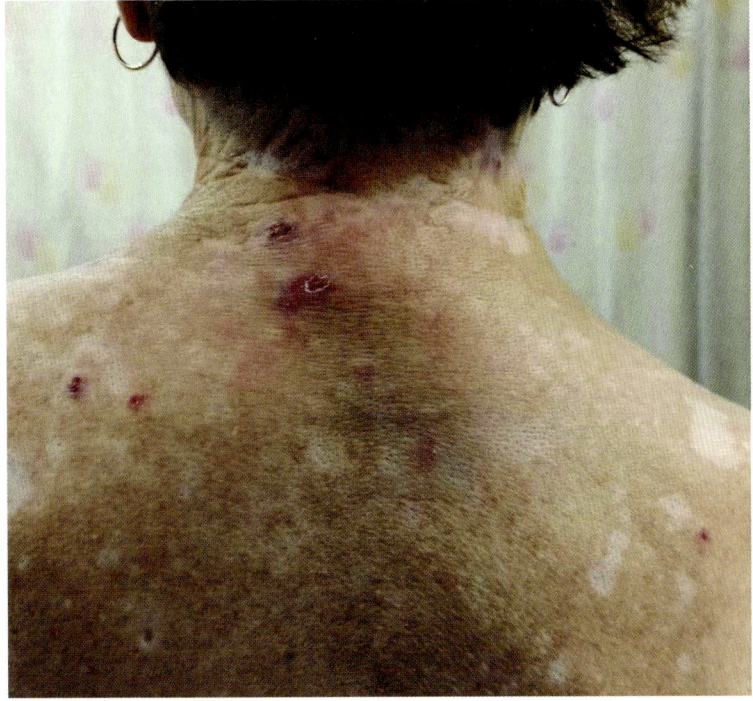

FIGURE 9–28. Numerous atrophic scars and eroded papules on the back.
Source. Dr. Mateusz Mateuszczyk.

Differential Diagnosis

In the differential diagnosis, primary consideration was given to pathological skin picking, dermatitis artefacta. However, the diagnostic scope was expanded to include dermatological and medical conditions associated with itch.

Diagnosis

All lab work was within normal limits, except hypothyroid state. Psychiatric consultation was conducted. Regarding her scratching behavior, she said, "I watch and scratch; I can't stop myself from doing it." A skin biopsy was taken from the lesion and was unremarkable. Based on the overall clinical picture and additional investigations, a diagnosis of excoriation disorder was established.

Management

After the psychiatric consultation, it was decided to switch from escitalopram 10 mg/day to paroxetine 20 mg/day and increase the frequency of quetiapine 25 mg from once to three times a day. Additionally, CBT was recommended.

Wound treatment was also applied. The patient did not follow up on the recommendations made, and she was later rehospitalized twice for worsening of her condition. Both times her psychotropic medications were adjusted, and special emphasis was placed on initiating psychotherapy.

Discussion

Pathological skin picking (excoriation or skin-picking disorder) is characterized by repetitive scratching, picking, rubbing, or squeezing of skin, resulting in the development of lesions that significantly impair quality of life (Odlaug et al. 2016). The patient is unable to refrain from the picking behavior because of increasing internal tension; engaging in the behavior brings relief and gratification. Patients may use nails, teeth, or sharp objects (Arnold et al. 2001). Unlike dermatitis artefacta, patients acknowledge self-inflicted skin damage and may report severe itching, but the symptoms cannot account for the severity of the lesions (Gieler et al. 2013).

The prevalence of pathological skin picking in the general population is 1.6%–5.4%, with female predominance. The age of onset for pathological skin picking varies, but the most common is during adolescence (93%), with the mean age being 13.6 years. However, there is also a smaller group with a later onset, with the mean age of 42.8 years (Ricketts et al. 2018). It is worth mentioning that the onset of the disorder during childhood is connected to prolonged duration of the condition and a lower inclination to seek treatment (Odlaug and Grant 2007).

The most prevalent comorbidities include anxiety disorders, depression, dissociative disorders, OCD, borderline personality disorder, substance dependence, and body dysmorphic disorder (Tomas-Aragones et al. 2017). The etiology of pathological skin picking is currently unclear. Neuroimaging techniques have suggested atypical brain activation in regions associated with habit formation, action monitoring, and inhibition (Odlaug et al. 2016). Clinically, a patient will typically exhibit polymorphic skin lesions of various sizes and severity, unlike the monomorphic eruptions often seen in dermatitis artefacta. Lesions are typically symmetrically localized within reach of the hands, the most common location being the face (Gieler et al. 2013).

Pathological skin picking can lead to significant body distortions that may require surgical correction, as well as serious skin, blood, and other infections, which can pose a direct threat to life (Odlaug and Grant 2007). Kim et al. (2013) described a near-fatal case of a 51-year-old woman with pathological skin picking who, using a knitting needle, caused tissue loss on the scalp, exposing the left frontal bone and leading to encephalomalacia. Patients suffering from pathological skin picking rarely seek medical help because of stigma and feelings of shame and guilt, along with the belief that their condition is incurable. Establishing good rapport and building trust are very important for better outcomes and compliance in therapy. A multidisciplinary treatment approach among dermatologists, psychiatrists, and psychologists plays a major role.

Along with wound management, the mainstay of therapy involves pharmacotherapy combined with CBT. SSRIs are used with good results (Tomas-Aragones et al. 2017). However, it is essential to remember that other factors, such as the involvement of the patient's support system (including family), the presence of coexisting medical conditions, and the age of onset, can also influence the effectiveness of treatment (Odlaug and Grant 2007; Tomas-Aragones et al. 2017).

TEACHING POINTS

- Skin picking typically exhibits polymorphic skin lesions of various sizes and severity, symmetrically localized within the reach of hands.

- Therapy requires close collaboration between a dermatologist, psychiatrist, the patient, and their support system (family, friends, or caregivers).

- Treatment typically involves the use of selective serotonin reuptake inhibitors and cognitive-behavioral therapy.

References

Arnold LM, Auchenbach MB, McElroy SL: Psychogenic excoriation: clinical features, proposed diagnostic criteria, epidemiology and approaches to treatment. CNS Drugs 15(5):351–359, 2001 11475941

Gieler U, Consoli SG, Tomás-Aragones L, et al: Self-inflicted lesions in dermatology: terminology and classification—a position paper from the European Society for Dermatology and Psychiatry (ESDaP). Acta Derm Venereol 93(1):4–12, 2013 23303467

Kim DI, Garrison RC, Thompson G: A near fatal case of pathological skin picking. Am J Case Rep 14:284–287, 2013 23919102

Odlaug BL, Grant JE: Childhood-onset pathologic skin picking: clinical characteristics and psychiatric comorbidity. Compr Psychiatry 48(4):388–393, 2007 17560962

Odlaug BL, Hampshire A, Chamberlain SR, et al: Abnormal brain activation in excoriation (skin-picking) disorder: evidence from an executive planning fMRI study. Br J Psychiatry 208(2):168–174, 2016 26159604

Ricketts EJ, Snorrason I, Kircanski K, et al: A latent profile analysis of age of onset in pathological skin picking. Compr Psychiatry 87:46–52, 2018 30199665

Tomas-Aragones L, Consoli SM, Consoli SG, et al: Self-inflicted lesions in dermatology: a management and therapeutic approach: a position paper from the European Society for Dermatology and Psychiatry. Acta Derm Venereal 97(2):159–172, 2017 27563702

Case 9–8

Clinical and Medical Treatment of a Woman With Skin-Picking Disorder

Etleva Jorgaqi, M.D.
Ermira Vasili, M.D.

Case Description

A 64-year-old woman was seen in our clinic with complaints of severe and generalized pruritus throughout the body, for which she felt an uncontrollable desire to scratch the skin. She stated that the sensation felt like "bee stings" and appearance of rash. She constantly complained of pruritus and admitted to skin scratching, after which she felt partial relief. She had seen several dermatologists and received various local treatments, but there was no improvement. Upon skin examination, the patient presented with localized lesions on the face, arms, legs, chest, and back. The lesions presented with erosions, excoriated papules with hemorrhagic crusts, postinflammatory hyperpigmentation, and scarring. The papules and erosions appeared in different stages of healing, distributed in a discrete manner, with clear borders and well demarcated from the healthy skin (Figure 9–29). Routine laboratory and imaging examinations were within the normal range. We sought psychiatric consultation to assess the psychoemotional status of the patient. The psychiatrist determined that the patient's mood was dysphoric and showed tendencies of obsessions and compulsions with prominent anxiety symptoms.

Differential Diagnosis

- Drug-induced rash
- Dermatitis artefacta
- Prurigo nodularis
- Insect bites
- Delusional infestation

Diagnosis

All lab work was within normal limits. Psychiatric consultation was conducted with the patient, indicating depression, anxiety, and obsessive and compulsive traits. Based on the overall clinical picture, thorough dermatological examination, and additional investigations, a diagnosis of skin-picking disorder concomitant with depression and anxiety was established.

Management

The patient was started on fluvoxamine maleate 50 mg at dinner for 6 days, increasing to 50 mg twice a day, and mexazolam 1 mg at dinner. The patient was also prescribed topical corticosteroids and antibiotics and recommended for psychotherapy. At 2-month follow-up, her raw skin lesions and excoriation had improved significantly, and her anxiety and depressive symptoms had decreased considerably.

Discussion

Although documented in the medical literature since the nineteenth century, skin-picking disorder has only recently been included as a distinct psychiatric entity. Prevalence estimates are 1.4%–5.4%. It may occur at any age, usually with onset in adolescence, and the majority of patients are female (Lochner et al. 2017).

The triggers that can precipitate an episode of skin picking can be emotional, perceptual, tactile, or environmental. Skin picking usually occurs in multiple sites, such as face, hands, fingers, arms, and legs. Lesions may arise from preexisting skin problems such as acne or urticated papules, or they may arise de novo. The most common sites of involvement are the face and back, followed by the neck, scalp, and ears. The butterfly sign on the back is a characteristic feature resulting from the reach of the patient's hand. Most patients use their fingernails to pick or squeeze lesions or use instruments such as tweezers and needles (Grant et al. 2012). Patients will usually admit that they are picking at their skin.

Skin-picking disorder is also associated with substantial comorbidity, including other BFRBDs, trichotillomania being the most common. OCD and body dysmorphic disorder are more prevalent in individuals with skin-picking disorder than in the general population. Mood and anxiety disorders are also common in skin-picking disorder, as in this case. Social embarrassment and avoidance and medical sequelae such as infections, lesions, scarring, and serious physical disfigurement have been reported (Odlaug and Grant 2008).

Both psychotherapy and pharmacologic treatment with SSRIs have been shown to be effective in the successful management of patients. Varying degrees of success with the use of antipsychotics, opioid antagonists, and glutamate modulators have been observed. SSRIs are the most widely used medication, with newer evidence of NAC also showing promise (Jafferany 2021). CBT and its variant HRT result in significant improvement in patient symptoms. A collaborative approach with a multidisciplinary team in providing psychotherapy and medication is recommended.

TEACHING POINTS

- A multidisciplinary approach of treatment has higher rates of success.
- The patient's support system, including family, friends, or caregivers, play a major role.
- Treatment usually comprises of the use of selective serotonin reuptake inhibitors and cognitive-behavioral therapy, particularly its variant habit-reversal training.

References

Grant JE, Odlaug BL, Chamberlain SR, et al: Skin picking disorder. Am J Psychiatry 169(11):1143–1149, 2012 23128921

Jafferany M: Handbook of Psychodermatology: Introduction to Psychocutaneous Disorders. New York, Springer, 2021

Lochner C, Roos A, Stein DJ: Excoriation (skin-picking) disorder: a systematic review of treatment options. Neuropsychiatr Dis Treat 13:1867–1872, 2017 28761349

Odlaug BL, Grant JE: Clinical characteristics and medical complications of pathologic skin picking. Gen Hosp Psychiatry 30(1):61–66, 2008 18164942

10

Cutaneous Sensory Syndrome

Dipali Rathod, M.D.
Farzana Ansari, M.D.

Introduction

Cutaneous sensory syndrome also goes by the names cutaneous sensory disorders (CSDs), chronic pain syndrome, mucocutaneous pain syndrome, and dysesthesic syndrome. It presents with disagreeable skin sensations such as itching, burning, stinging, or pain (allodynia) and sensory symptoms such as numbness and hypoesthesia. CSDs can involve any body region but are mostly confined to body sites with dense epidermal neural innervation such as the face, scalp, and perineum (Gupta and Gupta 2013). Thus, CSDs are described in the literature with region-specific terms such as burning mouth syndrome, glossodynia, carotidynia (also known as Fay syndrome or transient perivascular inflammation of the carotid artery [TIPIC syndrome]), coccygodynia (coccydynia), proctodynia, and genital dysesthetic syndromes such as vulvodynia, vestibulodynia, orchidynia, and penoscrotodynia (Gupta and Gupta 2013; Heymann 2004). Additionally, heightened sympathetic tone may result in excessive sweating with associated pruritus during sleep. Sleep deprivation or insomnia, somatization, and dissociation play a central role in the pathogenesis of CSDs.

CSDs are complex, and there is a poorly understood interplay of neurobiological factors associated with neuropathic pain, neuropathic itch, and neurologic/neuropsychiatric states (e.g., radiculopathies, stroke, depression, and PTSD). A common but unknown central or peripheral nervous system dysfunction underlies these disorders (Gupta and Gupta 2013). Patients may have associated psychiatric symptoms such as body dysmorphic disorder and drug misuse (Siddappa 2002). CSDs are more prevalent in females.

General management includes cognitive-behavioral therapy (CBT), tricyclic antidepressants (TCAs), selective serotonin reuptake inhibitors (SSRIs), and antipsychotics (e.g., pimozide) (Zakrzewska and Bewley 2016). Amitriptyline is preferred when pain, such as burning, stinging, biting, or chafing, is the primary sensation. Doxepin is preferred when pruritus is the primary symptom, as doxepin has histamine (H1) receptor affinity ~56 times that of hydroxyzine and 775 times that of diphenhydramine (Koo and Gambla 1996).

CSDs may be divided into two categories. Those in the first category have known causes, such as sensory mononeuropathies, notalgia paresthetica, meralgia paresthetica, postherpetic neuralgia (PHN), trigeminal trophic syndrome, erythromelalgia, and brachioradial pruritus. Those in the second category have no demonstrable neurological cause, such as scalp dysesthesia (allodynia), vulvodynia, penodynia, scrotodynia, prostatodynia, atypical trigeminal trophic syndrome, trigeminal neuropathic pain syndrome, and burning mouth syndrome (Zakrzewska and Bewley 2016). Other miscellaneous conditions and terminologies considered under mucocutaneous pain syndromes are skin ache syndrome, atypical facial pain, syndrome of oral complaints, perianal pain syndrome, pruritus ani/vulvae/scrotum, chronic perianal pain, perianal syndrome, and chronic skin pain (Siddappa 2002).

Burning Mouth Syndrome

Burning mouth syndrome is a sensation of continuous burning within the oral cavity, usually accompanied by altered taste with no clinical signs. No oral, dental, or systemic cause is identifiable. It is often a diagnosis of exclusion, with a prevalence of ~1%. It is common in perimenopausal females; peak age is 50–60 years, with a female-to-male ratio of ~20:1. There is often a history of associated mental health problems, most commonly anxiety and depression. It is hypothesized to be caused by neuropathic changes inside the taste neuronal connections that remove inhibitory control over somatic small-fiber afferents. The disorder may occur after wisdom tooth extraction following damage to the chorda tympani nerve.

Patients present with a history of several months to several years of increasing consistent oral burning pain or discomfort. The tongue is the most commonly affected intraoral region, with generally bilateral infliction. Burning mouth syndrome can also affect the lips and sometimes the entire oral mucosa without following any nerve distribution. The symptoms do not radiate outside the mouth. Altered taste (e.g., metallic or bitter) and altered salivation (mostly dryness) are also associated. Some patients identify certain triggers or exacerbating factors (usually spicy or acidic foods); most patients find relief with food or drink, at least temporarily. Some patients acquire a habit of thrusting their tongue against the lower anterior teeth in an attempt to alleviate symptoms. The oral mucosal examination is normal, with no objective evidence of xerostomia, although a normal fissured or geographic tongue may be found in some patients.

The management of burning mouth syndrome comprises thorough examination of the oral cavity to look for changes of lichen planus, candidiasis, xerostomia, or contact allergy and relevant investigations to rule out these differentials. Once the diagnosis is made, patients need to be reassured about the disease, that symptoms are real, and CBT can be given. Topical agents such as clonazepam, lidocaine gel, and benzydamine mouthwash and oral drugs such as α-lipoic acid and TCAs can be given (Siddappa 2002; Zakrzewska and Bewley 2016).

Vulvodynia and Penoscrotodynia

Vulvodynia can be subdivided into vestibulodynia and other dynias according to the affected vulval site. Similarly, peno- and scrotodynia can be site specific. Sexual or nonsexual touch may be a provoking factor in some patients. Common features of these disorders are idiopathic nature, chronicity, and nonresponse to simple analgesia. Significant psychological comorbidities may be associated with these conditions.

The prevalence among females is 8% and 2% among males, which may be due to underreporting from male patients. It can affect any age group but peaks in the third to fourth decade of life. Anxiety and depression may be associated but should not be straightforwardly blamed as the cause of the disease. Sexual dysfunction such as dyspareunia, erectile dysfunction, and ejaculatory disturbance are common. Patients have been reported more commonly to have irritable bowel syndrome, fibromyalgia, and chronic fatigue syndrome. Dysfunction of the peripheral or central sensory nerve pathways that innervate the genital areas is hypothesized to be the main pathophysiology. The role of infection or hormonal imbalance as the cause has been disregarded.

A history of severe, chronic sensations of burning, stabbing pain, rawness, and itching of the whole or specific part of the genital skin is described by the patient. Symptoms may be continuous or provoked by sexual/nonsexual touch. A genital examination is normal, except for localized or more generalized erythema of skin or mucosa, but this may be within the normal range and should not be overinterpreted. More commonly in women than men, point tenderness (with cotton wool tips) can be found. It is a diagnosis of exclusion. Other genital dermatoses can be ruled out clinically. Sometimes genital pain syndromes are part of generalized pain syndrome diseases.

The condition is usually recalcitrant without treatment. Treatment may take time to achieve remission or symptom amelioration, but it is usually successful. Clinicians and patients may have to search via trial and error for the treatment that best suits the individual patient. Patients can be offered CBT. Topical lidocaine gel or ointment and TCAs (amitriptyline, doxepin, imipramine, and desipramine) form the first line of therapy. The analgesic dosage (25–75 mg) of TCAs is much less than their antidepressant dosage (100 mg or more). SSRIs, gabapentin, and pregabalin may be tried as a second line of management. Anticonvulsants such as topiramate form the third line of drugs (Siddappa 2002; Zakrzewska and Bewley 2016).

Chronic Scalp Pain

In chronic scalp pain, the patient complains of severe chronic scalp or hair pain and tenderness with contact triggers (like combing of hair) without any scalp disease or other identifiable cause. Thalamus dysfunction has been proposed as the pathophysiology of scalp allodynia. The differential diagnosis includes all scalp dermatoses, which can be ruled out after clinical examination and appropriate history. Education and reassurance should be given after diagnosis. Gentle shampoos should be used, and overzealous styling and dying of the hair should be avoided. CBT can be offered, as in the treatment of other cutaneous sensory syndromes. Pharmacologically, TCAs form the first line of therapy. SSRIs, gabapentin, and pregabalin form the second line of therapy. Acupuncture has also been tried for this condition (Siddappa 2002; Zakrzewska and Bewley 2016).

Notalgia Paresthetica

Notalgia paresthetica is characterized by episodes of itching and burning sensation over the midscapular area. Electromyographic evidence suggests that it likely results from isolated peripheral sensory neuropathy affecting spinal nerves T2–T12. There is lichenification and postinflammatory pigmentation due to melanin induced within macrophages by trauma. Necrotic keratinocytes are observed in the epidermis, and features of macular amyloidosis may also be seen. Response to capsaicin suggests a role of neuropeptides in the pathogenesis of this condition (Siddappa 2002; Zakrzewska and Bewley 2016).

Postherpetic Neuralgia

PHN is neuropathic pain that occurs 3–6 months after infection with herpes zoster. Neuropathic pain is defined by the International Association for the Study of Pain as "pain arising as a direct consequence of a lesion or disease affecting the somatosensory system." In the updated International Classification of Headache Disorders, painful cranial neuropathies include trigeminal neuralgia, PHN, posttraumatic trigeminal neuropathy, and pain related to central causes such as multiple sclerosis, space-occupying lesions, and stroke (Zakrzewska and Bewley 2016). It can present with stabbing pain, spontaneous and continuous deep aching and throbbing pain, lancinating pain, or paroxysms of burning pain, which may have nontoxic provoking stimuli such as contact with clothes or temperature change and itching with sharp exacerbations. This pain is associated with autonomic instability and is exacerbated by stress and alleviated by relaxation. It mostly affects immunocompromised and elderly people.

Risk factors for PHN after herpes zoster are severe and disseminated rash, involvement of ophthalmic division of the trigeminal nerve, allodynia, poor mood, and viremia during the acute phase of herpes zoster. PHN can lead to disturbed sleep, depression, and isolation and has a significant impact on activities of daily living. Management includes topical lidocaine or capsaicin, TCAs, gabapentin, pregabalin, tramadol, and other opioids (Koo and Gambla 1996; Siddappa 2002; Zakrzewska and Bewley 2016).

Trigeminal Trophic Syndrome

Trigeminal trophic syndrome (TTS) is a neuropathic condition characterized by paresthesia, chronic burning, pain, and stinging sensations in the distribution of the trigeminal nerve, with an irreversible desire to pick, rub, and scratch uninvolved skin in an attempt to get rid of the unpleasant sensations. Disorders found to be causative are central sensory neuronal damage, postencephalitic parkinsonism, syringobulbia, posterior fossa tumor, occlusion of the posterior inferior cerebellar artery, leprous neuritis, brainstem infarct, damage to the trigeminal nerve by attempts to relieve intractable trigeminal neuralgia (by surgery or alcohol injections into the Gasserian ganglion), and neuritis related to herpes zoster or herpes simplex.

Because of the relative anesthesia of the skin, patients do not realize the damage they inflict on the skin; that damage can extend to destroy the nasal cartilage, cheek, and upper lip. Patients freely admit to their attempts to traumatize the area, and it can mimic dermatitis artefacta. TTS affects men twice as frequently as women, and scapular rim involvement is characteristic. Treatment measures include protective dressing of ulcers, use of gloves to limit repetitive picking of the area, TCAs, SSRIs, gabapentin, pregabalin, duloxetine, carbamazepine, CBT, and surgical interventions. Atypical TTS differs from TTS in distribution—it may be bilateral and involve the neck or two areas of the trigeminal nerve (Zakrzewska and Bewley 2016).

Brachioradial Pruritus

Brachioradial pruritis is a chronic itch induced by sunlight exposure over the outer aspects of bilateral elbows and upper and lower arms in the C6–C8 area. It is more prevalent in fair-colored people living in the tropics. Generalized pruritus due to chronic sun exposure, termed solar pruritus, is likely identical to brachioradial pruritus (Heymann 2004).

Erythromelalgia

Erythromelalgia is defined by an intense burning sensation of the extremities (usually the feet) together with persistent fixed erythema. It is also known as Mitchell disease, acromelalgia, red neuralgia, or erythermalgia. The mean age of presentation is 60 years, and it more commonly affects females. It is usually idiopathic; however, many patients have been found to have distal cutaneous small-fiber neuropathy, which reduces sympathetic vasoconstrictive response, resulting in increased acral blood flow. This ultimately leads to decreased oxygen supply to the skin and subcutaneous tissue, further provoking symptoms.

Secondary erythromelalgia may have an underlying hematological malignancy, peripheral neuropathies, connective tissue diseases, medications and poisons, and pregnancy. Familial cases of erythromelalgia are hypothesized to have an inherited neuron ion channelopathy. Diagnosis is clinical. The most affected sites are the feet, hands, ears, and neck, and the face may also be involved. Heat and exercise may induce and exacerbate episodes; cooling gives relief. Extremities seem normal in between attacks or may be slightly cool or cyanotic. Apart from the treatment used for other cutaneous sensory syndromes, intravenous lidocaine, sodium nitroprusside, or prostaglandins may be tried. For therapy-resistant cases, surgical intervention is possible, such as sympathetic blockade, sympathectomy, or dorsal cord stimulation. CBT is helpful in some cases (Zakrzewska and Bewley 2016).

Conclusion

Cutaneous sensory disorder is a term best used for patients presenting with a disturbance in the cutaneous sensation such as itching, crawling, burning, stinging, or biting, without an apparent diagnosable medical or dermatological condition. CSDs are neuropsychiatric or neurologic states that occur at a structural or functional level of modulating pain and itch perception by affecting their respective pathways.

Whether there is any connection between the sensory complaint and psychopathology is not known. If one finds a diagnosable psychiatric condition such as anxiety or depression, it is justified to refer the patient to a psychiatrist for further management. If no diagnosable psychiatric condition is found, it is reasonable to start the patient empirically on psychotropic medications for the control of various sensations, such as pain, itch, and burning, and monitor the patient properly while on treatment.

References

Gupta MA, Gupta AK: Cutaneous sensory disorder. Semin Cutan Med Surg 32(2):110–118, 2013 24049969

Heymann WR: Mucocutaneous pain syndromes. J Am Acad Dermatol 51(6):970–971, 2004 15583591

Koo J, Gambla C: Cutaneous sensory disorder. Dermatol Clin 14(3):497–502, 1996 8818559

Siddappa K: Cutaneous and mucosal pain syndromes. Indian J Dermatol Venereol Leprol 68(3):123–130, 2002 17656906

Zakrzewska JM, Bewley A: Mucocutaneous pain syndromes, in Rook's Textbook of Dermatology, 9th Edition. Edited by Griffiths C, Barker J, Bleiker T, et al. Oxford, UK, Wiley-Blackwell, 2016, pp 1–12

Case 10-1
The Key Role of Psychodermatology in the Understanding of Medically Unexplained Dermatologic Symptoms: A Case of Glossodynia

Bárbara Roque Ferreira, M.D.

Case Description

A 54-year-old woman, previously seen by an otolaryngologist, was referred to the department of dermatology due to burning oral pain, without objective clinical findings. Gastroesophageal reflux disease had been previously excluded, and she did not have any recent change of dentures. She exhibited an intermittent, daily burning sensation of the oral cavity that was localized at the anterior two-thirds of the tongue and lower lip, with a clinical evolution over 18 months. Dermatological examination showed no dental braces, no associated dermatosis, and no clinical evidence of xerostomia.

The patient's medical history was significant for left kidney stone and left carpal tunnel syndrome. Before her appointment, the patient was also seen by a neurologist for some vague symptomatology of her left hand, focusing on her finger joints. The patient reported being on sick leave for the last 2 years due to difficulty in movements in her left fingers, which made it impossible for her to work as a cleaner. She further reported that her boyfriend had oral dysesthesia. Her current medications included lormetazepam and trazodone for sleep disorders.

Differential Diagnosis

- Primary glossodynia
- Secondary glossodynia

Diagnosis

The diagnosis of secondary glossodynia could be considered, as the oral dysesthesia could result from local or systemic disorders. Considering this patient's clinical history and the associated clinical examination, the etiologies related to secondary glossodynia, such as contact allergy, infection, gastroesophageal reflux, and autoimmune diseases, were excluded. A laboratory evaluation was performed to rule out other important etiologies, including complete blood count with differential, serum folate, serum B_{12}, metabolic panel, thyroid-stimulating hormone, and free thyroxine. Only folic acid was not in the normal range at 2.9 ng/mL (reference range 3.1–20.5 ng/mL), but this value could not completely explain the symptoms.

Considering both the clinical examination and the laboratory tests, the diagnosis of primary glossodynia was retained. The symptoms were not attributable to any underlying systemic disease or an objective local condition. Furthermore, this patient also had psychiatric illness, which is commonly observed in association with a diagnosis of primary glossodynia and which could be placed in two groups, somatic symptom and related disorders (illness anxiety disorder/hypochondriasis) or sleep-wake disorders (insomnia disorder).

Management

A combination of a pharmacological approach, psychoeducation, and simple CBT was started. The patient's trazodone was discontinued, and duloxetine was started. α-Lipoic acid was added, and folic acid levels were corrected. Psychoeducation regarding glossodynia and medically unexplained dermatologic symptoms was provided. CBT was conducted to address her distorted thoughts, help her feel less self-conscious about her disorder, and better control the obsessions surrounding her disorder. Global improvement was observed after 2 months, which was maintained in follow-up, including her mood and physical symptoms. She had a significant improvement of the dysesthesic sensations.

Discussion

This patient exhibited dysfunctional coping skills due to excessive worrying and body checking related to burning mouth syndrome and the issue regarding the left hand. The patient's psychodynamic could link the dermatological symptoms and the psychiatric illness, and hence the oral dysesthesia, the sleep disorders, and the illness anxiety disorder. From her clinical history, there are relevant findings to understand this dynamic. Two years earlier, her partner had suffered from oral dysesthesia symptoms, without official diagnosis; at the time of presentation, she also had some disorders without a precise diagnosis, involving the tongue and the left hand. This probably has driven her to "hospital shopping," with the need to see several medical specialties not to understand her problems, but to perpetuate them. The psychodynamic was related to her inner conflict. She was fearful about the transmissibility of her oral symptoms, and her hand symptoms prevented her from working. CBT can be useful to develop adequate coping strategies and can be started during a dermatology consultation (Matsuoka et al. 2017; Williams and Garland 2002).

TEACHING POINTS

- Patients with glossodynia may exhibit multifactorial etiology; adequate clinical examination and laboratory tests should be performed to rule out local or systemic diseases.

- Different etiologies may coexist and contribute to oral dysesthesia symptoms.

- Medically unexplained dermatologic symptoms can induce significant patient distress, and the physician has a key role in providing adequate psychoeducation.

References

Matsuoka H, Chiba I, Sakano Y, et al: Cognitive behavioral therapy for psychosomatic problems in dental settings. Biopsychosoc Med 11(1):18, 2017 28630646

Williams C, Garland A: A cognitive-behavioural therapy assessment model for use in everyday clinical practice. Adv Psychiatr Treat 8(3):172–179, 2002

Case 10-2

Vulvodynia: A Diagnostic Dilemma

Saadia Tabassum, M.D.
Atiya Rahman, M.D.
Tazein Amber, M.D.

Case Description

A 51-year-old woman, a homemaker and mother of two children, presented to the dermatology outpatient clinic with complaints of a persistent burning sensation over the vulvar area for the past 8 months. She described it as a feeling of "rawness" over the lower part of the vulva near the vestibule. It was aggravated with friction, specifically during prolonged sitting and intercourse. However, she denied associated itch, pain, vaginal discharge, or dysuria. She was referred to a dermatologist by a gynecologist, who treated her for vulvovaginal candidiasis with repeated courses of oral and topical antifungals, with no relief.

Her medical history was relevant for a renal transplant 35 years earlier, for which she was on immunosuppressive drugs. Furthermore, she was diagnosed with high-grade B-cell lymphoma 2 years earlier, for which she had debulking surgery of a left paraspinal mass, followed by chemotherapy that had been completed 9 months earlier. Her regular medications included oral prednisolone, oral azathioprine, oral cyclosporine, and a multivitamin supplement. Additionally, she took bromazepam as an anxiolytic on an as-needed basis for disturbed sleep. She was perimenopausal and bled 5 days during a 60-day cycle with scanty flow. She was an ex-smoker with a 10-pack-year history who quit 2 years earlier.

On examination, a faint perceptible erythema on the right labia minora, near the posterior fourchette, was observed. The remaining mucosa had a normal, pink-colored, glistening appearance with normal surrounding skin.

Differential Diagnosis

Lichen planus was ruled out by detailed dermatological examination, and no other lesions were found on the body. The patient had no history of painful, grouped, vesicular eruption in the past; therefore, PHN was not pertinent. The possibility of recurrent vulvovaginal candidiasis existed, as she was on immunosuppressive medications, but the wet mount was negative, and she had taken repeated courses of antifungals without improvement. There were no signs of atrophic vaginitis. Results of a high vaginal swab and Pap test were negative.

Diagnosis

Keeping in view her persistent burning pain along with absence of clinical or laboratory evidence of infection or inflammation, the differentials narrowed down to a chronic neuropathic condition. On further inquiry, she reported limited daily activities due to constant preoccupation with her vaginal discomfort. She acknowledged having mood instability and chronic stress due to her past medical issues. The diagnosis of vulvodynia was made on clinical grounds.

Management

The patient was initially advised to use a neutral-pH vaginal wash along with the antihistamine ebastine 10 mg at night. She was also advised against the use of antiseptics and to pat dry the genital area with nonfragrant toilet roll after every wash. At a 2-week follow-up appointment, she denied any improvement and complained of a diffuse burning sensation over the vulva. She was then advised to take oral pregabalin 50 mg at bedtime. Her subsequent follow-up was scheduled at 4 weeks. She reported complete resolution of her symptoms, with resolution first becoming noticeable after 2 weeks of therapy. Apart from mild daytime sedation during the first week of therapy, no significant side effects were reported. On subsequent follow-up at 3 months, she reported a sense of well-being and resumed her routine social and sexual activities.

Discussion

Vulvodynia is defined as pain of at least 3-month duration, in the absence of a clear identifiable cause (Reed 2006). The vulvar discomfort ranges from burning pain, stinging, and rawness to mild irritation affecting either a localized area of the vulva or the whole vulva (Moyal-Barracco and Lynch 2004). Vulvodynia was first described in 1889 as "excessive sensitivity" of the vulva; however, it rarely was referred to in the medical literature until the 1980s. The International Society of Sexual and Venereological Diseases recently revised the definition to include two subgroups: generalized vulvodynia, in which the symptoms may spread to the whole vulva, and localized vulvodynia, in which only part of it is involved, e.g., the clitoris (clitorodynia) or the vestibule of the vagina (vestibulodynia) (Bornstein et al. 2016; Reed 2006). Nevertheless, generalized spontaneous vulvar pain and localized provoked vulvar pain may often overlap.

Vestibulodynia occurs in young women, whereas the generalized form is more common in older postmenopausal women. It is a diagnosis of exclusion with unknown etiology. The reported associations are other pain syndromes or conditions such as fibromyalgia, irritable bowel syndrome, migraines, back pain, and interstitial cystitis. Depression is frequently common, but it is difficult to ascertain whether this is a primary cause or a secondary effect of the symptoms. Chronic pain syndromes are rarely caused by primary psychiatric disorders but rather are the result of peripheral or central neuronal sensitization. Most patients affected by vestibulodynia are psychologically normal, but they do tend to have increased anxiety, as in this patient. A genetic predisposition with polymorphisms increases the risk of candidiasis or other vulvar infections.

Patients initially seek consultation with family physicians or gynecologists, who must exclude other causes of vulvar pain and collaborate with a dermatologist. For example, this patient was referred from a gynecologist after getting several courses of antifungals for presumed candidiasis. Affected individuals often disclose lack of intimacy and disaffection by their partners, yet ~40% of women never seek advice in their lifetime (Harlow and Stewart 2003). Of those who seek consultation, 60% are seen by more than three physicians to ascertain a final diagnosis (Harlow and Stewart 2003).

When doing the initial workup, it is important to exclude common vulvar infections, inflammatory disorders, neoplasia, and neurological conditions, e.g., PHN, nerve compression or injury, and neuromas. Obstetrical trauma or iatrogenic causes such as postoperative changes, chemotherapy, and radiation exposure should also be excluded. Hormonal deficiencies such as genitourinary syndrome of menopause and lactational amenorrhea are some other entities to be considered. This patient had had chemotherapy and radiation therapy; however, the temporal relationship was not in favor of these being the cause.

Although many therapeutic options are available, few systematic reviews and trials exist on effective treatments for vulvodynia. Approaches include vulvar care measures, psychological support, pharmacological treatment, surgical procedures, electrical nerve stimulation, and laser therapy, but there is no single treatment effective for all patients. The effective management of pain and distress warrants the treatment to be tailored and holistic, with a multidisciplinary approach (Vasileva et al. 2020). Oral treatment is preferred over vaginal because of the discomfort that can arise with vaginal treatments. First-line therapy for vulvodynia is the same as for neuropathic pain. SSRIs and anticonvulsants are commonly used. Amitriptyline has thus far been the most researched TCA, with oral doses of 10–225 mg daily. Desipramine, alone and in combination with topical lidocaine 5%, has shown good results (Loflin et al. 2019). Gabapentin has been used both orally and topically; the oral dose can be started from 100 mg, titrating to 3,000 mg each day in divided doses, with satisfactory results (Loflin et al. 2019). Topical compounded agents are buffered to pH 4.5 (equal to normal vaginal pH of 3–5.5) using a hydrophilic base. Amitriptyline in a mixture with baclofen cream, gabapentin cream in strengths of 2%–6%, and 2% topical lidocaine can be used up to six times per day without toxicity. Among injectable therapies, enoxaparin, botulinum toxin A, and corticosteroids have been used (Loflin et al. 2019). The last resort is surgery, typically consisting of vulvar excision and vestibulectomy. Alternative therapies include acupuncture, localized transcutaneous electrical nerve stimulation (TENS) therapy applied to the labia majora, and avoiding diets high in oxalates (Loflin et al. 2019).

This patient had taken several courses of antifungals with no relief. Additionally, neither of the patient's existing immunomodulators (azathioprine and cyclosporine) helped her symptoms, decreasing the possibility of inflammatory dermatoses. A temporal relationship with chronic stress also existed in this patient, as her symptoms started a month after her chemotherapy ended, ultimately suggesting vulvodynia.

Low-dose pregabalin improved her symptoms markedly within 3 weeks of therapy initiation. Pregabalin is a synthetic γ-aminobutyric acid approved for the treatment of fibromyalgia and several neuropathic conditions.

Vulvodynia is an underreported entity that often goes unrecognized despite having a negative impact on quality of life of the affected woman and her partner. Nonetheless, it can be successfully treated with a holistic approach and individualized plan.

> **TEACHING POINTS**
>
> - The effects of vulvodynia on a woman's quality of life can be physically devastating; it also carries a debilitating psychosocial impact. Women report lack of self-esteem and a loss in their personal relationships.
>
> - Apart from medical management, it is deemed necessary to educate the patient that their symptoms are valid and to make them understand that regardless of pain intensity, there is no physical damage to their genitalia.

References

Bornstein J, Bogliatto F, Haefner HK, et al: The 2015 International Society for the Study of Vulvovaginal Disease (ISSVD) terminology of vulvar squamous intraepithelial lesions. Obstet Gynecol 127(2):264–268, 2016 26942352

Harlow BL, Stewart EG: A population-based assessment of chronic unexplained vulvar pain: have we underestimated the prevalence of vulvodynia? J Am Med Womens Assoc (1972) 58(2):82–88, 2003 12744420

Loflin BJ, Westmoreland K, Williams NT: Vulvodynia: a review of the literature. J Pharm Technol 35(1):11–24, 2019 34861006

Moyal-Barracco M, Lynch PJ: 2003 ISSVD terminology and classification of vulvodynia: a historical perspective. J Reprod Med 49(10):772–777, 2004 15568398

Reed BD: Vulvodynia: diagnosis and management. Am Fam Physician 73(7):1231–1238, 2006 16623211

Vasileva P, Strashilov SA, Yordanov AD: Aetiology, diagnosis, and clinical management of vulvodynia. Prz Menopauzalny 19(1):44–48, 2020 32699543

Case 10–3
Gardner-Diamond Syndrome

İlknur Kıvanç Altunay, M.D.
İlayda Esna Gülsunay, M.D.

Case Description

A 20-year-old woman was referred to a dermatology clinic with a 2-year history of recurrent spontaneous bruising. She had arthroscopic meniscus sur-

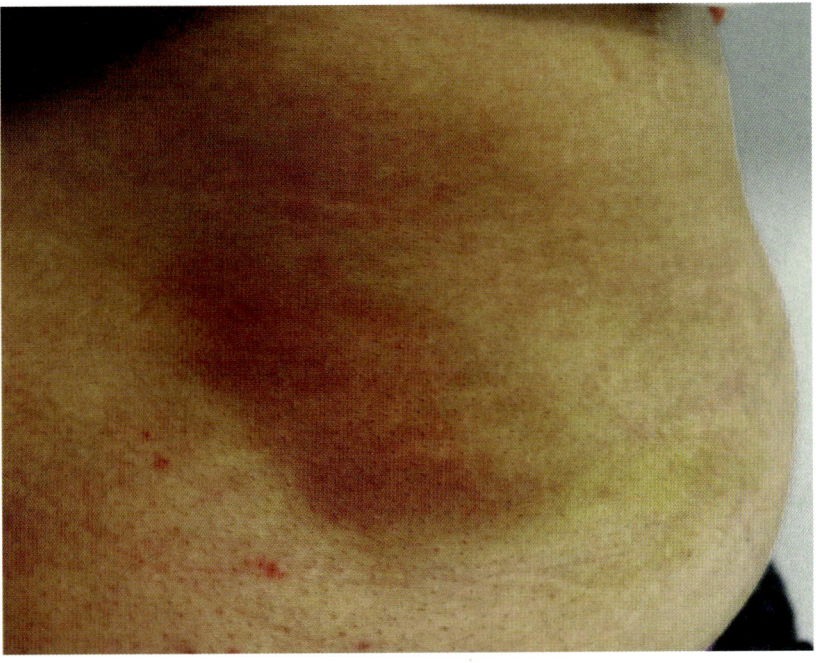

FIGURE 10–1. Resolving ecchymotic patch.
Source. Dr. Ilayda Gülsunay.

gery for a ligament tear on her knee that had caused pain and swelling for 2 years. Soon after the surgery, she developed painful large ecchymosis extending to the distal pretibial area in her operated knee. No cause was determined for the ecchymosis and pain, despite multiple tests. The ecchymosis healed spontaneously; however, she kept having episodes of painful bruises on other parts of her body, including her face, trunk, and extremities. During these 2 years, she was seen in multiple clinics including internal medicine and rheumatology with extensive lab work, yet there was no clear diagnosis. When she was referred to the dermatology clinic, she had a painful ecchymotic patch on her right gluteal region (Figure 10–1).

Differential Diagnosis

Because of the presence of spontaneous purpura and ecchymosis, bleeding disorders including abnormalities of platelet function, clotting factors, and the fibrinolytic system should be considered. Family history is also important to exclude inherited bleeding disorders. Some medications and unusual diets may cause increased bleeding; thus a detailed medical history should be taken. Connective tissue diseases and vascular disorders may also cause purpura or ecchymosis on the skin, and a skin biopsy may be performed to exclude these disorders. Physical abuse and self-inflicted injury should also be considered, and therefore a psychiatric evaluation is necessary.

Diagnosis

The patient and her family did not have any history of bleeding or coagulation disorders. She had no history of drug or food supplement use. The patient had been investigated by hematology and rheumatology clinics, and all necessary tests were performed, including complete blood count, bleeding time, prothrombin time, activated partial thromboplastin time, factor VIII, von Willebrand antigen and ristocetin cofactor, fibrinogen, D-dimers, thyroid profile, complement 3 and 4, protein C and S levels, antinuclear factor, anti-dsDNA antibody, and anticardiolipin antibody, but all results were within normal limits. A punch biopsy was performed from the eccyhmotic patch, which revealed erythrocyte extravasation without evidence of vasculitis or vasculopathy. An intradermal auto-erythrocyte sensitization skin test was also performed on the forearm with saline control. Within 24 hours, the patient developed erythema with a burning sensation, which transformed to painful ecchymosis in the autologous blood injection site (Figure 10–2); the saline control was negative. Considering all these results, with typical history and lesions, we diagnosed the patient with Gardner-Diamond syndrome (GDS).

Management

The patient was referred to psychiatry, and it was found that the patient showed histrionic personality traits. She was started on sertraline 50 mg/day in addition to psychotherapy sessions two times a week. During the psychotherapy, it was revealed that the patient had difficulty understanding and expressing negative emotions, such as anger. In the sessions, the patient was educated to recognize and express her emotions positively. Family interviews were also conducted. The patient did not have any new episodes of ecchymosis and was in remission during follow-up periods of 1 and 3 months.

Discussion

GDS is a rare psychodermatological condition that must be kept in mind in cases of spontaneous ecchymoses with recurrent pain, especially in adolescent females. It is a diagnosis made by exclusion of other causes of purpura and ecchymosis. Burning, stinging, or itching may precede the lesions, and systemic symptoms such as fever, malaise, nausea, and epigastric pain can also occur. Onset frequently follows emotional or physical stress, mechanical trauma such as surgery, injury, or a period of physical fatigue during the past 24 hours. Psychological stress is considered a major trigger. Our patient developed symptoms after arthroscopic meniscus surgery.

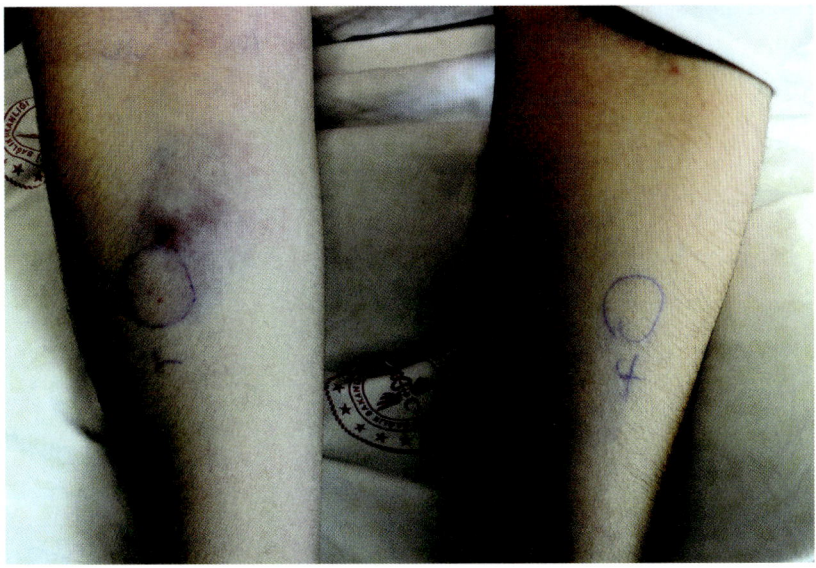

FIGURE 10–2. Positive result of intradermal auto-erythrocyte sensitization skin test with negative saline control.
Source. Dr. Ilayda Gülsunay.

The pathophysiology of the disease is not known; nevertheless, stress-related hemostatic and immune changes may play a role. Although an auto-erythrocyte sensitization skin test can be performed to support the diagnosis, this test is not validated, and negative results do not exclude the diagnosis of GDS (Sridharan et al. 2019). Our patient showed positive results of the auto-erythrocyte sensitization skin test and had a history of physical trauma as a precipitating factor. She also showed histrionic personality traits, which supports the diagnosis and is seen in many cases (Ivanov et al. 2009).

Different treatment modalities with different outcomes have been tried for GDS. Treatment approaches aim to manage symptoms and ameliorate psychological comorbidities. Psychopathologies include depression, anxiety, obsessive disorders, histrionic or borderline personality disorder, difficulty in addressing aggression and hostility, emotional instability, hypochondriasis, abnormal guilt, sexual problems, and masochism. Therefore, a detailed psychological evaluation is very important. The most successful treatment outcomes have been achieved with SSRIs, TCAs, and psychotherapy (Block et al. 2019). Additional treatments for the management of symptoms include antihistamines, anti-inflammatory drugs, corticosteroids, or other immunosuppressive agents (Block et al. 2019;

Sridharan et al. 2019). In this patient, sertraline was prescribed in association with psychotherapy, with beneficial results.

TEACHING POINTS

- Gardner-Diamond syndrome, also known as psychogenic purpura, is a rare disorder characterized by recurrent and spontaneous painful bruising.
- Comprehensive lab work is necessary to rule out other hematologic conditions.
- It is necessary to have a high index of clinical awareness and address psychiatric comorbidities.

References

Block ME, Sitenga JL, Lehrer M, et al: Gardner-Diamond syndrome: a systematic review of treatment options for a rare psychodermatological disorder. Int J Dermatol 58(7):782–787, 2019 30238440

Ivanov OL, Lvov AN, Michenko AV, et al: Autoerythrocyte sensitization syndrome (Gardner-Diamond syndrome): review of the literature. J Eur Acad Dermatol Venereol 23(5):499–504, 2009 19192020

Sridharan M, Ali U, Hook CC, et al: The Mayo Clinic experience with psychogenic purpura (Gardner-Diamond syndrome). Am J Med Sci 357(5):411–420, 2019 30879737

Case 10-4
A Case of Glossodynia (Burning Mouth Syndrome)

Polina G. Iuzbashian, M.D.
Andrey N. Lvov, M.D.
Dimitry V. Romanov, M.D.

Case Description

A 47-year-old woman presented with burning and tingling sensations on the palate and the tip of the tongue. She described the sensations "as if I had hot pepper on my tongue" and "as if I scalded my mouth with boiling water." She reported that she had a sensation of "plaque" on her tongue that interfered with talking and eating and distracted her from daily activities. She reported that the sensation constantly migrated along the upper surface and sides of the tongue, palate, and gums. The burning sensation was almost imperceptible in the morning and increased by the evening, especially when the patient was fatigued or in a conflict or stressful/irritating situation. At rest, the sensations subsided. The sensations did not disturb sleep and did not intensify during meals. The patient also complained of insomnia due to anxiety over the possibility of a serious illness. The patient reported having an itchy, urticarial-like rash all over the body after anxiety attacks, accompanied by elevation of blood pressure, nausea, and hot flashes. The condition had persisted for 7 months. The onset was triggered by a conflict at work. Shortly before the conflict, she went to her dentist to replace fillings and attributed the sensations to possible trauma to the mucosa.

She consulted dentists, general practitioners, and gastroenterologists, but no cause for her burning tongue had been identified. The patient categorically refused to have a tongue biopsy as suggested by a dentist and admitted that the thought of undergoing the procedure scared her even more than the sensations in her mouth. The patient was frustrated by the physicians' inability to diagnose her.

On examination, the vermillion area was unremarkable, and the lips were sufficiently moistened, without any erosion, cracks, or crusting. Labial, buccal, and hard and soft palate mucosae were pale pink and normally hydrated, with no edema. The dorsum of the tongue was clean, with no desquamation, cracking, or ulcers (Figure 10–3). Examination of the skin was unremarkable. A scrape of oral mucosae did not detect pathogens, and all other lab work was unremarkable.

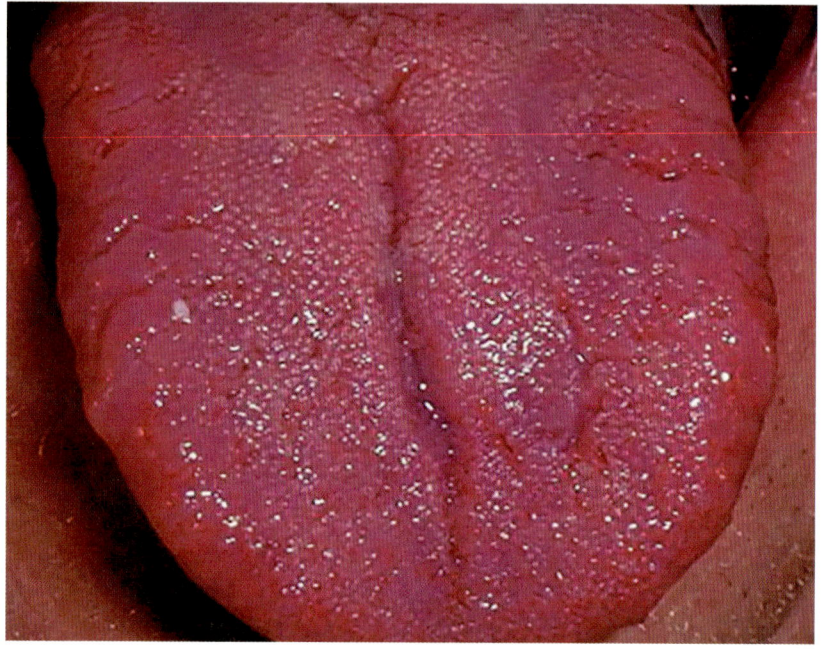

FIGURE 10-3. No visible abnormalities in tongue mucosa.
Source. Dr. A.V. Tereshchenko.

Differential Diagnosis

- Oral lichen planus
- Oral candidiasis
- Topical (dental products, toothpastes) or systemic (medicines, food) allergy
- Hypothyroidism
- Glossodynia

Diagnosis

Based on the patient's history, clinical examination, and lab tests being unremarkable, the diagnosis of glossodynia was made. The patient did not have white, linear lines or atrophic or erosive lesions on the oral mucosa, effectively ruling out oral lichen planus. The negative oral mucosa scrape test ruled out oral candidiasis. All allergen tests were negative, and hormone lab results were within normal limits.

Management

The patient was prescribed periciazine 0.3 mg (3 drops/day) in the morning and alimemazine 5 mg before bed, plus CBT. Within a month of therapy, her symptoms improved. The patient's sleep normalized, and she noted that she was less irritable and anxious. Within 3 months, the oral sensations completely resolved, and the patient no longer felt plaque on her tongue. She no longer feared cancer.

Discussion

The diagnosis of burning mouth syndrome in this case meets ICD-10 criteria, which includes unpleasant burning sensations on the oral mucosa without any dental or other medical cause (World Health Organization 2016). In this case, the onset and intensity of symptoms appeared to correlate with stress and workplace conflicts accompanied by anxiety and irritation. In addition to mucous membrane sensations, a hive-type rash, blood pressure fluctuations, nausea, and hot flashes are also induced by emotional distress.

Psychotherapy is the primary type of treatment for somatic symptom disorder (SSD) and medically unexplained symptoms, according to current recommendations (Allen et al. 2002). Data from most studies of SSD treatment indicate that CBT has the widest range of supporting scientific evidence (Kleinstäuber et al. 2011).

TEACHING POINTS

- Burning mouth syndrome is relatively common but underdiagnosed. Dermatologists need to be aware of the burning mouth syndrome diagnostic pattern to determine appropriate treatment.

- Oral mucosal dermatoses, gastrointestinal pathology, and endocrine disorders need to be ruled out before diagnosing burning mouth syndrome; however, comorbidity is also possible.

- Treatment of burning mouth syndrome requires a multidisciplinary team including psychiatrist, dermatologist, and primary care provider.

References

Allen LA, Escobar JI, Lehrer PM, et al: Psychosocial treatments for multiple unexplained physical symptoms: a review of the literature. Psychosom Med 64(6):939–950, 2002 12461199

Kleinstäuber M, Witthöft M, Hiller W: Efficacy of short-term psychotherapy for multiple medically unexplained physical symptoms: a meta-analysis. Clin Psychol Rev 31(1):146–160, 2011 20920834

World Health Organization: International Statistical Classification of Diseases and Related Health Problems, 10th Revision. Geneva, World Health Organization, 2016

Case 10–5
Psychogenic Itch: A Complex Phenomenon

Aleksandra Stefaniak, M.D.
Jacek C. Szepietowski, M.D.

Case Description

An 80-year-old man presented to the clinic for a follow-up appointment related to a chronic itch of 2 years' duration. The itching first appeared during a relationship with a new partner. This association significantly altered his lifestyle, leading to a reduction in social and recreational activities out of a fear of having a contagious disease.

Initially, the itch was localized to his feet but subsequently spread to cover his entire body. The itch was more severe in the evening and at night, leading to significant sleep disturbances. The itch was exacerbated by warmth, hot water, sweating, and periods of inactivity. Cold water seemed to provide some relief.

The patient's adherence to treatment regimens was inconsistent. Interestingly, the patient reported the most significant relief from his symptoms after receiving infusions of 0.9% NaCl, a placebo treatment. This response suggested a strong psychogenic component to his symptoms. The chronicity of his symptoms, the significant impact on his quality of life, and the lack of an identifiable somatic cause for his itch all pointed toward a psychodermatological condition. The patient's case was further complicated by his age, his living situation, and the psychological distress he was experiencing, all of which required careful consideration in the diagnosis and management of his condition.

Differential Diagnosis

- Atopic dermatitis
- Scabies
- Senile pruritus
- Neuropathic itch

Diagnosis

The patient underwent a thorough diagnostic evaluation including skin scrapings, mycological examinations, direct immunofluorescence (DIF), and histopathological examination. DIF results were nonspecific, and histopathological examination only revealed features of scratch skin lesions. Gastroscopy, colonoscopy, abdominal ultrasound, and electromyography did not reveal any pathology that could induce skin complaints. These investigations, the absence of primary skin lesions, the chronic duration of the symptoms, and the lack of a clear somatic cause, along with the patient's psychological profile and significant relief from placebo treatment, led to the consideration of a psychogenic itch.

The diagnosis was based on the patient's clinical presentation and history. The patient met the three mandatory criteria for a psychogenic itch according to the French Psychodermatology Group: localized or generalized itch without primary skin lesions, chronic itch (>6 weeks), and absence of a somatic cause (Misery et al. 2007). He also met three of the seven optional criteria: stress-related changes in intensity, nocturnal fluctuations, and an increase in symptoms during rest or inactivity. A psychiatric consultation confirmed a diagnosis of somatization disorder.

Management

The patient's treatment plan encompassed a blend of pharmacological and psychotherapeutic strategies. Pregabalin was reintroduced at a dose of 300 mg/day, later escalated to 600 mg/day, to address potential neuropathic mechanisms contributing to the itch and to serve as a mood stabilizer. Venlafaxine, a selective serotonin and norepinephrine reuptake inhibitor, was initiated at a dose of 75 mg/day. This medication was chosen for its potential benefits in managing chronic pain and pruritus. Psychotherapy was recommended to address the patient's health anxiety, improve adherence to the treatment plan, and assist in the development of healthier coping mechanisms. Initially, habit reversal training (HRT) was suggested to disrupt the itch-scratch cycle, which can exacerbate pruritus and contribute to a vicious cycle of itching and scratching.

Discussion

This case illustrates the complex interplay between psychological and dermatological symptoms, highlighting the importance of a holistic approach to patient care. The patient's chronic itch, initially suspected to be related to a physical condition, was eventually diagnosed as psychogenic in nature. This diagnosis was supported by the absence of primary skin lesions, the generalized nature of the itch, the chronic duration of the symptoms, and the lack of a clear somatic cause. The patient's psychological profile, including his health anxiety, the use of the itch as a distraction from age-related concerns, and the significant relief from placebo treatment, further supported this diagnosis (Misery et al. 2018).

The management of this patient's condition presented several challenges. His nonadherence to the recommended treatment regimen underscores the difficulties in managing such cases and highlights the importance of addressing psychological factors in treatment planning. The patient's significant relief from receiving infusions of 0.9% NaCl, a placebo treatment, underscores the complex interplay between psychological and dermatological symptoms in his case (Weisshaar et al. 2012). The use of pregabalin and venlafaxine in the patient's treatment plan illustrates the importance of considering the patient's individual needs and concerns in treatment planning. Psychotherapy, particularly HRT, played a crucial role in the patient's treatment plan. This nonpharmacological approach aimed to help the patient develop healthier coping mechanisms, improve his adherence to the treatment regimen, and address any underlying psychological issues that might be contributing to his symptoms (Shenefelt 2010). In conclusion, this case underscores the importance of a comprehensive approach to the management of psychodermatological conditions, considering both the physical and psychological aspects of the patient's symptoms.

TEACHING POINTS

- Psychogenic itch is a diagnosis of exclusion. It is essential to rule out other dermatological conditions and internal diseases before arriving at this diagnosis. This may involve extensive diagnostic evaluations, including skin scrapings, mycological examinations, direct immunofluorescence, histopathological examination, and investigations to rule out internal diseases.

- Treatment plans for psychodermatological conditions should be individualized, considering the patient's specific needs and concerns. This may involve a combination of pharmacological treatments, psychotherapy, and lifestyle modifications.

- Psychotherapy, particularly habit reversal training, can play a crucial role in the management of psychodermatological conditions. It can help patients develop healthier coping mechanisms and improve their adherence to the treatment regimen.

- The significant relief from placebo treatments in some patients underscores the strong psychogenic component of their symptoms. This highlights the importance of addressing psychological factors in the management of psychodermatological conditions.

References

Misery L, Alexandre S. Dutray S, et al: Functional itch disorder or psychogenic pruritus: suggested diagnosis criteria from the French Psychodermatology Group. Acta Derm Venereol 87(4):341–344, 2007

Misery L, Dutray S, Chastaing M, et al: Psychogenic itch. Transl Psychiatry 8(1):52, 2018 29491364

Shenefelt PD: Psychological interventions in the management of common skin conditions. Psychol Res Behav Manag 3:51–63, 2010 22110329

Weisshaar E, Szepietowski JC, Darsow U, et al: European guideline on chronic pruritus. Acta Derm Venereol 92(5):563–581, 2012 22790094

Case 10–6

Gardner-Diamond Syndrome in a 5-Year-Old Girl

Ines Lahouel, M.D.
Asmahane Souissi, M.D.
Hichem Belhadjali, M.D.
Mohammad Jafferany, M.D.
Jameleddine Zili, M.D.

Case Description

A 5-year-old girl presented to dermatology clinic with recurrent spontaneous painful bruises on the upper and lower limbs developing over 5 months. Her mother reported that the first episode occurred a few weeks

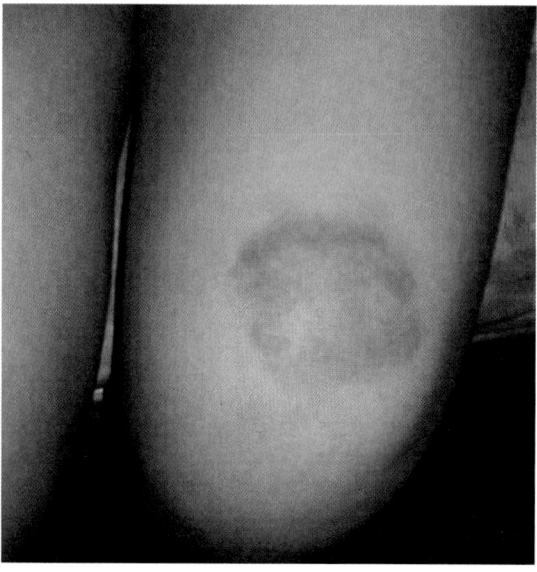

FIGURE 10–4. Ecchymotic plaque on the left knee.
Source. Dr. Hichem Belhadjali.

after a surgical procedure (tonsillectomy) ~5 months earlier. During those 5 months, the patient suffered from burning sensation and edema in the lower legs, along with walking difficulty. No fever, pain in abdomen, or vomiting were noticed. There was no history of any recent new medication intake or drug reactions. The mother stated that the bruises usually healed spontaneously within a week then appeared on other sites without any known precipitating factor. Physical examination showed numerous ecchymotic patches localized on the forearms, thighs, and legs (Figures 10–4 and 10–5). Systemic examination was normal. The patient and her mother denied any possible trauma or self-mutilation attempts. During the interview, the mother acknowledged that the patient has an estranged relationship with her father, and she is always afraid of her father's anger, although no physical abuse was reported. The father was not happy with patient's constant irritability, concentration difficulties, and tantrums. Sometimes the father used to scream at the child and compare her with other children, including her siblings and cousins.

Differential Diagnosis

- Idiopathic thrombocytopenic purpura
- Coagulation disorders such as acquired VIII factor inhibitor
- Panniculitis

Cutaneous Sensory Syndrome

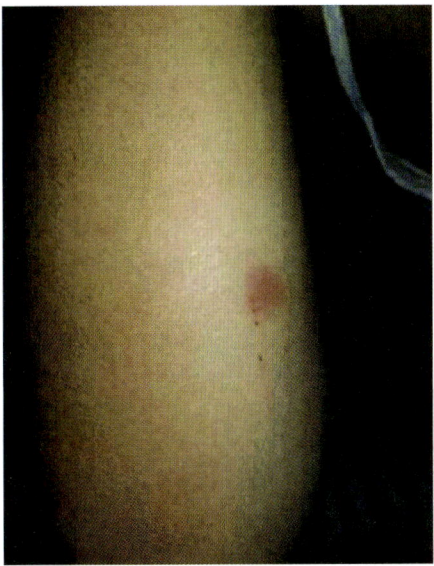

FIGURE 10–5. Ecchymotic plaque on the right forearm.
Source. Dr. Hichem Belhadjali.

- Child abuse
- Gardner-Diamond syndrome

Diagnosis

Routine lab work revealed normal complete blood cell count, platelet count, and platelet aggregation test. Coagulation tests revealed normal values for prothrombin time, partial thromboplastin time, factor VIII, fibrinogen, D-dimers, anti-thrombin III, and protein C and S levels. Antinuclear antibodies, anticardiolipin antibodies, Coomb test, and cryoglobulins were negative. Skin biopsy of the lesion showed superficially extravasated erythrocytes and a superficial infiltrate of inflammatory cells that extended from the subcutaneous level down to the deep dermis. An intradermal erythrocyte sensitization test was considered, but it was not available in the area where the patient resided. Although it is a commonly performed test in these patients, it is not confirmatory. The test has limited specificity and sensitivity, and positive responses to the control or negative responses to plasma do not rule out GDS. Therefore, we did not pursue this test further.

The patient was referred to the psychiatry department for assessment and management. During the psychiatric evaluation, the patient's mood instability, anger, and attentional difficulties were confirmed. There was no history suggestive of child abuse. The above data led us to suspect the diagnosis of GDS.

Management

The patient was started on low-dose sertraline 7.5 mg daily in liquid preparation, and she was recommended for regular counseling sessions along with her parents. Subsequently, the skin lesions improved dramatically, and anxiety symptoms notably decreased. The patient's relationship with her father also improved.

Discussion

GDS, also known as psychogenic purpura or auto-erythrocyte sensitization syndrome, is a rare and poorly understood clinical condition in which patients develop unexplained painful bruises, mostly on the extremities and or face, during times of stress. It is predominantly seen in women but rarely in children (Khadke et al. 2022).

GDS is characterized by recurrent occurrence of painful bruises preceded by a burning sensation and followed by erythema and edema. It is a diagnosis of exclusion after ruling out other causes of bleeding by performing relevant testing and investigations. GDS often occurs after severe emotional stress. In this case, symptoms started few weeks after a surgical procedure and perpetuated after developing an estranged relationship with the father. Despite typical lesions and pain, investigations were normal. Biopsy of the lesions is not essential, and histological signs are not specific. Intradermal testing helps to confirm the diagnosis, but it is not specific and sensitive (Dick et al. 2019).

There is no specific treatment for this condition. Symptoms are treated on case-by-case basis and symptomatically. Psychiatric follow-up is essential to address the underlying psychiatric disorder. Many patients, particularly adults, may require SSRIs for comorbid depression and anxiety.

TEACHING POINTS

- Gardner-Diamond syndrome is a rare disorder that should be considered in patients with bruises or purpuric lesions of unknown etiology.

- Gardner-Diamond syndrome is a diagnosis of exclusion. All lab work and investigation must be completed to rule out other causes before declaring the diagnosis.

- The treatment is directed at the underlying psychological cause to prevent recurrence.

- Intradermal test of auto-erythrocytes is not confirmatory, as it may appear negative in certain cases.

References

Dick MK, Klug MH, Gummadi PP, et al: Gardner-Diamond syndrome: a psychodermatological condition in the setting of immunodeficiency. J Clin Aesthet Dermatol 12(12):44–46, 2019 32038765

Khadke RR, Joshi AV, Kulkarni GL: Gardner-Diamond syndrome in an adolescent girl. Indian Pediatr 59(8):658, 2022 35962664

Case 10-7
A Young Woman With Painful Indurated Erythematous Plaques

Meriem Amouri, M.D.
Zeineb Amouri, M.D.
Choumous Kallel, M.D.
Sonia Boudaya, M.D.
Mohammad Jafferany, M.D.
Hamida Turki, M.D.

Case Description

An otherwise healthy 29-year-old woman presented with painful ecchymotic lesions on the right lower limb developing over 1 week. There was no history of local trauma, injury, or medication intake. Physical examination revealed firm edema and painful ecchymotic noninfiltrated plaques on the right lower limb (Figure 10–6). There were no injuries, scars, hyperpigmentation, or depigmentation, as an indicator for previous or current self-inflicted injury. Complete hemogram, platelet count, complete coagulation profile, and antinuclear antibodies were within normal limits. Upon further detailed interview, the patient acknowledged that she recently broke up with her boyfriend of 3 years. This breakup devastated her, and she stopped going out or engaging in social activities. She slept most of the day and night and had no appetite.

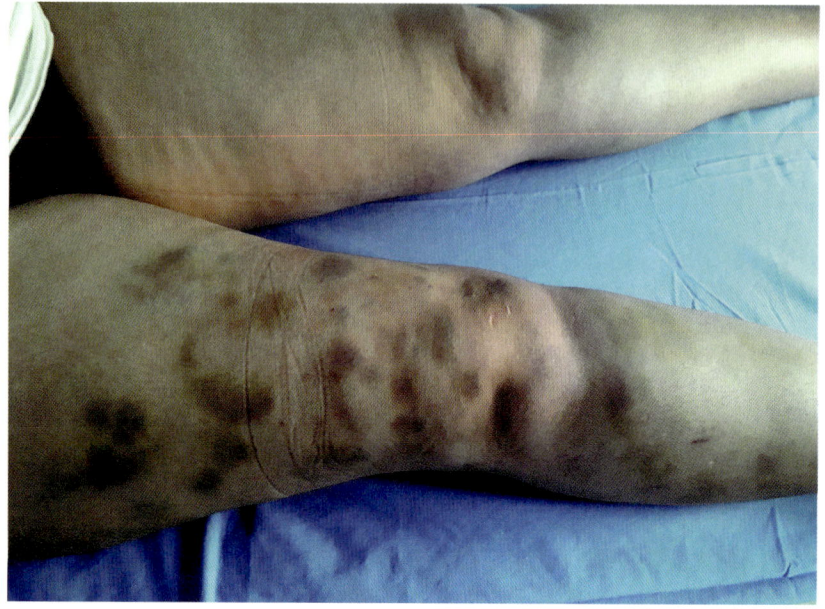

FIGURE 10–6. Ecchymotic noninfiltrated plaques on the right lower limb.

Source. Dr. Meriem Amouri.

Differential Diagnosis

- Skin manifestations of coagulation disorders
- Vasculitis
- Munchausen syndrome
- Factitious purpura
- Gardner-Diamond syndrome

Diagnosis

The diagnosis of GDS was considered based on the all-negative workup for bruising. In an auto-erythrocyte self-sensitization test, 0.1 mL from a panel of autologous erythrocytes with different hematocrits (40%, 50%, 60%, and 70%) was injected intradermally on the left forearm, which caused the development of erythema that transformed to painful ecchymosis within 24 hours. On the other arm intradermal injection of 0.1 mL autologous plasma and saline solution caused no reaction (Figure 10–7). This confirmed our suspicion of GDS.

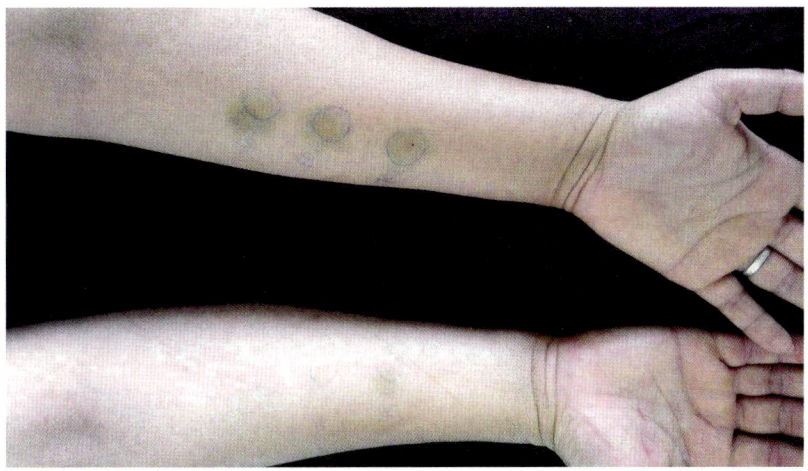

FIGURE 10–7. Positive result of intradermal auto-erythrocyte sensitization skin test with negative saline control.
Source. Dr. Meriem Amouri.

Management

No specific treatment has been effective for GDS patients. This patient required SSRIs and CBT, which significantly improved her skin symptoms and mood stability. The patient started to socialize again and return to normal. She acquired various abilities through CBT to handle periods of stress and her depressive symptoms.

Discussion

GDS is characterized by spontaneous development of painful edematous skin lesions progressing to ecchymosis over the next 24 hours. Severe stress and emotional trauma always precede the skin lesions. The condition is commonly seen in women, but isolated cases have been reported in adolescents and in males (Jafferany and Bhattacharya 2015). The most consistent associations with GDS are psychological disorders (Hällström et al. 1969). A wide range of psychological disturbances have been reported, including depression, anxiety, difficulty in addressing aggression and hostility, emotional instability, adjustment issues, hypochondriasis, abnormal guilt, sexual problems, masochism, and histrionic and borderline personalities, as well as conversion and obsessive disorders (Ratnoff 1980). This patient reported increasing depression, anxiety, and emotional instability after a breakup.

Overall prognosis in GDS is quite good, although in many patients, relapses and remissions are common. Biopsy has never been conclusive and is considered an unreliable method for diagnosis. An auto-erythrocyte injection test involves injecting the patient with their own plasma, using normal saline as the control. Bruising occurring at the site of plasma injection is considered a positive result supporting a GDS diagnosis. However, this test has limited specificity and sensitivity, and positive responses to the control or negative responses to plasma do not completely rule out GDS (Dick et al. 2019).

No specific treatment has proven helpful. A multidisciplinary approach focused on improving underlying psychological conditions plays an integral role in effective management of these cases. Most patients benefit from a combination of CBT and SSRIs. This patient responded well with psychotherapy and low-dose antidepressant treatment.

TEACHING POINTS

- Psychogenic purpura can be a diagnostic dilemma and requires thorough investigation.
- Proper diagnosis of psychogenic purpura could save many unnecessary procedures.
- The role of stress in psychogenic purpura should not be ignored.

References

Dick MK, Klug MH, Gummadi PP, et al: Gardner-Diamond syndrome: a psychodermatological condition in the setting of immunodeficiency. J Clin Aesthet Dermatol 12(12):44–46, 2019 32038765

Hällström T, Hersle K, Mobacken H: Mental symptoms and personality structure in autoerythrocyte sensitization syndrome. Br J Psychiatry 115(528):1269–1276, 1969 5352663

Jafferany M, Bhattacharya G: Psychogenic purpura (Gardner-Diamond syndrome). Prim Care Companion CNS Disord 17(1), 2015 26137346

Ratnoff OD: The psychogenic purpuras: a review of autoerythrocyte sensitization, autosensitization to DNA, "hysterical" and factitial bleeding, and the religious stigmata. Semin Hematol 17(3):192–213, 1980 7006087

Case 10–8
Gardner-Diamond Syndrome in an Adolescent Girl

Piotr K. Krajewski, M.D.
Jacek C. Szepietowski, M.D.

Case Description

A 16-year-old girl was admitted to the department of dermatology after the appearance of recurrent, spontaneous skin lesions. According to her medical history, the first lesions appeared 3 years earlier, shortly after major psychological trauma caused by finding out that she was adopted. The girl was informed about the adoption from a teacher, and she had regrets that she did not receive this message from her adoptive parents. The erythematous patches with ecchymoses were initially localized on the right side of the face and right arm. The lesions healed spontaneously after 3 months without leaving a scar. The patient stated that the lesions would appear without any inducing factor and would always be associated with malaise and pain of very high severity (9 out of 10 points according to the 0–10 point numeric rating scale), which she compared to the feeling of being burned. According to the patient's parents, the lesions tended to appear in periods of increased stress. After being informed about the adoption, she also presented with impulsive behavior, including cutting of both forearms.

On admission, a physical examination revealed a big erythematous patch with ecchymoses localized on the patient's left periorbital area (Figure 10–8). A similar, longitudinal erythematous patch was localized transversally on the left thigh. Several transverse scars were seen on both forearms.

Differential Diagnosis

The differential diagnosis included mostly factitious disorders, self-inflicted or stress-induced lesions, and physical abuse. Moreover, dermatological disorders, including autoimmunological blistering diseases, had to be excluded due to the atypical presentation of the lesions.

Diagnosis

During the hospitalization, laboratory tests did not show any abnormalities. The patient had two punch skin biopsies taken from the lesion on the right shin, and no abnormalities were observed on direct immunofluorescence. The histological examination revealed hyperkeratosis, hypergranulosis, and focal edema of the basal layer. Sparse perivascular lymphocytic infiltrates with single eosinophils and extravascular erythrocytes were visualized in the

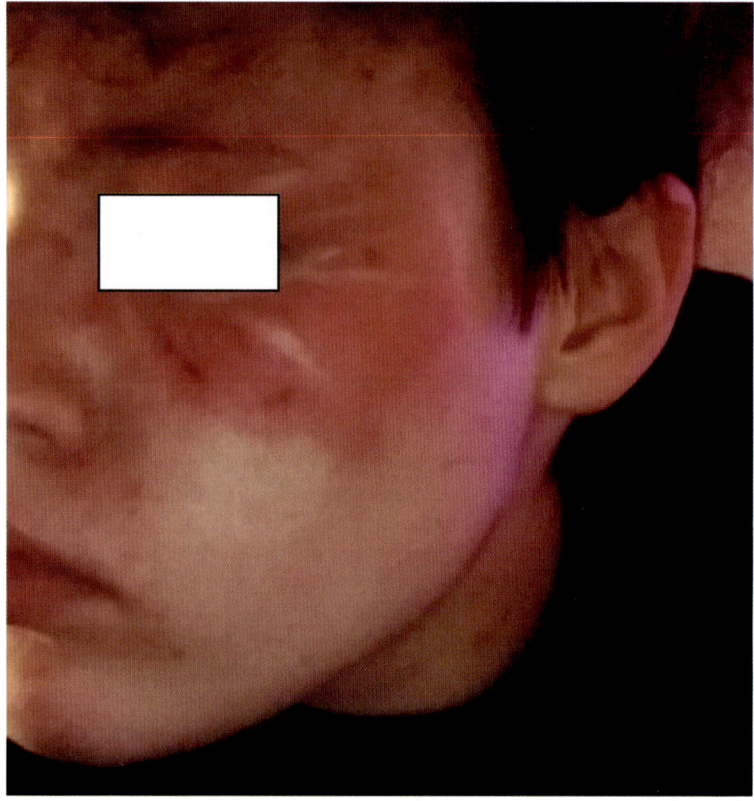

FIGURE 10–8. Widespread erythematous lesions on patient's face.
Source. Dr. Piotr Krajewski.

dermis. The patient saw a psychiatrist and psychologist, who observed traits of personality disorder and mild depression. Because of the history of major psychological trauma associated with the appearance of skin lesions, traits of personality disorders, and depression, as well as the exclusion of underlying dermatological disorders, GDS was diagnosed.

Management

After the exclusion of underlying dermatological disorders and according to the recommendations of the consulting psychiatrist, the patient was started on antidepressants, psychotherapy, and psychological guidance. Because of the high severity of associated pain, the drug of choice was duloxetine 30 mg daily. The persistent lesions were treated with topical corticosteroids and hydrocolloid dressings. Unfortunately, the parents decided to discontinue all oral medication after 10 days of administration.

Discussion

Psychogenic purpura or GDS is an uncommon clinical syndrome characterized by the spontaneous appearance of petechiae or ecchymosis (Ratnoff 1980; 1989). The condition is alternatively referred to as painful ecchymosis syndrome, bruising syndrome, or painful bruising syndrome. Gardner and Diamond first described the syndrome in 1955 (Gardner and Diamond 1955). Although several similar cases were reported afterward, a proper diagnosis was not established until Ratnoff (1989) published a description of 71 patients with similar symptoms and introduced the term *psychogenic purpura*.

The pathogenesis of this syndrome remains poorly understood. Current evidence suggests that the symptoms may arise due to a factitious disorder, in which skin changes are artificially induced by patients with psychological or psychiatric issues (Harth et al. 2010). However, some researchers have postulated that the eruption of lesions could be attributed to the release of kinins in the nervous system in response to emotional stimuli, abnormal complement activation, platelet defects, or erythrocyte membrane abnormalities (Merlen 1987).

The actual prevalence of this disease is difficult to estimate, as the available literature primarily consists of case reports and two larger case series (Sridharan et al. 2019). The syndrome primarily affects young women 20–30 years old, but cases have also been reported in males and children (Block et al. 2019).

The skin changes in GDS are usually preceded by prodromal sensations at the lesion site. They may present as pain, burning, itching, or stinging. Systemic symptoms, such as headaches and myalgia, have been described before the appearance of lesions. The size and location of GDS lesions can vary, with the lower extremities being the most affected site, although lesions on the trunk and face have also been reported. Identifying potential triggering factors is crucial in preventing lesion occurrence. Recent surgery (32% of cases) or trauma (29%) are the most common causes of spontaneous petechiae or ecchymosis, but emotional events, such as psychological stress, trigger almost a quarter of occurrences (Sridharan et al. 2019).

The psychiatric background of this disorder is significant and must be emphasized. Although individuals with diagnosed GDS may appear otherwise healthy, psychiatric disturbances are common, with depression (up to 56%), anxiety, and personality disorders being among the most frequent observations (Sridharan et al. 2019, Block et al. 2019).

The diagnosis of GDS is entirely clinical, as no definitive laboratory or histopathological tests confirm it. Psychiatric and psychological evaluations are necessary for accurate diagnosis and future management (Jafferany and

Bhattacharya 2015; Gieler et al. 2020). Various medications, including corticosteroids, antihistamines, and immunosuppressive drugs, have been used in GDS treatment without satisfactory response. Because of the association of GDS with psychological and psychiatric problems, systemic treatment should be based on SSRIs or tricyclic antidepressants. This treatment regimen has shown the best efficacy in managing symptoms and preventing future relapses, even after the medication is discontinued (Çelik-Göksoy et al. 2017). Referring patients to psychological counseling or therapy is crucial, as it can aid in GDS management.

TEACHING POINTS

- Gardner-Diamond syndrome is a diagnosis of exclusion.
- The treatment is directed at the underlying psychological cause to prevent recurrence.
- Intradermal test of auto-erythrocytes, although helpful in diagnosis, is not a confirmatory test, as it may appear negative in certain cases.
- All lab work and investigation must be completed to rule out other causes before declaring the diagnosis.
- Childhood abuse, neglect, and trauma must be considered in children and adolescents.

References

Block ME, Sitenga JL, Lehrer M, Silberstein PT: Gardner-Diamond syndrome: a systematic review of treatment options for a rare psychodermatological disorder. Int J Dermatol 58(7):782–787, 2019 30238440

Çelik-Göksoy Ş, Kılınçaslan A, Kaya İ: Psychogenic purpura successfully treated with antidepressant therapy. Turk J Haematol 34(3):274–275, 2017 28270377

Gardner FH, Diamond LK: Autoerythrocyte sensitization; a form of purpura producing painful bruising following autosensitization to red blood cells in certain women. Blood 10(7):675–690, 1955 14389581

Gieler U, Gieler T, Peters EMJ, Linder D: Skin and psychosomatics—psychodermatology today. J Dtsch Dermatol Ges 18(11):1280–1298, 2020

Harth W, Taube KM, Gieler U: Facticious disorders in dermatology. J Dtsch Dermatol Ges 8(5):361–372, quiz 373, 2010 20163503

Jafferany M, Bhattacharya G: Psychogenic purpura (Gardner-Diamond syndrome). Prim Care Companion CNS Disord 17(1): 2015 26137346

Merlen JF: Ecchymotic patches of the fingers and Gardner-Diamond vascular purpura [in French]. Phlébologie (Paris) 40(2):473–487, 1987

Ratnoff OD: The psychogenic purpuras: a review of autoerythrocyte sensitization, autosensitization to DNA, "hysterical" and factitial bleeding, and the religious stigmata. Semin Hematol 17(3):192–213, 1980 7006087

Ratnoff OD: Psychogenic purpura (autoerythrocyte sensitization): an unsolved dilemma. Am J Med 87(3N):16N–21N, 1989 2486528

Sridharan M, Ali U, Hook CC, et al: The Mayo Clinic experience with psychogenic purpura (Gardner-Diamond syndrome). Am J Med Sci 357(5):411–420, 2019 30879737

Case 10–9
Gardner-Diamond Syndrome in an Adult Woman

Shahrukh Raza, M.D.
Diptarup Ray, M.D.
Sambit Chatterjee, M.D.
Mohammad Jafferany, M.D.
Anupam Das, M.D.

Case Description

A 49-year-old woman presented to the dermatology outpatient clinic with chief complaints of multiple bruising of varying size on her hamstrings and calves (Figures 10–9 and 10–10). The skin lesions were preceded by a burning, stinging, and itching sensation that gradually progressed into ecchymosis. Upon inquiry, she denied any history of trauma and insisted that they occurred spontaneously, especially with stress and sadness, and resolved gradually without any treatment within a couple of weeks. The lesions were usually associated with headache. She denied a history of any regular oral medication intake including anticoagulants or antiplatelet drugs. She denied having any history of fever, nausea, vomiting, diarrhea, blood in urine or stool, or recurrent abdominal pain. She had a normal menstrual history. No one else in her family had a history of any similar episodes, menstrual abnormalities, or bleeding disorders. She denied having addiction to tobacco, alcohol, or any other substances.

On physical examination, her general status was well, and her vital signs were stable. She had ecchymoses on the dorsum of both hamstrings and

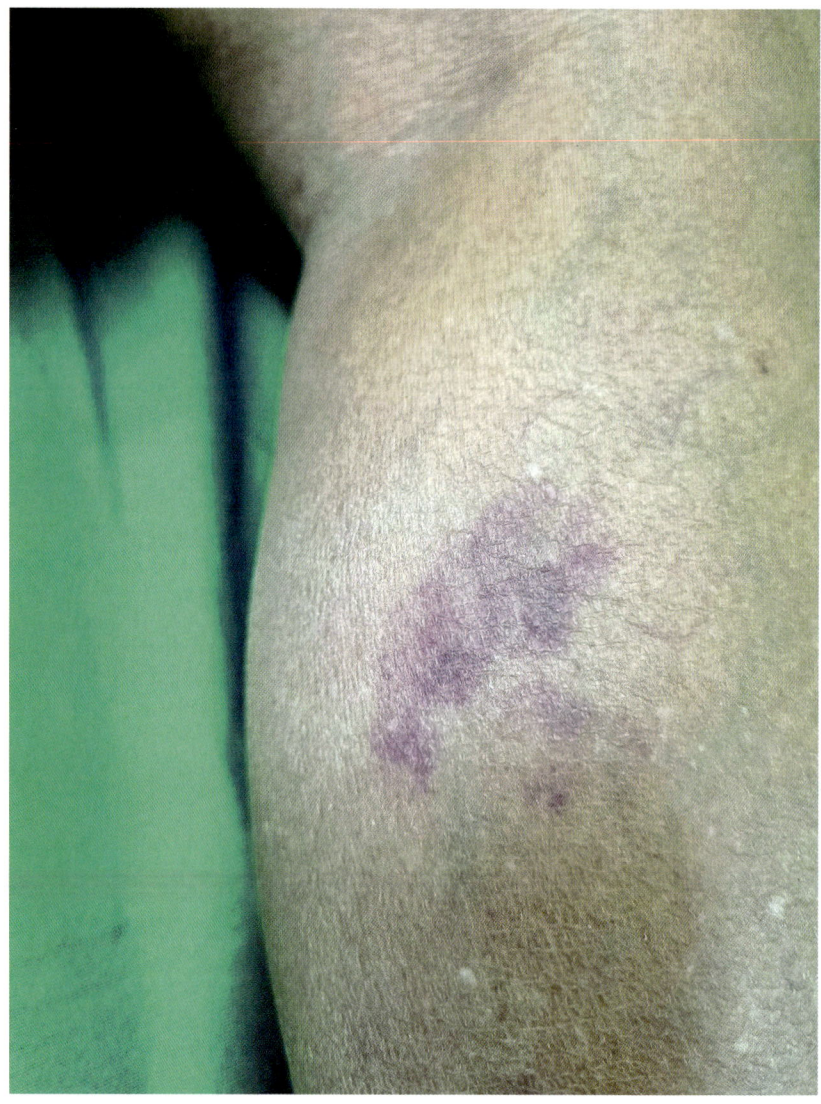

FIGURE 10–9. Erythematous lesions on the legs.
Source. Dr. Anupam Das.

calves. The lesion on the left hamstring was most prominent and was round, smooth on the surface, and yellow in the middle and had a spotted appearance. The lesion was painful on palpation. No pathological finding (epistaxis) was found on otolaryngological examination.

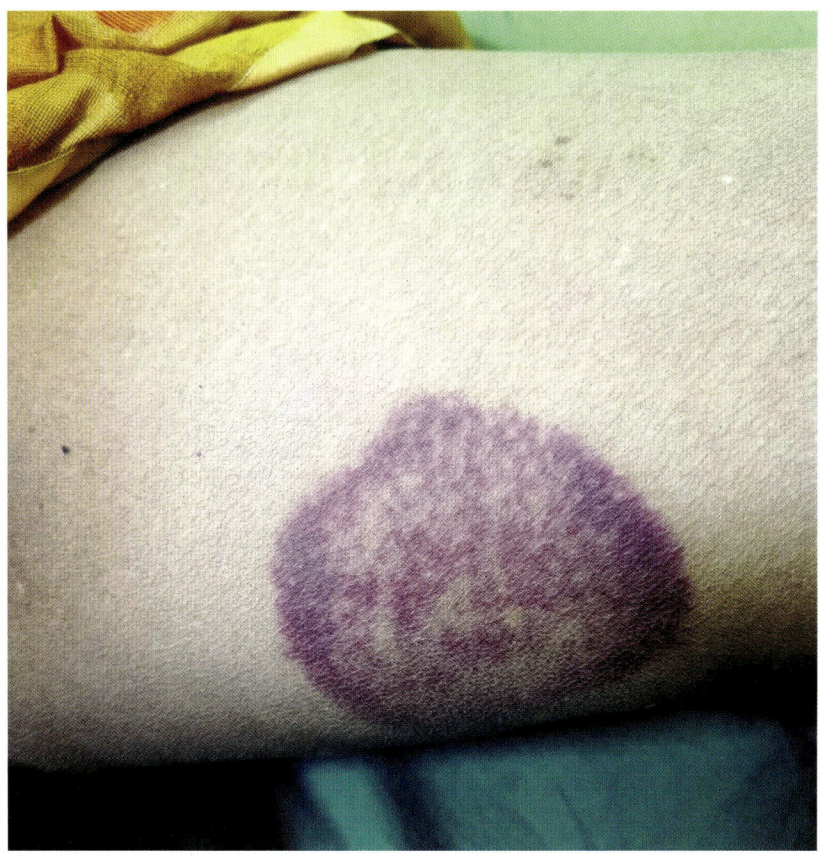

FIGURE 10–10. Erythematous lesions on the legs.
Source. Dr. Anupam Das.

Differential Diagnosis

- Disseminated intravascular coagulation
- Idiopathic thrombocytopenic purpura
- Henoch-Schoenlein purpura
- von Willebrand disease
- Ehlers-Danlos syndrome
- Dermatitis artefacta
- Systemic lupus erythematosus
- Cellulitis
- Compartment syndrome
- Factor XIII deficiency

- Weber-Christian panniculitis
- Polyarteritis nodosa
- Gardner-Diamond syndrome
- Munchausen syndrome
- Ecchymosis related to copper-containing intrauterine devices
- Glomerulonephritis

Diagnosis

Investigations done in this case were a complete blood count and tests for bleeding time, clotting time, prothrombin time, and activated partial thromboplastin time, results of which were within normal limits. The patient's own washed erythrocytes were injected intradermally on her left forearm. It was observed that ecchymoses developed 1 hour after the erythrocyte injection, which eventually subsided within the course of her next visit 72 hours later. Thus, after taking a thorough history and clinical examination and relevant investigations, the diagnosis of GDS was made.

Management

The patient was prescribed oral vitamin C supplements and given topical anticoagulants alongside liberal application of emollients. The patient was referred to psychiatry for psychological counseling and antidepressant therapy.

Discussion

Psychogenic purpura (GDS) is a rare disease that is difficult to diagnose and may progress with recurrent attacks and variable intervals between attacks (Dick et al. 2019). Symptoms may be observed in the whole body but are especially common in the extremities, and they usually resolve spontaneously within a couple of weeks. The lesions may be associated with headache, paraesthesia and syncope, blurred vision or diplopia, arthralgia, myalgia, and bleeding in the nose, eye, ear, and genitourinary system (Jafferany and Bhattacharya 2015). There is an underlying psychological component to the syndrome, which is usually triggered by severe stress or emotional trauma. Psychiatric disorders including mood disorders, anxiety disorder, personality disorder, and somatoform and dissociative disorders may be observed (Silny et al. 2010). Because this condition can be easily overshadowed by other differential diagnoses of recurrent ecchymosis and bleeding, complete psychodermatologic evaluation is of vital importance for diagnosis and management (Vun and Muir 2004).

> **TEACHING POINTS**
>
> - Gardner-Diamond syndrome is a psychodermatological condition characterized by painful, ecchymotic, purpuric lesions developing following stress or trivial trauma.
> - It is mostly seen in young women, although men and adolescents may also present with this condition.
> - It is a diagnosis of exclusion after ruling out bleeding disorders.
> - A multidisciplinary approach targeting the underlying psychological condition is pivotal in the treatment.

References

Dick MK, Klug MH, Gummadi PP, et al: Gardner-Diamond syndrome: a psychodermatological condition in the setting of immunodeficiency. J Clin Aesthet Dermatol 12(12):44–46, 2019 32038765

Jafferany M, Bhattacharya G: Psychogenic purpura (Gardner-Diamond syndrome). Prim Care Companion CNS Disord 17(1): 2015 DOI: 10.4088/PCC.14br01697 26137346

Silny W, Marciniak A, Czarnecka-Operacz M, et al: Gardner-Diamond syndrome. Int J Dermatol 49(10):1178–1181, 2010 20883407

Vun YY, Muir J: Periodic painful purpura: fact or factitious? Australas J Dermatol 45(1):58–63, 2004 14961912

11

Miscellaneous Case Reports

Case 11-1
Hallucinations and Delusions of Vitiligo: A Case Report of Stress-Induced Symptoms

Tanyo Tanev, M.Sc.

Case Description

A 63-year-old who self-identified as a woman and an ethnic Bulgarian was seen at a psychotherapist practice. Initially, the patient was hesitant to provide any information. She would cross her hands and stare at the window, allowing time to pass and ignoring questions from the therapist. The first session provided no assessment information, as the patient refused to communicate. Therefore, that session was used as an introduction and psychoeducation. This included providing the patient with extensive information about confidentiality and her rights in therapy. Because the patient did not want to talk, the therapist spent part of the session explaining CBT rationale. This was a private session scheduled by the patient, and thus it was surprising that she refused to communicate the nature of her issue. Because of her behavior, there were no expectations for her to return for the second session, scheduled a week later.

Surprisingly, the patient returned for the second session. She reported feeling comfortable and was happy with the information that was provided during the first session. At that time, she shared that the initial session was not her idea—that she was asked to attend by her children. Following this admission, the assessment phase began. The patient reported not being diagnosed with physical or mental conditions, and she was not taking any medication. She reported that she did not take any drugs and did not drink coffee. She smoked one to two packs of cigarettes a day and drank a glass of wine every other night for the last 20 years. The patient reported having a son (42) and a daughter (35) who were both in touch with her regularly and provided her with various forms of help. She also stated that she had a stable circle of friends that she met with regularly.

The reason for her visit was vitiligo that was "ruining her life." The session took place in a well-lit office, and there was no indication of pigmentary changes on the patient's face or arms. The patient reported that vitiligo spots of various sizes and forms would appear on her arms and legs. Those spots would grow and shrink and "behave erratically." She spoke about those spots as entities and not simply discoloration. The patient denied applying any concealing products. She diagnosed herself from internet articles without consultation with a medical professional. The patient was advised to consult with a dermatologist for examination and treatment suggestions, but she refused the idea of such consultation as "pointless."

At this point, the patient was conceptualized as experiencing hallucinations that she identified as vitiligo spots. She also had delusions that those spots were providing warnings about difficult life situations. The next two sessions focused on identifying situations in which the spots caused problems for the patient. A link was established between moments of psychological stress and symptoms becoming stronger. The patient reported that the spots would increase in size and pulsate right before difficult events. She interpreted them as signs that warned her of trouble. When she stopped an activity that exacerbated the spots, they would disappear. The patient dismissed any connection between stress and the perceived spots and instead insisted that it was a manifestation of a condition with a suggestion of supernatural causes. It is important to note that although not religious, the patient reported being spiritual. She believed that the spots would appear as warnings and prevent her from making wrong choices. A consultation with a psychiatrist was suggested, with an emphasis on the increased efficacy of combining pharmacotherapy and psychotherapy. The patient refused the consultation with a psychiatrist.

The patient had a complex relationship with the symptoms of her condition. On one hand, they were highly bothersome and caused her physical and psychological distress. On the other hand, she saw them as a warning system. This was important and was identified early during the goal-setting phase of treatment. At that time, the patient decided that despite their perceived usefulness, she would prefer not to have the spots at all. Using cognitive restructuring, the patient identified several negative automatic thoughts and changed them to more adaptive ones. The most prevalent thought was, "there are spots, something bad will happen!," which typically resulted in a strong stress response that made her avoid the activity. The patient found the thought, "the spots don't bother me," to be an appropriate alternative thought. After discussing and listing difficult situations where she did not see the spots, she became more accepting of that thought.

Additionally, the patient was instructed in a combination of muscle relaxation and breathing techniques to use during times of stress or when spots started to appear. The patient terminated her treatment after eight sessions stating that she had come to use the techniques and that her vitiligo did not bother her anymore. The patient continued to believe that the vitiligo spots and their perceived effect were real.

Discussion

Primary psychiatric conditions can manifest in various ways and affect patient functioning differently. Here we have an example of a patient who believed a manifestation of vitiligo was giving her warning signs about future events. Despite the lack of visible changes to skin pigmentation, the patient was convinced that the condition was in fact vitiligo. Researchers have noted that there is a direct relationship between stress and the prognosis of skin disease (Jafferany et al. 2020). In the current case, stress appeared to cause symptoms that mimicked the presence of skin disease. It is not uncommon to have patients in dermatology who have a primary psychiatric disease (Bewley 2017). There has been insufficient evidence for an evidence-based recommendation to be made for the treatment of delusions (Skelton et al. 2015). Nevertheless, CBT proved successful in contributing to the patient's goal of managing the uncomfortable symptoms that she was experiencing. This case demonstrates a patient who, while functioning in society, is suffering from complex symptoms that could have been worsened by inaccurate disease presentation on the internet. Stigmatization of dermatological conditions in society is a problem significantly affecting those afflicted (Dimitrov and Szepietowski 2017). This case brings forth the danger of misinformation and self-diagnosis and the effects they can have on patient symptoms.

TEACHING POINTS

- Patients need to be properly informed of a condition and have the option to call back with further questions. When information is provided online, it needs to be peer reviewed and evidence based. Online information should also refrain from guiding patients to self-diagnose but instead advise them to seek professional help if concerned about their health.

- Psychodermatological conditions might not have a dermatological component that is visible. The presence of a multidisciplinary team becomes crucial when the patient holds unchangeable beliefs about a dermatological condition.

- Somatic manifestation in this case shows a less-known form of symptom presentation. Although psychiatric referral is beneficial, clinicians should be prepared for its refusal and instead work with patients to find other appropriate solutions.

References

Bewley A: The neglected psychological aspects of skin disease. BMJ 358:j3208, 2017 28684435

Dimitrov D, Szepietowski JC: Stigmatization in dermatology with a special focus on psoriatic patients. Postepy Hig Med Dosw 71(0):1115–1122, 2017 29225203

Jafferany M, Ferreira BR, Abdelmaksoud A, et al: Management of psychocutaneous disorders: a practical approach for dermatologists. Dermatol Ther 33(6):e13969, 2020 32621633

Skelton M, Khokhar WA, Thacker SP: Treatments for delusional disorder. Cochrane Database Syst Rev 2015(5):CD009785, 2015 25997589

Case 11–2

Pemphigus Vulgaris and Psychological Percussion

Harrison W. Loftus, B.A.
Mohammad Jafferany, M.D.

Case Description

A previously healthy 31-year-old woman suddenly developed painful, recurring oral lesions that would rupture with light pressure. In the following weeks, the patient also developed pain with bowel movements, lesions on the external genitalia that would periodically desquamate, and episodes of serosanguinous epistaxis. The oral lesions progressed into a cycle of scabbing, eroding, and bleeding whenever the patient ate solid foods or spoke. Because of the physical tension created by the scabs, the patient began habitually picking and manipulating them to achieve temporary pain relief. Soon after, the patient began reporting severe exhaustion and social anxiety related to the lesions, which began interfering with her personal and professional life.

The patient began using maladaptive lifestyle changes to avoid social interactions that required eating in public or speaking for extended periods of time. The patient reported that she ignored phone calls, canceled plans with friends, stopped going to after-work events with coworkers, and avoided intimacy with her spouse to avoid triggering pain. The patient also began eating a strictly liquid diet, which caused rapid, unwanted weight loss. The patient reported that after work she would immediately fall asleep and only wake up to eat a liquid dinner before going back to sleep. This new sleep pattern created additional strain on the patient's mental health and close relationships. Family members would make remarks such as "You're so lazy," and "How could you ever raise kids if you can't get through a day without taking a nap?," which further affected the patient's declining self-esteem. Over time, the patient lost her sense of control and sense of self from these undesired lifestyle changes, as she completely eliminated key aspects of her social identity.

Unable to eat the foods she wanted and unable to engage in normal activities, the patient became socially isolated and began experiencing anhedonia and depression. With the swift loss of primary social supports, the patient's reported depression levels worsened significantly. Without an explanation for the symptoms, the patient also began feeling hopeless. The patient admitted to contemplating suicide out of an overwhelming combination of physical pain, exhaustion, social withdrawal, depression, and undesired lifestyle changes.

During the diagnostic process, the patient was evaluated by a dentist, followed by a gastroenterologist, an internist, a gynecologist, and a maxillofacial specialist. At no point was the patient screened for symptoms of depression or suicidal ideation, even though she admitted to extreme psychological distress throughout the entire diagnostic process and treatment course. The patient stated that the constant referrals and lack of provider continuity made it difficult to express her feelings of depression and suicidal ideation.

Additionally, the patient reported that some of the providers' comments worsened her feelings of shame and stigmatization surrounding her symptoms. During a dentist visit, the lesions were mistaken for aphthous stomatitis, and the patient was accused of poor dental hygiene and poor diet. During a gynecological evaluation of the patient's genital lesions, the patient was accused of being promiscuous by a provider, even though she was in a monogamous relationship with her spouse. After this encounter, the patient reported feeling significantly embarrassed and judged, and did not feel comfortable discussing her mental health. During a dermatology follow-up appointment, the patient was reassured that she was getting better, since some of the lesions appeared smaller, even though her reported pain level and quality of life were worsening. Months later, the patient was diagnosed with pemphigus vulgaris after getting a biopsy during an appointment with a maxillofacial specialist.

Differential Diagnosis

- Treatment-resistant aphthous stomatitis and anal fissures secondary to undiagnosed Crohn's disease or colitis
- Abnormal presentation of Behçet's disease with unexplained oral involvement
- Sexually transmitted infection

Diagnosis

In this case, the diagnosis of pemphigus vulgaris was made by exhausting other possibilities. The patient's colonoscopy was negative for colitis. Her bloodwork was negative for HIV, hepatitis B, syphilis, and herpes simplex. Swabs were negative for gonorrhea and chlamydia. Of note, the patient had markedly elevated antinuclear antibodies and a moderately elevated eosinophil count, both of which can be indicative of an underlying autoimmune disease. After referral to a maxillofacial specialist, punch biopsies of active oral lesions, under H&E stain and direct immunofluorescence, resulted in the diagnosis of pemphigus vulgaris.

Management

The patient was simultaneously started on a course of prednisone 80 mg qam, mycophenolate mofetil 1.5 g bid, and clobetasol propionate 0.05% gel to apply twice a day. While on prednisone, the patient reported increased food cravings, weight gain, hot flashes, inability to fall asleep, episodes of mania, and worsening depression. These symptoms amplified the patient's negative self-image and a reduced sense of self-control.

Further into the treatment course, the patient developed a lung infection that required an inhaler, cessation of the mycophenolate mofetil, and follow-up with a pulmonologist. The patient continued the course of prednisone, and resolution of all lesions occurred ~3 months after treatment was initiated. The patient reported that it took several weeks for most of the corticosteroid side effects to dissipate. After the lesions resolved, the patient reported that her psychological symptoms began to rapidly improve, as she was able to start reintroducing foods, social events, and activities that she had enjoyed before disease onset. The patient also became involved with a patient support organization, which provided her with a supportive environment to validate her experience and build new social supports.

Discussion

Even after receiving her diagnosis, this patient reported that she sometimes wished she had cancer instead, because cancer is something that most people understand. The rarity of pemphigus vulgaris made it difficult for the patient to explain her symptoms and experience to others. The patient felt that her experience and pain were being minimized by those around her, which they were unable to combat without those individuals having a clear understanding of what pemphigus vulgaris is.

Before starting treatment, the patient was informed that pemphigus vulgaris could interfere with fertility, and that none of the treatments are pregnancy-safe. This meant that the patient would be unable to attempt to conceive unless she went into remission or discontinued treatment. This created significant stress on the patient, who was hoping to have children in the near future. After this, comments such as "When are you going to have kids?" from the patient's parents became triggering and began damaging the patient's self-image again.

If this patient had been evaluated for psychiatric disease, many of her somatic symptoms (exhaustion, weight changes, sleep disturbance) would appear to overlap with psychiatric symptoms. Corticosteroid side effects further confounded symptom manifestation, making it extremely difficult to determine etiology. For example, the exhaustion from the disease paired with an inability to sleep from the prednisone made the patient susceptible to episodes of emotional lability and impaired decision-making abilities, which affected her personal relationships, further harming her mental health.

The General Health Questionnaire-28 (GHQ-28), Dermatology Life Quality Index (DLQI), Beck Anxiety Inventory (BAI), Beck Depression Inventory (BDI), and EuroQol Five Dimensions Questionnaire (EQ-FD) are all useful measures to consider implementing when screening patients for psychological symptoms associated with chronic blistering diseases such as pemphigus vulgaris (Matthews and Ali 2022; Wang et al. 2023). Studies show that the incidence of both depression and anxiety are statistically higher in those with pemphigus than the general population or those with other chronic skin disorders (Hsu et al. 2020; Matthews and Ali 2022).

TEACHING POINTS

- It is necessary to repeatedly screen and monitor patients with suspected blistering diseases for symptoms of depression or suicidal ideation, both during the initial workup phase and throughout treatment.

- The somatic and psychological symptoms that manifest from pemphigus vulgaris and those that are a result of medication side effects have a complicated, potentially bidirectional relationship that needs to be addressed during treatment.

- Treatment with corticosteroids may inadvertently worsen symptoms of depression in patients with pemphigus vulgaris, which may interfere with compliance and intended treatment outcomes.

- Patient support organizations can serve as a protective factor to reduce hopelessness, address isolation, support social support development, and assist patients in regaining their sense of control over their daily lives.

References

Hsu YM, Fang HY, Lin CL, et al: The risk of depression in patients with pemphigus: a nationwide cohort study in Taiwan. Int J Environ Res Public Health 17(6):1983, 2020 32192212

Matthews R, Ali Z: Comorbid mental health issues in patients with pemphigus vulgaris and pemphigus foliaceus. Clin Exp Dermatol 47(1):24–29, 2022 34459019

Wang J, Wu H, Cong W, et al: Psychological morbidity in patients with pemphigus and its clinicodemographic risk factor: a comparative study. J Dermatol 50(10):1237–1245, 2023 37381772

12

Psoriasis, Depression, and Suicide

Harrison W. Loftus, B.A.
Cemre Busra Turk, M.D.
Mohammad Jafferany, M.D.

Introduction

Psoriasis is a chronic inflammatory condition that classically presents with scaly plaques and pruritus predominantly involving the elbows, knees, and scalp. The physical manifestations of the disease are well described, but its effects on mental health are underestimated. Depression, social stigmatization, social withdrawal, and overall poor quality of life have all been reported at increased levels by patients with psoriasis compared with the general population (Liang et al. 2019), and estimates of suicidality in patients with psoriasis are increased by as much as 40% (Kurd et al. 2010). Psychological factors are known to affect the course of many diseases, and the same is true for psoriasis. Low self-esteem, shame, sexual dysfunction, and social stigma have been shown to impact the treatment course and long-term quality of life of those with psoriasis.

The driving mechanism behind psoriasis is an overactive immune response mediated by T cells and dendritic cells (Tashiro and Sawada 2022). At the cellular level, proinflammatory cytokines, such as tumor necrosis factor-α (TNF-α), interleukin (IL)-17, and IL-23, are responsible for triggering an inflammatory cascade that produces the characteristic plaques seen in psoriasis (Tashiro and Sawada 2022). Internally, this cascade causes systemic inflammation very similar to what is observed in depression, suggesting that psoriasis may potentiate depression.

There is currently no permanent cure for psoriasis, but many newer effective treatment modalities have emerged. Long-term outcomes for patients with psoriasis are variable but appear to depend largely on quality-of-life measures and treatment adherence, both of which may be impeded by psychiatric comorbidity. Therefore, routine screening for depression and the implementation of psychological interventions may greatly improve the health outcomes of these patients.

Psychiatric Epidemiology

Psychiatric comorbidities associated with psoriasis are increasingly recognized. Among them, suicidality—which encompasses suicidal ideation (SI), suicide attempts, and completed suicide—has been highlighted as an area of particular concern for individuals with psoriasis (Liang et al. 2019; Nock et al. 2008). Numerous recent studies have explored the relationship between psoriasis and various forms of suicidality, but findings are inconsistent (Chi et al. 2017; Singh et al. 2017). Moreover, some studies fail to make important clinical distinctions between SI, suicide attempts, and actual suicides, often focusing only on limited aspects of this complex issue.

In individuals with psoriasis, the rate of suicidality has been documented at 0.9 per 1,000 person-years, compared with 0.7 per 1,000 person-years in the general population (Kurd et al. 2010; Liang et al. 2019). In a comprehensive multicenter study involving 626 psoriasis patients across 13 European countries, the prevalence of SI was markedly elevated at 17.3%, compared with 8.3% in the control group of healthy individuals. Notably, 67.6% of those experiencing SI explicitly attributed their suicidal thoughts to their psoriasis condition (Dalgard et al. 2015). Studies indicate that the lifetime history of SI in psoriasis patients is remarkably high (up to 37.4%) compared with patients without psoriasis (16.7%) (Pompili et al. 2016). Regarding suicide attempts, psoriasis patients have a rate of 1.43 per 10,000 person-years versus 1.00 in the general public (Egeberg et al. 2016a). The distinction became even more evident in a study in which 6.6% of those with psoriasis reported past suicide attempts, versus 0.0% in the group with other skin conditions (Pompili et al. 2016). The completed suicide rate is 2.03 per 10,000 person-years for psoriasis patients compared with 1.64 in the general population (Egeberg et al. 2016a; Svedbom et al. 2015). Singh et al. (2017) showed that psoriasis patients are more likely to attempt and complete suicides (pooled odds ratio 1.26; 95% CI 1.13–1.40) than control subjects without psoriasis. Two nationwide studies from Taiwan and South Korea evaluated the relationship between psoriasis and suicidality (Kim et al. 2023; Wang et al. 2020). The studies arrived at slightly divergent conclusions. The Taiwanese study found no significant association between suicidal behavior and psoriasis or psoriatic arthritis (Wang et al. 2020), and the Korean study reported an elevated risk of suicidality in the psoriasis group compared with controls (Kim et al. 2023). Notably, Kim et al. (2023) emphasized that the risk was particularly heightened among those with accompanying psoriatic arthritis.

Current data show that age is a determining factor. Younger psoriasis patients (in their 20s) exhibited a pronounced risk across the spectrum of suicidality, in contrast to psoriasis patients in their 60s or older (hazard ratio 1.83; 95% CI 1.64–2.05) (Kurd et al. 2010; Singh et al. 2017).

The role of disease severity in suicidal tendencies remains ambiguous. Wu et al. (2017) showed that there is no direct correlation between the severity of psoriasis and suicidality risk. Conversely, several studies proposed a stronger inclination for self-inflicted injuries and unsuccessful suicide attempts in patients with severe psoriasis compared with milder cases (Dalgard et al. 2015; Egeberg et al. 2016a; Singh et al. 2017). Still, the rates of confirmed completed attempts did not seem to vary based on psoriasis severity (Koo et al. 2017). According to Koo et al. (2017), if patients with psoriatic arthritis are excluded, suicidality risk and disease severity are not associated. Consistent with this, Chi et al. (2017) did not find a significant relationship between psoriasis and suicide. This phenomenon implies that the matrix of factors leading to suicidality in psoriasis patients may be more multifaceted than initially assumed, with coexistent conditions, such as psoriatic arthritis or other biopsychosocial factors, potentially playing a crucial role.

Concomitant depression seems to be linked with suicide in psoriasis. In a UK-based study of 607 psoriasis patients, those with major depressive disorder (MDD) had a rate of suicidal thoughts 10 times higher than the overall study population (35% vs. 3.5%) (Koo et al. 2017; Wang et al. 2020). In a study analyzing various factors linked to SI in psoriasis patients, having depression or a related disorder was the most significant predictor of SI, with an odds ratio of 12.8 (95% CI 6.3–26.1) (Picardi et al. 2006).

Psychiatric Comorbidities

As previously discussed, psoriasis is a condition that intersects with a host of comorbidities that affect virtually every organ system. For instance, psoriasis has been associated with malignancies, infections, kidney disorders, metabolic syndromes, and mood disorders (Monks et al. 2021). Psychiatric comorbidities have been gaining increased recognition in recent years. The chronic nature of psoriasis and lack of a definitive cure compound the lifetime risk for psoriatic patients to experience psychiatric comorbidities. Therefore, the extent of this relationship and the pursuit of effective treatments require further attention.

As the complex relationship between psoriasis and psychiatric comorbidity continues to be untangled, evidence keeps suggesting a high prevalence of depressive symptoms, SI, schizophrenia, and anxiety in those with psoriasis (Hedemann et al. 2022). The inflammatory pathways observed in psoriasis, as well as those observed in depression, schizophrenia, and anxiety, seem to lie at the center of this relationship (Liang et al. 2019). The pathophysiological similarities linking psoriasis and depression suggest the existence of a similar relationship between psoriasis and suicide.

Depression is a common disorder that can manifest through depressed mood, low energy levels, sleep disturbances, changes in diet, slow mentation, psychosis, and suicidality. The occurrence of depression in a patient with psoriasis may also be influenced indirectly through the previously discussed social burdens of the disease, primarily social stigma and social isolation. Furthermore, the presence of psychiatric comorbidity in the context of any disease requiring long-term treatment raises concerns for nonadherence and poor outcomes without proper management.

Psoriatic patients with comorbid depression appear to be at increased risk of myocardial infarction, stroke, and cardiovascular death (Egeberg et al. 2016b). These patients are additionally 10 times more likely to experience suicidal thoughts versus psoriatic patients without depression (Koo et al. 2017; Wang et al. 2020). Studies have also shown that low levels of estrogen, vitamin D_3, and melatonin in psoriatic patients may mediate the relationship between psoriasis and depression (An et al. 2021; Sahi et al. 2020). Whether these suicidal thoughts are related to the underlying disease pathophysiology or diminished quality of life requires further investigation. Regardless, these associations highlight vulnerable populations that may require additional screening and treatment.

While there is irrefutable evidence of a connection between psoriasis and psychiatric comorbidities, the directionality of this relationship is still being explored. Although the association of psoriasis with depression is often linked to external psychological stigma from visible skin lesions, there is growing evidence that suggests immunological factors are responsible for a common pathogenesis (Hölsken et al. 2021). This theory is complicated: some studies postulate that depression and SI may precede a diagnosis of psoriasis (Pompili et al. 2016, 2017). More research is required to better understand this relationship.

Pathophysiology of Depression and Suicidal Thoughts in Psoriasis

Immunopathogenesis of Psoriasis

Psoriasis is characterized by an abnormal immune response in which dendritic cells, T helper 1 (Th1)/Th17 lymphocytes, and keratinocytes engage in a pathological interplay. Activation of dendritic cells releases cytokines such as interferons (IFNs) and TNF, which subsequently stimulate T cells, including Th1 and Th17 subsets. This results in a further cascade of cytokines, with IL-12 promoting Th1 cell differentiation and IL-23 enhancing Th17 responses. These T cell subsets then release their signature cytokines: Th1 cells produce IFN-γ, and Th17 cells release IL-17 and IL-22 (Arican et al. 2005; Di Cesare et al. 2009; Grossman et al. 1989; Kimura and Kishimoto 2010; Koo et al. 2017; Singh et al. 2021). Keratinocytes, the primary epidermal cells, respond to these cytokines, particularly IL-17 and IL-22, by proliferating excessively, leading to the thickened, scaly plaques typical of psoriasis (Singh et al. 2021).

Inflammation and Depression

Chronic inflammation has emerged as a pivotal player in the pathogenesis of depression. Patients with MDD frequently have an activated inflammatory response system, marked by increased circulating levels of proinflammatory cytokines, especially IL-6, and acute-phase proteins such as C-reactive protein (Dowlati et al. 2010; Howren et al. 2009; Miller and Raison 2016; Raison et al. 2006). At a molecular level, cytokines activate the enzyme indoleamine-2,3-dioxygenase, which catabolizes tryptophan (a serotonin precursor) into kynurenine. This shift in metabolic pathways results in decreased serotonin synthesis, potentially contributing to depressive symptoms (Chourbaji et al. 2006; Dantzer and Kelley 2007; Dunn et al. 2005; Schiepers et al. 2005; Sublette et al. 2011; Weiss et al. 1999). Moreover, proinflammatory cytokines can exert direct neurotoxic effects and hyperstimulate the hypothalamic-pituitary-adrenal axis, a primary neuroendocrine system governing stress responses (Fonseka et al. 2015; Koo et al. 2017; Pariante and Lightman 2008; Raber et al. 1997; Young et al. 2014).

Psoriasis, Cytokines, Depression, and Suicide

Psoriasis has profound systemic implications mediated through a web of cytokines in addition to skin changes. This cytokine milieu drives skin pathology and interlinks with neuropsychiatric processes.

A common thread linking psoriasis and depression appears to be inflammatory cytokines. Several studies emphasize the relationship between proinflammatory cytokines such as IL-6, IL-1, IL-17, and TNF-α with depression and suicide (Pandey 2013; Raison et al. 2006; Tsai et al. 2011). In particular, elevated systemic levels of IL-6, observed in psoriasis and depression, can penetrate the blood-brain barrier, influencing central neurotransmitter dynamics and brain function; individuals diagnosed with depression, even without inflammatory skin conditions like psoriasis, exhibit augmented levels of these cytokines in their blood and cerebrospinal fluid (CSF) (Levine et al. 1999; Tonelli et al. 2008). This suggests a broader systemic role of cytokines in modulating neuropsychiatric conditions, possibly by influencing serotonin metabolism (Lindqvist et al. 2011). Lindqvist et al. (2009) proposed that IL-6 in the CSF might influence the manifestations of suicidal behavior, potentially by modulating dopamine and serotonin metabolism. They showed that the CSF of people who have attempted suicide has higher IL-6 levels than those who have not. These findings suggest potential cytokine-mediated neuromodulation, but the precise biologic mediators orchestrating this intricate association remain under rigorous investigation.

Furthermore, it is intriguing that while cytokines such as IL-17 play a pivotal role in psoriatic pathogenesis, with elevated IL-17 levels tied to anxiety in rheumatoid arthritis patients, such links have yet to be explored deeply in psoriasis patients (Gniadecki et al. 2012; Liu et al. 2012). Nevertheless, the potential role of IL-17 in mental health cannot be overlooked, as evidenced by reports of a positive correlation between IL-17 serum levels and MDD (Davami et al. 2016), as well as suicide among patients in clinical trials for brodalumab, an anti-IL-17RA antibody (Papp et al. 2016). Clinical reports of suicidal behavior in patients treated with IL-17 inhibitors underscore the importance of thoroughly elucidating these connections (Danesh and Kimball 2016).

Management

Treatment options for psoriasis have drastically expanded over the past century and include topical corticosteroids, phototherapy, nonbiological systemic medications, and biologic agents. The preferred treatment modality depends largely on the severity and extent of body surface area affected. Increased attention is being placed on addressing concomitant psychiatric conditions alongside the cutaneous and systemic manifestations of psoriasis.

Topical corticosteroids have long been a mainstay treatment for psoriatic plaques owing to their anti-inflammatory, vasoconstrictive, and immunosuppressive characteristics. These agents typically require 4 weeks of consistent use to resolve plaques, although administration for up to 12 weeks under careful physician monitoring has been demonstrated to prevent unwanted side effects such as skin thinning and striae (Elmets et al. 2021). Nonsteroidal medications such as tacrolimus and pimecrolimus have also been used off-label to treat psoriasis owing to their inhibitory effect on cytokine synthesis.

Historically, broadband ultraviolet B (UVB) followed by narrowband UVB has been used to treat psoriasis, but these treatments are becoming less common due to their phototoxic and carcinogenic effects (Elmets et al. 2019).

Low-dose methotrexate has been shown to effectively treat psoriasis by reducing lymphoid cell proliferation. Supplemental treatment with folic acid is recommended to decrease the risk of adverse effects. Methotrexate is currently preferred over cyclosporine, a more potent immunosuppressant that decreases the activation of T cells through calcineurin inhibition. In 2014, the FDA approved apremilast, a phosphodiesterase 4 inhibitor, for the treatment of psoriasis. More recently, oral Janus kinase (JAK) inhibitors approved for psoriatic arthritis have been used off-label to treat psoriasis (Menter et al. 2020). In 2022, deucravacitinib was the first JAK inhibitor to be approved for the treatment of moderate to severe plaque psoriasis.

Several biologic agents have been successfully used to treat moderate to severe plaque psoriasis and can be used either as monotherapy or in combination with other treatments. This class includes TNF-α inhibitors such as etanercept and monoclonal antibodies such as infliximab, adalimumab, and certolizumab. In the past decade, more targeted IL-17 and IL-23 human monoclonal antibodies have been approved for adults with plaque psoriasis. Ustekinumab and adalimumab have shown ability to decrease depressive symptoms, potentially owing to the shared inflammatory pathways observed in both depression and psoriasis (Fleming et al. 2015). Whether the improvement is directly due to reduced inflammation or indirectly due to improved psoriasis leading to improved quality of life has not been determined (Patel et al. 2017).

As the relationship between psoriasis and psychiatric comorbidity becomes clearer and more recognized, additional emphasis has been placed on psychological evaluation and targeted psychotherapeutic treatment in conjunction with traditional therapeutic management of psoriasis. The 9-item Patient Health Questionnaire (PHQ-9) is a widely used and validated screening tool to assess for depression and is useful in monitoring the psychological manifestations of SI, hopelessness, and anhedonia in the context of psoriasis (Bardazzi et al. 2022). Additional instruments that may be used to assess depression and SI include the Beck Depression Inventory (BDI-II), Hamilton Rating Scale for Depression (HAM-D), Center for Epidemiologic Studies Depression Scale (CES-D), Montgomery-Åsberg Depression Rating Scale (MADRS), Columbia Suicide Severity Rating Scale (C-SSRS), and the Ask Suicide Screening Questions (ASQ). In clinical settings where the PHQ-9 is not routinely administered, physicians may consider initial screening with the 2-item PHQ-2 to identify patients who require additional depression screening measures (McDonald et al. 2018). A timely diagnosis may reduce the risk of psychological manifestations, improve quality of life, and improve overall prognosis.

Psychological treatments such as mindfulness-based stress reduction, CBT, and problem-solving therapy may alleviate symptoms of anxiety and depression in patients with psoriasis. These treatments have all shown efficacy in improving quality-of-life measures in those with psoriasis (Kabat-Zinn et al. 1998; Xiao et al. 2019). These psychological interventions spotlight promising nonpharmaceutical treatments that may attenuate the psychological impact psoriasis has on quality of life, and potentially psychiatric comorbidities as well.

A multidisciplinary approach to treating psoriasis that includes psychological and dermatological interventions is key in improving long-term patient outcomes. Whether or not the exact relationship between psoriasis, depression, and suicide is fully understood, the seriousness and potential life-threatening consequences of these psychiatric comorbidities must be addressed. Therefore, psychological assessment within dermatologic practices is crucial in identifying patients who are at risk of having or developing depression or SI.

Conclusion

Knowledge surrounding the complex relationship between psoriasis and psychiatric comorbidity is improving but is still inadequate. SI, suicide attempts, and completed suicide remain very real concerns for individuals with psoriasis. The pathophysiological commonalities underpinning psoriasis, depression, and suicide as consequences of an inappropriate inflammatory response appear promising. Regardless, patients with psoriasis are more likely to have psychiatric comorbidities that require acute attention than the general population.

A multidisciplinary approach to treating psoriasis is invaluable, especially for patients experiencing psychiatric comorbidities. Tools for assessing depression in this population are particularly useful and should be administered routinely and frequently in dermatologic contexts. The spectrum of disease severity coupled with the spectrum of depression and SI puts this population at an increased risk for extremely poor health outcomes.

To date, most studies linking psoriasis and suicidal behaviors are limited by sample size and study design. Additionally, many studies fail to differentiate SI, suicide attempts, and completed suicide, making the relationship between suicide and psoriasis severity less clear. Further research on the effects of specific treatments and interventions is needed to better understand this relationship. Currently, psychological interventions have shown effectiveness in addressing quality of life, and some biologic agents appear to decrease depressive symptoms owing to their anti-inflammatory effects. By appropriately addressing the psychological burden of patients with psoriasis and psychiatric comorbidities, depression and suicide risk can be greatly reduced. Improving these patients' quality of life may also encourage long-term treatment adherence and improved outcomes.

References

An X, Yao X, Li B, et al: Role of BDNF-mTORC1 signaling pathway in female depression. Neural Plast 2021:6619515, 2021 33628219

Arican O, Aral M, Sasmaz S, et al: Serum levels of TNF-alpha, IFN-gamma, IL-6, IL-8, IL-12, IL-17, and IL-18 in patients with active psoriasis and correlation with disease severity. Mediators Inflamm 2005(5):273–279, 2005 16258194

Bardazzi F, Bonci C, Sacchelli L, et al: Suicide risk and depression in patients with psoriasis. Ital J Dermatol Venereol 157(6):497–501, 2022 36651203

Chi CC, Chen TH, Wang SH, et al: Risk of suicidality in people with psoriasis: a systematic review and meta-analysis of cohort studies. Am J Clin Dermatol 18(5):621–627, 2017 28409490

Chourbaji S, Urani A, Inta I, et al: IL-6 knockout mice exhibit resistance to stress-induced development of depression-like behaviors. Neurobiol Dis 23(3):587–594, 2006 16843000

Dalgard FJ, Gieler U, Tomas-Aragones L, et al: The psychological burden of skin diseases: a cross-sectional multicenter study among dermatological out-patients in 13 European countries. J Invest Dermatol 135(4):984–991, 2015 25521458

Danesh MJ, Kimball AB: Brodalumab and suicidal ideation in the context of a recent economic crisis in the United States. J Am Acad Dermatol 74(1):190–192, 2016 26702804

Dantzer R, Kelley KW: Twenty years of research on cytokine-induced sickness behavior. Brain Behav Immun 21(2):153–160, 2007 17088043

Davami MH, Baharlou R, Ahmadi Vasmehjani A, et al: Elevated IL-17 and TGF-β serum levels: a positive correlation between T-helper 17 cell-related pro-inflammatory responses with major depressive disorder. Basic Clin Neurosci 7(2):137–142, 2016 27303608

Di Cesare A, Di Meglio P, Nestle FO: The IL-23/Th17 axis in the immunopathogenesis of psoriasis. J Invest Dermatol 129(6):1339–1350, 2009 19322214

Dowlati Y, Herrmann N, Swardfager W, et al: A meta-analysis of cytokines in major depression. Biol Psychiatry 67(5):446–457, 2010 20015486

Dunn AJ, Swiergiel AH, de Beaurepaire R: Cytokines as mediators of depression: what can we learn from animal studies? Neurosci Biobehav Rev 29(4–5):891–909, 2005 15885777

Egeberg A, Hansen PR, Gislason GH, et al: Risk of self-harm and nonfatal suicide attempts, and completed suicide in patients with psoriasis: a population-based cohort study. Br J Dermatol 175(3):493–500, 2016a 27038335

Egeberg A, Khalid U, Gislason GH, et al: Impact of depression on risk of myocardial infarction, stroke and cardiovascular death in patients with psoriasis: a Danish Nationwide Study. Acta Derm Venereol 96(2):218–221, 2016b 26280176

Elmets CA, Lim HW, Stoff B, et al: Joint American Academy of Dermatology-National Psoriasis Foundation guidelines of care for the management and treatment of psoriasis with phototherapy. J Am Acad Dermatol 81(3):775–804, 2019 31351884

Elmets CA, Korman NJ, Prater EF, et al: Joint AAD-NPF Guidelines of care for the management and treatment of psoriasis with topical therapy and alternative medicine modalities for psoriasis severity measures. J Am Acad Dermatol 84(2):432–470, 2021 32738429

Fleming P, Roubille C, Richer V, et al: Effect of biologics on depressive symptoms in patients with psoriasis: a systematic review. J Eur Acad Dermatol Venereol 29(6):1063–1070, 2015 25490866

Fonseka TM, McIntyre RS, Soczynska JK, et al: Novel investigational drugs targeting IL-6 signaling for the treatment of depression. Expert Opin Investig Drugs 24(4):459–475, 2015 25585966

Gniadecki R, Robertson D, Molta CT, et al: Self-reported health outcomes in patients with psoriasis and psoriatic arthritis randomized to two etanercept regimens. J Eur Acad Dermatol Venereol 26(11):1436–1443, 2012 22035157

Grossman RM, Krueger J, Yourish D, et al: Interleukin 6 is expressed in high levels in psoriatic skin and stimulates proliferation of cultured human keratinocytes. Proc Natl Acad Sci USA 86(16):6367–6371, 1989 2474833

Hedemann TL, Liu X, Kang CN, et al: Associations between psoriasis and mental illness: an update for clinicians. Gen Hosp Psychiatry 75:30–37, 2022 35101785

Hölsken S, Krefting F, Schedlowski M, et al: Common fundamentals of psoriasis and depression. Acta Derm Venereol 101(11):adv00609, 2021 34806760

Howren MB, Lamkin DM, Suls J: Associations of depression with C-reactive protein, IL-1, and IL-6: a meta-analysis. Psychosom Med 71(2):171–186, 2009 19188531

Kabat-Zinn J, Wheeler E, Light T, et al: Influence of a mindfulness meditation-based stress reduction intervention on rates of skin clearing in patients with moderate to severe psoriasis undergoing phototherapy (UVB) and photochemotherapy (PUVA). Psychosom Med 60(5):625–632, 1998 9773769

Kim SM, Ahn J, Cho YA, et al: Increased risk of suicidality in patients with psoriasis: a nationwide cohort study in Korea. J Eur Acad Dermatol Venereol 37(1):75–84, 2023 36028994

Kimura A, Kishimoto T: IL-6: regulator of Treg/Th17 balance. Eur J Immunol 40(7):1830–1835, 2010 20583029

Koo J, Marangell LB, Nakamura M, et al: Depression and suicidality in psoriasis: review of the literature including the cytokine theory of depression. J Eur Acad Dermatol Venereol 31(12):1999–2009, 2017 28681405

Kurd SK, Troxel AB, Crits-Christoph P, et al: The risk of depression, anxiety, and suicidality in patients with psoriasis: a population-based cohort study. Arch Dermatol 146(8):891–895, 2010 20713823

Levine J, Barak Y, Chengappa KN, et al: Cerebrospinal cytokine levels in patients with acute depression. Neuropsychobiology 40(4):171–176, 1999 10559698

Liang SE, Cohen JM, Ho RS: Psoriasis and suicidality: a review of the literature. Dermatol Ther 32(1):e12771, 2019 30315629

Lindqvist D, Janelidze S, Hagell P, et al: Interleukin-6 is elevated in the cerebrospinal fluid of suicide attempters and related to symptom severity. Biol Psychiatry 66(3):287–292, 2009 19268915

Lindqvist D, Janelidze S, Erhardt S, et al: CSF biomarkers in suicide attempters: a principal component analysis. Acta Psychiatr Scand 124(1):52–61, 2011 21198458

Liu Y, Ho RC, Mak A: The role of interleukin (IL)-17 in anxiety and depression of patients with rheumatoid arthritis. Int J Rheum Dis 15(2):183–187, 2012 22462422

McDonald K, Shelley A, Jafferany M: The PHQ-2 in dermatology-standardized screening for depression and suicidal ideation. JAMA Dermatol 154(2):139–141, 2018 29282453

Menter A, Gelfand JM, Connor C, et al: Joint American Academy of Dermatology-National Psoriasis Foundation guidelines of care for the management of psoriasis with systemic nonbiologic therapies. J Am Acad Dermatol 82(6):1445–1486, 2020 32119894

Miller AH, Raison CL: The role of inflammation in depression: from evolutionary imperative to modern treatment target. Nat Rev Immunol 16(1):22–34, 2016 26711676

Monks G, Rivera-Oyola R, Lebwohl M: The psoriasis decision tree. J Clin Aesthet Dermatol 14(4):14–22, 2021 34055182

Nock MK, Borges G, Bromet EJ, et al: Suicide and suicidal behavior. Epidemiol Rev 30(1):133–154, 2008 18653727

Pandey GN: Biological basis of suicide and suicidal behavior. Bipolar Disord 15(5):524–541, 2013 23773657

Papp KA, Reich K, Paul C, et al: A prospective phase III, randomized, double-blind, placebo-controlled study of brodalumab in patients with moderate-to-severe plaque psoriasis. Br J Dermatol 175(2):273–286, 2016 26914406

Pariante CM, Lightman SL: The HPA axis in major depression: classical theories and new developments. Trends Neurosci 31(9):464–468, 2008 18675469

Patel N, Nadkarni A, Cardwell LA, et al: Psoriasis, depression, and inflammatory overlap: a review. Am J Clin Dermatol 18(5):613–620, 2017 28432649

Picardi A, Mazzotti E, Pasquini P: Prevalence and correlates of suicidal ideation among patients with skin disease. J Am Acad Dermatol 54(3):420–426, 2006 16488292

Pompili M, Innamorati M, Trovarelli S, et al: Suicide risk and psychiatric comorbidity in patients with psoriasis. J Int Med Res 44(1)(suppl):61–66, 2016 27683142

Pompili M, Innamorati M, Forte A, et al: Psychiatric comorbidity and suicidal ideation in psoriasis, melanoma and allergic disorders. Int J Psychiatry Clin Pract 21(3):209–214, 2017 28326880

Raber J, O'Shea RD, Bloom FE, et al: Modulation of hypothalamic-pituitary-adrenal function by transgenic expression of interleukin-6 in the CNS of mice. J Neurosci 17(24):9473–9480, 1997 9391003

Raison CL, Capuron L, Miller AH: Cytokines sing the blues: inflammation and the pathogenesis of depression. Trends Immunol 27(1):24–31, 2006 16316783

Sahi FM, Masood A, Danawar NA, et al: Association between psoriasis and depression: a traditional review. Cureus 12(8):e9708, 2020 32944430

Schiepers OJ, Wichers MC, Maes M: Cytokines and major depression. Prog Neuropsychopharmacol Biol Psychiatry 29(2):201–217, 2005 15694227

Singh R, Koppu S, Perche PO, et al: The cytokine mediated molecular pathophysiology of psoriasis and its clinical implications. Int J Mol Sci 22(23):12793, 2021 34884596

Singh S, Taylor C, Kornmehl H, et al: Psoriasis and suicidality: a systematic review and meta-analysis. J Am Acad Dermatol 77(3):425–440.e2, 2017 28807109

Sublette ME, Galfalvy HC, Fuchs D, et al: Plasma kynurenine levels are elevated in suicide attempters with major depressive disorder. Brain Behav Immun 25(6):1272–1278, 2011 21605657

Svedbom A, Dalén J, Mamolo C, et al: Increased cause-specific mortality in patients with mild and severe psoriasis: a population-based Swedish register study. Acta Derm Venereol 95(7):809–815, 2015 25766866

Tashiro T, Sawada Y: Psoriasis and systemic inflammatory disorders. Int J Mol Sci 23(8):4457, 2022 35457278

Tonelli LH, Stiller J, Rujescu D, et al: Elevated cytokine expression in the orbitofrontal cortex of victims of suicide. Acta Psychiatr Scand 117(3):198–206, 2008 18081924

Tsai TF, Wang TS, Hung ST, et al: Epidemiology and comorbidities of psoriasis patients in a national database in Taiwan. J Dermatol Sci 63(1):40–46, 2011 21543188

Wang SH, Wang J, Chi CC, et al: Risk for suicidal behavior among psoriasis patients: a nationwide cohort study. Am J Clin Dermatol 21(3):431–439, 2020 31782075

Weiss G, Murr C, Zoller H, et al: Modulation of neopterin formation and tryptophan degradation by Th1- and Th2-derived cytokines in human monocytic cells. Clin Exp Immunol 116(3):435–440, 1999 10361231

Wu JJ, Penfold RB, Primatesta P, et al: The risk of depression, suicidal ideation and suicide attempt in patients with psoriasis, psoriatic arthritis or ankylosing spondylitis. J Eur Acad Dermatol Venereol 31(7):1168–1175, 2017 28214371

Xiao Y, Zhang X, Luo D, et al: The efficacy of psychological interventions on psoriasis treatment: a systematic review and meta-analysis of randomized controlled trials. Psychol Res Behav Manag 12:97–106, 2019 30799963

Young JJ, Bruno D, Pomara N: A review of the relationship between proinflammatory cytokines and major depressive disorder. J Affect Disord 169:15–20, 2014 25128861

Index

Page numbers printed in **boldface** *type refer to tables or figures.*

AAT (approach avoidance therapy), 251
Acceptance and commitment therapy (ACT)
    for body-focused repetitive behaviors (BFRBs), 102, 251
    for prurigo nodularis, 183
    for trichotillomania, 86
Acitretin, 27
Acne excoriée, **13**
Acneiform eruptions, 21, 24
Acupuncture, 182–183, 251, 298, 307
Adalimumab, for psoriasis, 355
ADHD
    alopecia areata, 213–214
    comorbid psychiatric conditions, 245–246
    prurigo nodularis, 179
Alexithymia, 214, 223, 231
Alimemazine, for burning mouth syndrome, 315
Alopecia, drug reaction associated, 21–24
Alopecia areata, 209–241
    case reports, 218–241
        case 5-2 (journey to trichotemnomania), 103–109
        case 8-1 (trichotillomania with), 218–222, **219–221**
        case 8-2 (psychological comorbidity), 222–228, **224–227**
        case 8-3 (holistic management), 228–232, **229–231**
        case 8-4 (in an infant), 233–237, **234–236**
        case 8-5 (anxiety and depression associated), 237–241, **239–240**
    clinical course and prognosis, 212
    clinical features, 210, **211**
    dermoscopy, 219, **220–221**, 226
    diagnosis, 210
    differential diagnosis, **213**
    epidemiology, 209, 239
    etiology and pathogenesis, 209–210
    introduction, 209
    misdiagnosis, 105
    as primary skin lesion, 11, **12**
    psychodermatologic perspective, 212–214
    treatment, 214–216, **215**
    trichoscopy, 90, 108, 120–121, 124, 210, **212**, 218–221, 223, **225–227**, 229, 233, 235, **235**, 238
Alopecia areata totalis, 209–210, **211**, 213–214
Alopecia areata universalis, 209–210, 213–214
Amitriptyline
    for cutaneous sensory disorders, 296
    for onychotillomania, 259
    for prurigo nodularis, 183
    for vulvodynia, 298, 307
Angioedema, 23
Anhedonia, 341, 355
Anticonvulsants, for vulvodynia, 298, 307
Antidepressants
    for alopecia areata, 215
    cutaneous adverse drug reactions (CADRs), 23
    for delusional disorders, 65
    for delusional infestation, 47–49
    examples and uses, 14
    for Gardner-Diamond syndrome, 326, 328

Antidepressants *(continued)*
  for onychotillomania, 259
  for prurigo nodularis, 183
Antiepileptics, 14
Antihistamines
  for prurigo nodularis, 197, 201
  psychiatric side effects, 25
Antioxidant-oxidant imbalance, 210
Antipsychotics
  for body-focused repetitive behavior disorders (BFRDs), 251
  cutaneous adverse drug reactions (CADRs), 23–24
  for cutaneous sensory disorders, 296
  for delusional disorders, 65–66
  for delusional infestation, 47, 53–54
  for dermatitis artefacta, 134, 164
  examples and uses, 14
  for onychophagia, 268
  for onychotillomania, 259
  for prurigo nodularis, 183
  for trichotillomania, 87–88
Antisocial personality disorder, 214
Anxiety
  alopecia areata, 214, 225, 230, 237–240
  breath work to control, 86
  comorbid psychiatric conditions, 245
  dermatitis artefacta, 162, 166
  Gardner-Diamond syndrome, 322, 325, 329
  onychophagia, 247–248, 266, 268
  onychotillomania, 257
  pemphigus vulgaris, 341
  prevalence of, 3
  prurigo nodularis, 179, 196, 203–209
  psoriasis, 352
  psychobiotics for, 15
  skin picking, 247, 276–277, 292–293
Anxiolytics
  cutaneous adverse drug reactions (CADRs), 24
  for dermatitis artefacta, 155
  for prurigo nodularis, 183
Approach avoidance therapy (AAT), 251

Apremilast, 25
Aprepitant, for prurigo nodularis, 182, 197
Apripiprazole, for trichotillomania, 87–88
Arthritis, psoriatic, 351, 355
Ask Suicide Screening Questions (ASQ), 356
Assessment, functional, 3
Atopic dermatitis, 2
  alopecia areata associated with, 210
  prurigo nodularis association with, 177–178, 197
Auto-erythrocyte sensitization syndrome. *See* Gardner-Diamond syndrome
Auto-erythrocyte sensitization test, 311, **311**, 321, 323–324, **325**, 326
Autoimmune disorder, 178, 209–210. *See also* Alopecia areata
Awareness training, 85

Baricitinib, 230
Beard, trichoteiromania of (case report), 109–115, **110–111**
Beck Anxiety Inventory (BAI), 347
Beck Depression Inventory (BDI), 347, 355
Behavior Assessment System for Children, 2nd Edition, Behavioral and Emotional Screening System (BASC-2 BESS), 249
Behavioral therapy
  for body-focuses repetitive behavioral disorders, 102, 251
  cognitive (*see* cognitive behavioral therapy)
  for onychotillomania, 259
Benzodiazepines
  drug reaction, 24
  therapeutic uses, 14
Besnier prurigo, 197
BFRBs (body-focused repetitive behaviors), 100
BFRDs. *See* Body-focused repetitive behavior disorders
Biopsy
  alopecia areata, 210

Index

prurigo nodularis, 181, 188, **190**, 195, 203–204
Bipolar disorder
    with dermatitis artefacta, 153
    negative association with alopecia areata, 213
Body dysmorphic disorder
    alopecia areata, 213
    comorbid psychiatric conditions, 245
    cutaneous sensory disorder associated, 296
Body-focused repetitive behavior disorders (BFRDs), 243–297
    case reports, 254–297
        case 9-1 (onychotillomania), 254–264, **255–256, 258–263**
        case 9-2 (treatment-resistant onychophagia), 264–268, **265–266**
        case 9-3 (pseudo-knuckle pads), 269–273, **270–271**
        case 9-4 (chronic wound secondary to skin picking), 274–279, **275–277**
        case 9-5 (OCD with repeated hand washing and fingernail onychomycosis), 279–283, **280–283**
        case 9-6 (onychophagia and dermatotillomania), 284–287, **285–286**
        case 9-7 (long-term pathological skin picking), 287–292, **288–289**
        case 9-8 (skin picking disorder in 64-year-old woman), 292–294
    classification, 246
    clinical features, 247–249, **248**
    comorbid psychiatric conditions, 245–246
    complications, 249–250
    epidemiology, 244–245
    introduction, 243
    measurement of severity, 249
    OCD compared, 249
    psychopharmacology, 251
    psychotherapy, 251

treatment, 250
Body-focused repetitive behaviors (BFRBs), 100
Borderline personality disorder, with dermatitis artefacta, 155, 163, 166
Brachioradial pruritus, 300
Breath work, 86
Brodalumab, 27
Broom hairs, **92**, 91–92, 109, **111**, 112–115, 118, **120**
Bruxism. See Teeth grinding
Bupropion, 23
Burning mouth syndrome. See also Glossodynia
    case report, 313–316, **314**
    overview, 296–297
Buspirone, 138
Butterfly sign, 180, 293

C-SSRS (Columbia Suicide Severity Rating Scale), 356
Cadaver hair, 210
CADRs. See Cutaneous adverse drug reactions
Calcineurin inhibitors, 228
Calcipotriol, for prurigo nodularis, 182
Cannabinoids, for prurigo nodularis, 182
Capsaicin, 299
Carbamazepine, 21–22, **22**
Carotidynia, 299
Casts, pigmented, 79, 119
CBT. See Cognitive behavioral therapy
Center for Epidemiologic Studies Depression Scale (CES-D), 355–356
Certolizumab, for psoriasis, 355
CGI-S (Clinical Global Impression-Severity), 249
Cheek biting/chewing, 245, 248, 273
Child abuse, 135, 163, 321
Children
    alopecia areata, 209, 213–214, 233–237
    body-focused repetitive behavior disorders (BFRDs), 244–245, 248–249, 265–266, 268, 273
    prurigo nodularis, 199–203
Chronic wound secondary to skin picking (case report), 274–279

Citalopram
    for alopecia areata, 215
    for body-focused repetitive behavior disorders (BFRDs), 251
Classification of psychocutaneous disorders, 8–9, **9**
Clinical Global Impression-Severity (CGI-S), 249
Clobetasol propionate, 223, 228, 342
Clomipramine
    for onychotillomania, 259
    for trichotillomania, 87
Clonazepam
    for burning mouth syndrome, 297
    for prurigo nodularis, 205
Clopidogrel, 56
Clozapine, 24
Coccygodynia, 295
Cognitive behavioral therapy (CBT)
    for alopecia areata, 214, 230
    for body-focused repetitive behaviors (BFRBs), 102, 249
    for burning mouth syndrome, 297, 315
    for cutaneous sensory disorders, 296
    for delusional disorders, 65
    for dermatitis artefacta, 150, 160, 171
    for erythromelalgia, 300
    for Gardner-Diamond syndrome, 325–326, 326
    for glossodynia, 303
    for hallucinations and delusions of vitiligo (case report), 337–340
    HRT (*see* Habit reversal training)
    for OCD, 249
    for onychophagia, 265, 268
    for onychotillomania, 258
    for prurigo nodularis, 183, 206
    for pseudo-knuckle pads, 272
    for psoriasis, 356
    for scalp pain, 298
    for skin picking, 289, 291, 294–297
    for trichoteiromania, 93, 112
    for trichotemnomania, 123
    for trichotillomania, 120
    for trichotillomania comorbid with trichotemnomania, 115
    for vulvodynia, 298
Cognitive bias dysfunction, 249
Cognitive restructuring
    for body-focused repetitive behaviors (BFRBs), 102
    for hallucinations and delusions of vitiligo (case report), 339
Coiled hair, 78, **79**, 90
Columbia Suicide Severity Rating Scale (C-SSRS), 356
Competing response practice, 85
Conversion disorder, 133
Coping strategies
    assessment of, 10
    nail biting, 248
    psychotherapy for improvement in, 14
    self-harm as emotional, 128
    trichotillomania as, 76
Corticosteroids
    for alopecia areata, 105, 218, 228, 233
    for Gardner-Diamond syndrome, 328
    for prurigo nodularis, 199–200
    for psoriasis, 354–355
    side effects, 28, 342–347
    for skin picking disorders, 293
Coudability hair, 238
CSDs (cutaneous sensory disorders), 295–335
Cutaneous adverse drug reactions (CADRs), 19–24
    antidepressants, 23
    antipsychotics, 23–24
    anxiolytics, 24
    immune-mediated, 20
    mood stabilizers, 21–22
    overview, 20–21
    prevalence, 20
Cutaneous sensory disorders (CSDs), 295–335
    brachioradial pruritus, 300
    burning mouth syndrome, 296–297
    case reports, 302–335
        case 10-1 (glossodynia in 54-year-old woman), 302–304
        case 10-2 (vulvodynia), 304–308

Index

case 10-3 (Gardner-Diamond syndrome in 20-year-old woman), 308–312, **309, 311**
case 10-4 (glossodynia in 47-year-old woman), 313–316, **314**
case 10-5 (psychogenic itch), 316–319
case 10-6 (Gardner-Diamond syndrome in 5-year-old girl), 319–323, **324–321**
case 10-7 (Gardner-Diamond syndrome in 29-year-old woman), 323–326, **324–325**
case 10-8 (Gardner-Diamond syndrome in 16-year-old girl), 327–331, **328**
case 10-9 (Gardner-Diamond syndrome in 49-year-old woman), 331–335, **332–333**
categories, 296
classification, 8, **9**
erythromelalgia, 300
introduction, 295–296
notalgia paresthetica, 298–299
penoscrotodynia, 297–298
postherpetic neuralgia (PHN), 299
scalp pain, chronic, 298
trigeminal trophic syndrome (TTS), 299–300
vulvodynia, 297–298
Cyclosporine, 25
Cytokines, 353–354

Dapoxetine, for onychomycosis co-morbid OCD, 281
Dapsone, 27
Decoupling, 249
Delusional disorder
 diagnostic criteria, 63–64
 Morgellons disease (case report), 66–69
 treatment, 65
Delusional infestation, 31–74
 case reports, 43–73
  case 4-1 *(folie à famille)*, 43–45
  case 4-2 (delusional parasitosis in 50-year-old woman), 45–48, **46**
  case 4-3 (58-year-old woman), 48–51, **49–50**
  case 4-4 (65-year-old woman), 51–55, **52, 54**
  case 4-5 (shrimp-infested nails), **57**, 56–58
  case 4-6 *(folie à deux)*, 59–62, **61**
  case 4-7 (delusions of sexually transmitted disease), 62–66
  case 4-8 (Morgellons disease), 66–69
  case 4-9 (delusional scalp infestation and *folie à deux*), 69–74, **70–72**
 clinical features, 35, **36–38**
 complications, 41
 definition, 63
 diagnosis, 53–54
 differential diagnosis, 35–39, **40**
 drug-induced, 56–58
 enhancing outcomes, 42
 etiology and epidemiology, 32
 evaluation, 34
 folie à deux/famille, 32, 35, 43–45, 59–62, 69–73
 Koo-Brownstone staging system, **61**, 61–62
 overview, 31–32
 pathophysiology, 33
 prognosis, 41
 as prurigo nodularis complication, 179
 treatment, 39–41
Delusional parasitosis. *See* Delusional infestation
Delusions of vitiligo (case report), 337–340
Dependent personality disorder, 214
Depression
 alopecia areata, 213–216, 223–227, 230, 237–240
 dermatitis artefacta, 166
 drug-associated, 26–28
 Gardner-Diamond syndrome, 322, 325, 328–329
 onychophagia, 266, 268

Depression *(continued)*
  onychotillomania, 257
  pemphigus vulgaris, 341–348
  prurigo nodularis, 179, 196, 203–209
  psoriasis, 349–357
  psychobiotics for, 15
  screening tools, 355–356
  skin picking, 247, 276–277
  vulvodynia, 306
Dermatitis artefacta, 127–178
  case reports, 136–178
    case 6-1 (case mimicking palmoplantar keratoderma), 136–139, **137–138**
    case 6-2 (53-year-old woman), 140–142, **141**
    case 6-3 (27-year-old woman), 142–145, **143**
    case 6-4 (51-year-old woman), 145–149, **147**
    case 6-5 (54-year-old man), 149–151, **150**
    case 6-6 (26-year-old woman), 151–154, **152**
    case 6-7 (diagnostic and therapeutic challenge), 154–157, **155**
    case 6-8 (complication of PTSD), 157–161, **158–159**
    case 6-9 (giant facial ulcer), 162–164, **163**
    case 6-10 (factitious hand lymphedema), 165–168, **166–167**
    case 6-11 (occupational in a soldier), 169–172, **170**
    case 6-12 (27-year-old woman), 172–178, **173**
  clinical features, **128**, 128–129
  diagnosis and differential diagnosis, 129, **131**, 131–133, **133**
  epidemiology, 128
  etiology and pathogenesis, 128
  findings that merit suspicion of, **131**
  introduction, 127
  management, 133–134, **134**

Munchausen syndrome by proxy, 135
  of nail unit, 257, **258**
  prognosis, 135
Dermatologic examination in psychodermatology, 11–12
Dermatological disorders with psychiatric symptoms, 2
Dermatological drugs, psychiatric adverse effects from, 24–28, **26**
  antihistamines, 25
  apremilast, 25
  corticosteroids, 28
  cyclosporine, 25
  dapsone, 27
  hydroxychloroquine, 25
  interferon α2β, 26
  interleukin inhibitors, 27
  intravenous immunoglobulin, 27
  isotretinoin and acitretin, 27
  methotrexate, 27
  tetracycline, 28
  tumor necrosis factor α inhibitors, 28
Dermatology Life Quality Index (DLQI), 3, 15, 228–230, 276, 284, 347
Dermatotillomania, onychophagia concomitant with, 284–287, **285–286**
Dermoscopy
  alopecia areata, 219, **220–221**, 226
  onychomycosis, 281
  onychophagia, 263, 267, **267**
  onychotillomania, 257, **259**, 262, **264–265**
  prurigo nodularis, 180, 199, **201**, 202
Desipramine, for vulvodynia, 298, 307
Dialectical behavior therapy, 102
DLQI (Dermatology Life Quality Index), 3, 15, 228–230, 276, 284, 347
Doctor-patient relationship, 2–3
Dopamine, 33
Doxepin
  for alopecia areata, 215
  for cutaneous sensory disorders, 296
  for prurigo nodularis, 183

Index

for vulvodynia, 298
Doxycycline, 28
DPCP, 238–240
Drug reaction with eosinophilia and systemic symptoms (DRESS), 20–21, **22**, 23–24
Duloxetine
  for Gardner-Diamond syndrome, 328
  for glossodynia, 303
Dupilumab, for prurigo nodularis, 182, 197

Ecchymosis, **309**, 309–310, 324–325, 329, 331, 334
Ekbom syndrome, 31
Emotional regulation theory, 245
Endocrine disorders, prurigo nodularis association with, 178
Erythema multiforme, 22–24
Erythematous plaques (case report), 323–326, **324–325**
Erythromelalgia, 300
Escitalopram
  for alopecia areata, 230
  for body-focused repetitive behavior disorders (BFRDs), 251
  for delusional infestation, 49
  for prurigo nodularis, 195
  for skin picking, 276, 278, 288–289
  for trichoteiromania, 112, 123
  for trichotemnomania, 123
Etanercept, 28
EuroQol Five Dimensions Questionnaire (EQ-FD), 347
Exclamation mark hairs, 90, 105, 108, 121, 122–124, 210, **212**, 218, **220**, 220, 222, **226**, 229, 233, 235, **235**
Excoriation disorders
  clinical features, 247
  diagnostic criteria, 246
  prevalence, 244
  psychopharmacology, 251
Exfoliative dermatitis, 23–24
Exposure response prevention, 273
Eye movement desensitization and reprocessing, for prurigo nodularis, 183

Eyebrows, trichotemnomania of (case report), **123**, 122–127

Factitial dermatitis. *See* Dermatitis artefacta
Factitious disorders
  dermatitis artefacta, 127–178
  diagnostic criteria for, 131–132
  differential diagnostic of, **133**
  hand lymphedema (case report), 165–168, **166–167**
  introduction, 127
Family Dermatology Life Quality Index, 284
Family therapy
  for alopecia areata, 214
  for dermatitis artefacta, 138, 160
Fay syndrome, 295
Fibromatosis disorders, 271
Fixed drug eruptions, 21–24
Flame hair, 78, 90, 92, 97, **98**, 108, 114, **117, 119,** 118–121
Fluocinonide, for prurigo nodularis, 195
Fluoxetine
  for alopecia areata, 223–224, 225
  for body-focused repetitive behavior disorders (BFRDs), 251
  for dermatitis artefacta, 155
  drug reactions, 23
  for onychomycosis, 280–281
  for onychophagia, 265
  for prurigo nodularis, 205
  for trichotillomania, 87, 120
Fluvoxamine, 251, 294
Folie à deux/famille
  case reports, 43–45, 59–62, **61**, 69–73
  overview, 32
  prevalence, 35
Friar Tuck sign, 77–78, **119**, 120
Functional assessment, 3
Fungal infection, skin-picking wounds mistaken for, 274–279

Gabapentin
  drug reactions, 21–22
  for postherpetic neuralgia, 299

Gabapentin *(continued)*
  for prurigo nodularis, 195, 197
  for scalp pain, 298
  for vulvodynia, 298, 307
Gabapentinoids, for dermatitis artefacta, 164
GAD-7 (generalized anxiety disorder/7 item), 229–230, 276
Gardner-Diamond syndrome (GDS) case reports
  case 10-3 (20-year-old woman), 308–312, **309, 311**
  case 10-6 (5-year-old girl), 319–323, **324–321**
  case 10-7 (29-year-old woman), 323–326, **324–325**
  case 10-8 (16-year-old girl), 327–331, **328**
  case 10-9 (49-year-old woman), 331–335, **332–333**
General Health Questionnaire-28 (GHQ-28), 347
Generalization training, 85–86
Generalized anxiety disorder, 3–4
  alopecia areata comorbidity, 213
  prurigo nodularis comorbidity, 195
Generalized anxiety disorder/7 item (GAD-7), 229–230, 276
Genital dysesthetic syndromes, 295, 297–298
GHQ-28 (General Health Questionnaire-28), 347
Glossodynia case reports
  case 10-1 (54-year-old woman), 302–304
  case 10-4 (47-year-old woman), 313–316, **314**
Glucocorticoids, for trichoteiromania, 93
Group behavior therapy, for BFRDs, 251
Gut microbiota dysfunction, 15

Habit control motivation, 85
Habit reversal training (HRT)
  for body-focused repetitive behaviors (BFRBs), 102, 251–252, 285–287
  for onychomycosis, 280–281
  for onychophagia, 268
  for onychophagia and dermatotillomania, 284–287, **286**
  for onychotillomania, 255
  for prurigo nodularis, 183, 205
  for pseudo-knuckle pads, 272
  for psychogenic itch, 317–319
  for skin picking, 252, 294–297
  for trichotillomania, 85–86
Hair loss. *See also* Alopecia areata; Trichotillomania
  case 5-2 (journey from alopecia areata to trichotemnomania), 103–109, **104, 106–107**
  stigmatization, 75
Hair pull test, 78, 89, 91, 94, 114, 118, 228, 233
Hair pulling. *See also* Trichotillomania
  automatic, 76–77
  clinical features, 247
  epidemiology, 244
  focused, 76–77, 120
Hallucinations of vitiligo (case report), 337–340
Hamilton Rating Scale for Depression (HAM-D), 355
Hand lymphedema, factitious (case report), 165–168, **166–167**
Hepatitis C, prurigo nodularis association with, 179
Herpes zoster, 299
History
  dermatitis artefacta patients, 129–130, 150, 159, 173
  hollow, 128–129
Histrionic personality traits, 310–311
HIV
  delusional infection, 65
  prurigo nodularis association with, 179
HLP (hypertrophic lichen planus), 180
Hook hairs, 79, **80**, 90, 92, 97, **98, 119,** 118–120
Hopelessness, 41, 119, 341, 348, 355
Hormones, 2
Hospital Anxiety and Depression Scale, 3
HRT. *See* Habit reversal training
Hydroxychloroquine, 25

Index

Hydroxyzine, for prurigo nodularis, 190
Hyperhidrosis, 22
Hypertrichosis, 23
Hypertrophic lichen planus (HLP), 180, 189

I-hairs, 100
IL-6, 353–354
IL-17, 353–355
IL-23, 353, 355
Imipramine
    for alopecia areata, 215
    for vulvodynia, 298
Immunoglobulin G, 27
Immunosuppressive agents
    for alopecia areata, 214
    for prurigo nodularis, 197
Infliximab, 28, 355
Inositol, 251
Interferon α2β, 26
Interleukin inhibitors, 27
Intestinal microflora, 15
Isotretinoin, 27
Itch-scratch-itch cycle, 93, 195, 197
Ixekizumab, 27

Janus kinase (JAK) inhibitor, 182, 230–231, 240, 355

Knuckle pads, 270–271
Koo-Brownstone staging system, **61**, 61–62

Lamotrigine
    drug reactions, 21–22
    for skin picking, 278
Lichen simplex chronicus, 195, 197
Lichenoid reactions, 21, 24
Lidocaine
    for cutaneous sensory disorders, 299
    for vulvodynia, 298, 307
Lip biting, 245, 247, 272
α-Lipoic acid, 297, 303
Lithium, 21–22
Loratadine, for prurigo nodularis, 195
Lupus erythematosus, 22
Lymphedema, factitious hand (case report), 165–168, **166–167**

Maculopapular exanthema, 20
Major depressive disorder (MDD)
    alopecia areata comorbidity, 213
    concomitant dermatitis artefacta, 143–144
    IL-17, levels in, 354
    inflammation, 353
Malingering, 171
Managing percutaneous disorders, 7–16
Mania, drug-associated, 26–28
Marie Antoinette syndrome (canities subita), 210
Massachusetts General Hospital Hair-pulling Scale (MGH-HPS), 249
Matchbox sign, 31, 34–35, 39, **46**, 51, 68
MDD. *See* Major depressive disorder
Medication side effects, 19–28
    dermatological drugs, 24–28, **26**
    psychiatric drugs, 20–24
Medications. *See also specific drug classes; specific drugs*
    for dermatitis artefacta, 134
    for prurigo nodularis, 182
    for skin picking, 290–291
Memantine, for trichotillomania, 88
Mental health assessment, 9–10, **11**
Menthol, for prurigo nodularis, 190
Methotrexate
    for psoriasis, 355
    psychiatric side effects, 27
    side effects, 25
Mexazolam, 294
MGH-HPS (Massachusetts General Hospital Hairpulling Scale), 249
Microneedling, 86–87
Milk thistle, 251
Milwaukee Inventory for Subtypes of Trichotillomania, **83**
Mindfulness-based stress reduction, 356
Minocycline, 28
Minoxidil, for alopecia areata, 223
Mitchell disease, 300

Montgomery-Åsberg Depression Rating Scale (MADRS), 356
Mood stabilizers, 21–22
Morgellons disease (case report), 66–69
Mucocutaneous pain syndrome, 295–296
Munchausen syndrome, 152, 158, 324, 334
Munchausen syndrome by proxy, 135
Mycophenolate mofetil, 197, 342

N-acetylcysteine (NAC)
  for body-focused repetitive behavior disorders (BFRDs), 256
  for delusions of infestation, 3
  for hair pulling, 251
  for onychophagia, 268
  for onychotillomania, 259
  for skin picking, 278, 294
  for trichoteiromania, 93
  for trichotillomania, 88, 120
Nail biting. *See also* Onychophagia
  clinical features, 247–248, **248**
  epidemiology, 244
Nail disorders
  with alopecia areata, 210, 213
  onychodystrophy, 100, **101**, 255, 258, 284
  shrimp-infested nails (case report), **57**, 56–58
Naltrexone, 3, 251, 278
Nefazodone, 23
Nemolizumab, for prurigo nodularis, 182
Nervous system, 1–2
Neurokinin-1 receptor antagonists, 182
Neurolinguistic programming, for prurigo nodularis, 183
Neuropathic pain, 296, 299, 307
Neuropathy, 27, 298–300
NIMH's Trichotillomania Symptom Severity Scale (NIMH-TSS), 81, **83**
Nonsecret self-inflicted skin lesions, 9
Nose picking (rhinotillexomania), 248–249
Notalgia paresthetica, 298–299

Obsessive-compulsive and related disorders (OCRD), 243, 246
Obsessive-compulsive disorder (OCD)
  alopecia areata comorbidity, 213
  body-focused repetitive behavior disorders (BFRDs) compared, 249
  comorbid psychiatric conditions, 245
  onychomycosis associated with, 281–283
  onychotillomania comorbidity, 257
  prurigo nodularis association with, 196
  with repeated hand washing and fingernail onychomycosis (case report), 279–284, **280–283**
Occupational dermatitis artefacta (case report), 169–172, **170**
Olanzapine
  for delusional disorders, 65
  for dermatitis artefacta, 147
  drug reaction, 24
  for hair pulling, 251
  for trichotillomania, 87–88
Onychodaknomania, 257
Onychodystrophy, 100, **101**, 255, 258, 279, **280–282**, 284
Onychomycosis, 280–282
Onychophagia (nail biting)
  clinical features, 247–248, **248**
  dermatotillomania concomitant with, 284–287, **285–286**
  onychotillomania compared, 256
  prevalence, 247–248
  psychiatric comorbidities, 265–266
  treatment-resistant (case report), 263–269, **265–266**
Onychoteiromania, 257
Onychotemnomania, 257
Onychotillomania
  case report, 254–261, **255–256, 258–263,**
  coexisting trichotillomania, 97–103, **98–99, 101**
  comorbidities, 255
  definition, 255
Ophiasis pattern, 210, 228
Oppositional defiant disorder, 245

Index

Oxcarbazepine, 21–22

Palmoplantar keratoderma, dermatitis artefacta mimicking (case report), 136–14, **137–138**
Parasitosis, delusional. *See* Delusional infestation
Paroxetine
  for alopecia areata, 215
  drug reactions, 23
  for skin picking, 289
PASI (Psoriasis Area Severity Index), 15
Patient Health Questionnaire/9 item (PHQ-9), 229–230, 276, 355–356
Pemphigus vulgaris (case report), 340–348
Penoscrotodynia, 297–298
Periciazine, for burning mouth syndrome, 315
Petechiae, 23, 329
Pharmacological interventions, 3
Pharmacotherapy. *See* Medications; *specific drugs*
Phenobarbital, 21
Phenothiazines, 23
Phenytoin, 21
PHN (postherpetic neuralgia), 299
Photosensitivity/phototoxicity, 21–24, 355
Phototherapy
  for prurigo nodularis, 182, 197, 199
  for psoriasis, 355
PHQ-9 (Patient Health Questionnaire/9 item), 229–230, 276, 355–356
Pigmentary changes, 21–23, 338
Pigtail hairs, 238
Pimecrolimus
  for prurigo nodularis, 182
  for psoriasis, 355
Pimozide
  for cutaneous sensory disorders, 296
  for delusional disorders, 65
  for delusional infestation, 3, 50, 53, 60
  for onychotillomania, 259
PITS (Psychiatric Institute Trichotillomania Scale), 81, **83**

Placebo treatments, 88, 316–319
Postherpetic neuralgia (PHN), 299
Posttraumatic stress disorder. *See* PTSD
Prebiotics, 15
Prednisolone, for alopecia areata, 223–224, 226, 228
Prednisone, for pemphigus vulgaris, 341
Pregabalin
  for dermatitis artefacta, 162
  for postherpetic neuralgia, 299
  for prurigo nodularis, 197
  for psychogenic itch, 317–318
  for scalp pain, 298
  for vulvodynia, 298, 305, 307
Primary delusional infestation
  definition, 32, 67
  diagnosis, 38–39, **40**, 49, 54, 60, 71–73
  overview, 32, 72
  prognosis, 41
  treatment, 39–41, 51, 53–54
Primary psychiatric disorders, classification of, 8–9, **9**
Primary skin lesions, 11
Problem-solving therapy, 356
Proctodynia, 295
Prurigo nodularis, 177–209
  case reports, 187–209
    case 7-1 (45-year-old-woman), 187–192, **188–190**
    case 7-2 (55-year-old-woman), 193–198, **194**
    case 7-3 (frustrating malady), 199–203, **200–202**
    case 7-4 (anxiety and depression with), 203–209, **204**
  clinical features, 179–180, **180–181**
  comorbidities, 179
  complications, 179
  dermoscopy, 180, 199, **201**, 202
  epidemiology, 178
  histopathology, 181, 195–196
  introduction, 177
  management, 181–183
  pathophysiology, 177–178, 196
Pruritus. *See also specific disorders*
  brachioradial, 300

Pruritus *(continued)*
  differential diagnosis, 36
  prurigo nodularis, 177–209
  solar, 300
Pseudo-knuckle pads (case report), 269–273, **270–271**
Psoriasis, 349–357
  cytokines, role of, 353–354
  depression and suicide, 349–357
  drug reactions, 21–25
  immunopathogenesis, 353
  introduction, 349–350
  management, 354–356
  pathophysiology, 353–354
  prurigo nodularis association with, 177–178
  psychiatric comorbidities, 351–352
  psychiatric epidemiology, 350–351
  quality of life, 15
  stigma, 8
Psoriasis Area Severity Index (PASI), 15
Psoriasis Symptom Inventory, 15
Psychiatric adverse effects from dermatological drugs, 24–28, **26**
Psychiatric comorbidity in dermatology, 10
Psychiatric disorders with dermatologic symptoms, 2
Psychiatric drugs. *See also specific drugs*
  cutaneous adverse drug reactions (CADRs), 19–24
  side effects, 20–24
Psychiatric Institute Trichotillomania Scale (PITS), 81, **83**
Psychoanalytic psychotherapy, for dermatitis artefacta, 171
Psychobiotics, 15
Psychocutaneous disorders
  classification and terminology, 8–9, **9**
  range of disorders, 2
  treatment, 2–3
Psychodermatology clinic, 4
Psychodynamic therapy
  for dermatitis artefacta, 134
  for trichotillomania, 86
Psychoeducation
  for glossodynia, 303
  for prurigo nodularis, 183
Psychogenic itch (case report), 316–319
Psychogenic purpura. *See* Gardner-Diamond syndrome
Psychopharmacology, for BFRDs, 251
Psychophysiological disorders, 2, 8, **9**
Psychosocial issues, assessment of, 10
Psychotherapy. *See also specific disorders; specific therapeutic modalities*
  for alopecia areata, 214–215, 225
  for dermatitis artefacta, 134
  for Gardner-Diamond syndrome, 310–312, 326, 328
  for prurigo nodularis, 183, 191, 201
  for psychogenic itch, 317–319
  for somatic symptom disorder (SSD), 315
Psychotropic drugs, 14–15
  for alopecia areata, 214
  for dermatitis artefacta, 171
  for pseudo-knuckle pads, 273
PTSD
  alopecia areata, 213
  dermatitis artefacta, 157–161, **158–159**, 163
Purpura, psychogenic. *See* Gardner-Diamond syndrome
Pyoderma gangrenosum, 140, 142

Quality of life
  Dermatology Life Quality Index (DLQI), 3, 15, 228–230
  impact on, 7–8, 10, 14
  prurigo nodularis, 179, 191, 196, 205
  psoriasis, 349, 353, 355–357
  vulvodynia, 307–308
Questionnaires, 3–4, 10

Rapunzel syndrome, 84
Relaxation training, for alopecia areata, 214–215
Renal disease, prurigo nodularis association with, 178
Repetitive Body-Focused Behavior Scale (RBBS), 249
Response inhibition training, 249
Riluzole, for skin picking, 278

Index

Risk assessment, 10
Risperidone, for delusional disorders, 44, 63, 65–67

SALT (Severity of Alopecia Tool), 228, 230
Scales, 10
Scalp
   delusional infestation of, 69–74, **70–72**
   pain, chronic, 298
Schizophrenia
   negative association with alopecia areata, 213
   psoriasis, 352
Screen for Anxiety-Related Disorders (SCARED), 284
Screening tools, 3–4
Secondary delusional infestation
   case reports, 57
   causes, **33**
   definition, 32, 67–68
   diagnosis, 39, **40**, 54
   overview, 32, 72
   prognosis, 41
   treatment, 39, 51, 54
Secondary psychiatric disorders, 8, **9**
Secondary skin lesions, 11–12
Secret self-inflicted skin lesions, 9
Selective serotonin reuptake inhibitors (SSRIs)
   for alopecia areata, 215, 224, 225
   for body-focused repetitive behavior disorders (BFRDs), 251
   for cutaneous sensory disorders, 296
   for delusional disorders, 65
   for dermatitis artefacta, 134, 160, 164, 166
   drug reactions, 23
   for Gardner-Diamond syndrome, 311, 322, 325–326, 326, 330
   for interferon α2β side effects, 26
   for onychomycosis comorbid OCD, 281
   for onychophagia, 268
   for prurigo nodularis, 182–183, 206
   for scalp pain, 298
   for skin picking, **277**, 278, 291, 294
   for trichotillomania, 87
   for vulvodynia, 298, 307
Self-inflicted cutaneous lesions. *See* Dermatitis artefacta
Serlopitant, for prurigo nodularis, 182, 197
Sertraline
   for Gardner-Diamond syndrome, 310, 312, 322
   for onychomycosis comorbid OCD, 281
   for onychotillomania, 26
Serum sickness-like reactions, 23
Severity of Alopecia Tool (SALT), 228, 230
Sexually transmitted disease, delusions of, 62–66
Shrimp-infested nails (case report), **57**, 56–58
Side effects of drugs, 19–28
   dermatological drugs, 24–28, **26**
   psychiatric drugs, 20–24
Skin picking
   acne excoriée, **13**
   case reports
      case 9-4 (chronic wound secondary to), 274–279, **275–277**
      case 9-7 (long-term pathological), 287–292, **288–289**
      case 9-8 (64-year-old woman), 293–297
   classification, 246
   clinical features, 247
   comorbidities, 247, 293–294
   diagnostic criteria, 246
   epidemiology, 244
   onychophagia and dermatotillomania, 284–287
   prevalence, 4, 290
   psychopharmacology, 251
   secondary skin lesions, 12, **13**
   terminology, 9
   triggers, 293
Skin Picking Scale (SPS), 249, 284
Skindex Questionnaire, 3
Sleep disorders
   depression, 352

Sleep disorders *(continued)*
  as medication side effect, 28, 347
  medications for, 14, 302
  prevalence, 10
  prurigo nodularis, 179
  psychogenic itch, 316
Social anxiety
  pemphigus vulgaris, 341
  trichotillomania, 250
Social avoidance
  alopecia areata, 218, 224
  body-focused repetitive behavior disorders (BFRDs), 250
  pemphigus vulgaris, 341
  skin picking, 294
Social isolation
  alopecia areata, 213
  prurigo nodularis, 201
  psoriasis, 352
  psychocutaneous conditions, 3
Social phobia, as alopecia areata co-morbidity, 213
Social withdrawal
  alopecia areata, 213, 223
  pemphigus vulgaris, 341
  percutaneous conditions, 3
  psoriasis, 349
Solar pruritus, 300
Somatic symptom disorder (SSD), 315
Somatization, 138–139, 318
Somatoform disorders, 132–133, 146–148, 334
Specimen sign, 31, 68, **71,** 73
SPS (Skin Picking Scale), 249, 284
SSRIs. *See* Selective serotonin reuptake inhibitors
Steroids, topical for prurigo nodularis, 182, 190, 195, 197, 201
Stevens-Johnson syndrome (SJS), 20–21, 23–24
Stigmatization, 3, 8, 339, 341, 349, 353
Stigmatization scale, 285
Stimulants, alopecia areata associated with use, 213
Stress
  alopecia areata, 210, 212–214, 223, 225–226, 234, 238–240
  as Gardner-Diamond syndrome trigger, 310–311, 322, 325, 329, 331, 334

  hallucinations and delusions of vitiligo (case report), 337–340
  pemphigus vulgaris, 341, 347
  posttraumatic stress disorder (PTSD), 157–161, **158–159,** 163, 213
Suicidality
  alopecia areata comorbidity, 213, 225, 229, 231
  depression as common cause, 225
  pemphigus vulgaris, 341, 348
  psoriasis, 349–357
  psychiatric epidemiology, 350–351
  screening tools, 355–356

Tacrolimus
  for prurigo nodularis, 190
  for psoriasis, 355
TCAs. *See* Tricyclic antidepressants
Teeth grinding (bruxism)
  clinical features, 248
  epidemiology, 244
  prevalence, 248
TEN (toxic epidermal necrolysis), 20–21, 23–24
Terminology, 8–9
Tetracycline, 28
Therapeutic intervention
  basic principles, 12–15
  combination of dermatology treatments with psychotherapy, 14
  components of, 13–14
  fields of knowledge involved, 12, **13**
  psychobiotics, 15
  psychotropic medications, 14–15
Thioridazine, for onychotillomania, 259
Thumb sucking, 245
Tinea capitis, trichoscopy of, 120–121
Tofacitinib, for prurigo nodularis, 197
Topiramate
  drug reactions, 22
  for skin picking, 278
  for vulvodynia, 298
Toxic epidermal necrolysis (TEN), 20–21, 23–24
Tramadol, for postherpetic neuralgia, 299
Transcutaneous electrical nerve stimulation (TENS) therapy, 307

Index

Transient perivascular inflammation of the carotid artery (TIPIC syndrome), 295
Trazodone, for delusional infestation, 48
Triamcinolone
   for alopecia areata, 215, 223–224, 226
   for prurigo nodularis, 182
Trichobezoar, 84, 250
Trichodaganomania, 94
Trichomalacia, 79, 90, 119
Trichophagia, 84, 250
Trichoptilosis, 79, **80**, 90, 108, 112, **119**, 118–120
Trichorrhexis nodosa, 92, **93**
Trichoscopy
   alopecia areata, 90, 108, 121, 124, 210, **212**, 218–221, 223–224, **225–227**, 229, 233, 235, **235**, 238
   delusional infestation, 71, **72**
   tinea capitis, 120–121
   trichoteiromania, 91–94, **91–93**, 109, 111, **111**, 112
   trichotemnomania, 90, **90**, 105, **106–107**, 108, **123**, 122–124
   trichotillomania, 78–79, **79–80, 82**, 97, **98, 119–120**, 119–121
   trichotillomania comorbid with trichotemnomania, 114–116, **116–117**
Trichoteiromania
   of the beard (case report), 109–115, **110–111**
   clinical features, 91, **91**
   definition, 91
   differential diagnosis, 93
   management, 93
   overview, **91–93**, 91–93
   trichoscopy, 91–93, **92–93**, 109–109, **111**, 112
Trichotemnomania
   case 5-2 (journey from alopecia areata to), 103–109, **104, 106–107**
   case 5-4 (association with trichotillomania), 114–117, **115–117**
   case 5-6 (of the eyebrows), **123**, 122–127
   clinical features, 89, **89**
   definition, 89
   differential diagnosis, 90
   of eyebrows (case report), **123**, 122–127
   overview, 89–90, **89–90**
   treatment, 90
   trichoscopy, 90, **90**, 105, **106–107**, 108, **123**, 122–124
Trichotillomania
   classification, 246
   clinical features, 247
   comorbid psychiatric conditions, 245, 247
   complications, 250
   habit reversal training (HRT), 102, 251–252
   skin picking, 293
Trichotillomania (TTM), 75–127
   assessment tools, 81, 83, **83**
   case reports, 97–127
      case 5-1 (coexisting TTM and onychotillomania), 97–103, **98–99, 101**
      case 5-2 (journey from alopecia areata to trichotemnomania), 103–109, **104, 106–107**
      case 5-3 (trichoteiromania of the beard), 109–115, **110111–111**
      case 5-4 (association of TTM and trichotemnomania), 114–117, **115–117**
      case 5-5 (TTM as more than hair-pulling disorder), **118–120**, 118–121
      case 5-6 (trichotemnomania of eyebrows), **123**, 122–127
      case 8-1 (alopecia areata associated with), 218–222, **219–221**
   clinical features, 77–78, **77–78**
   comorbidities and complications, 83–84
   diagnosis, 81
   differential diagnosis, 83
   early-onset, 85
   epidemiology, 75–79

Trichotillomania *(continued)*
  etiology, 76
  histopathology, 79
  pathogenesis, 76
  philosopher comments on, 1
  prevalence, 75
  prognosis, 84
  psychopathological features, 76–77
  treatment, 84–88
    acceptance and commitment therapy (ACT), 86
    antipsychotics, 87–88
    habit reversal training (HRT), 85–86
    memantine, 88
    microneedling, 86–87
    N-acetylcysteine (NAC), 88
    nonpharmacological, 85–87
    overview, 84–85
    pharmacological, 87–88
    psychodynamic therapy, 86
    SSRIs, 87
    tricyclic antidepressants, 87
  trichoscopy, 78–79, **79–80, 82,** 97, **98, 119–120,** 119–121
  variants, 88–94
    trichodaganomania, 94
    trichoteiromania, **91–93,** 91–93
    trichotemnomania, 89–90, **89–90**
Tricyclic antidepressants (TCAs)
  for burning mouth syndrome, 297
  for cutaneous sensory disorders, 296
  for Gardner-Diamond syndrome, 330
  as Gardner-Diamond syndrome trigger, 311
  for onychophagia, 268
  for postherpetic neuralgia, 299
  for prurigo nodularis, 182–183
  for scalp pain, 298
  for trichotillomania, 87
  for vulvodynia, 298, 307
Trigeminal trophic syndrome (TTS), 299–300
Trihexyphenidyl, for delusional infestation, 44
TTM. *See* Trichotillomania
TTS (trigeminal trophic syndrome), 299–300
Tulip hairs, 79, 92, 114, **116,** 119–120, **120**
Tumor necrosis factor α inhibitors, 28

Ultraviolet B (UVB), 355
Urticaria, 23
Ustekinumab, for psoriasis, 355

V sign, 79, **82, 119,** 119–120
Valproic acid, 21–22
Vasculitis, drug reaction and, 23–24
Vellus hairs, 108, 119, **120,** 124, 220, 223, **226–227,** 229, 235, 238
Venereophobia, 63, 65
Venlafaxine, for psychogenic itch, 317–318
Vestibulodynia, 297, 306
Visible skin lesions, 11–12
Vitiligo, hallucinations and delusions of (case report), 337–340
Vulvodynia
  case report, 304–308
  definition, 305
  overview, 297–298

Yale-Brown Obsessive-Compulsive Scale-Trichotillomania (Y-BOCS-TM), 81, **83**